Home Care
Positioning the Hospital for the Future

Edited by Dan Lerman

Division of Ambulatory Care
of the American Hospital Association

American Hospital Publishing, Inc.,
a wholly owned subsidiary of the
American Hospital Association

Library of Congress Cataloging-in-Publication Data

Home care.

Bibliography: p.
1. Home care services.   2. Hospitals—Home care
programs.   3. Home care services—United States.
4. Hospitals—United States—Home care programs.
I. Lerman, Dan. [DNLM: 1. Home Care Services—
United States.   WY 115 H765]
RA645.3.H646   1987   362.1'4   86-30220
ISBN 1-55648-000-8

Catalog no. 016138

Text printed in English Times
2.5M—2/87-0143

Sandra L. Weiss, Project Editor
Wayne S. Brown, Managing Editor
Peggy DuMais, Production Coordinator
Marcia Vecchione, Designer
Brian W. Schenk, Books Division Director

Contents

List of Figures

Acknowledgments

To publish a book of this scope required the invaluable contribution of numerous individuals.

I want to thank Diane Howard, director of the Division of Ambulatory Care of the American Hospital Association, as well as other members of the division's professional staff—Ted Matson, Susan Nathanson, Gary Rahn, and Ed Zimmerman—for providing the stimulating, challenging, and dynamic work environment that was necessary for the completion of this project. Cheryl Allen, Nina Cooper, Trina Ealy, and Gilda Mitchell provided superb support in the production of the manuscript. I also want to thank Joseph Kubal and Charles Schreiber from AHA's Data Center, for their assistance in providing key national hospital home care survey data used in the manuscript. Sandy Weiss, editor, American Hospital Publishing, Inc., and other staff provided excellent editorial assistance.

My parents, grandparents, brother, and sister instilled in me dual passions: a passion for caring and a passion for analytical thinking and business commonsense. I hope that these passions are woven throughout the fabric of this book.

I must also acknowledge and thank the richness and diversity of home care clients that I have served at the grass-roots level. These clients-friends enriched my life, personally and professionally.

Finally, I want to thank the contributing authors for articulating so well the key patient care and business issues involved in hospital home care development, management, and expansion.

Dan Lerman

Contributors

Larry Brothers is vice-president of Kensington Health Enterprises, a for-profit subsidiary of St. Joseph Health System, Flint, Michigan, and president of Metro Duramed, a durable medical equipment (DME) company based in the Detroit area. Mr. Brothers is currently responsible for DME operations, retail pharmacy, and the medical-surgical supply and consultant divisions at Kensington Health Enterprises. His staff is also responsible for external project development and management services for St. Joseph Health System. Mr. Brothers developed one of the first hospital-based DME programs and a network of hospital-related DME programs to compete for HMO and PPO contracts.

Dorothy Buckels, R.N., is director of the St. Clair Home Care Department, a hospital-based agency affiliated with South Hills Health System/Home Health Agency of Pittsburgh, Pennsylvania. Mrs. Buckels manages a staff of 34 employees who provide home care to a daily census of 300 to 350 patients. Mrs. Buckels has a broad and varied nursing background encompassing 40 years.

William D. Cabin, J.D., M.A., is an independent health care consultant affiliated with Home Health Associates, Totowa, New Jersey. Prior to establishing his independent practice, Mr. Cabin was director of regulatory affairs and research for the National Association for Home Care and senior editor of *Caring* magazine for three years. Mr. Cabin specializes in the areas of HMO management and contracting, corporate reorganization, joint ventures, mergers, acquisitions, management audits, budgeting, and home care regulatory affairs. He has written extensively in the health care field, with articles in *Caring* magazine, *Home Health Line, Hospital Home Health* newsletter, and *Outreach*, the newsletter of the Division of Ambulatory Care of the American Hospital Association.

Roberta N. Clarke, M.B.A., D.B.A., is an associate professor at Boston University and a lecturer at the Harvard School of Public Health. She received her master's degree in business administration and her doctorate from Harvard Business School. Her 12 years of teaching experience in the field of health care marketing and her extensive consulting experience with many types of health care organizations has made her a recognized authority on the marketing of health care services. She was the first person to be honored as Health Care Marketer of the Year, an award presented by the American College of Health Care Marketing. Professor Clarke also serves on the Board of Directors of the Society for Hospital Planning and Marketing of the American Hospital Association.

Kaye Daniels, R.N., M.B.A., vice-president of Kokua Home Nursing Agency in Honolulu, Hawaii, is a nurse with a business background. She served for 16 years as president of Hospital Home Health Care of California, a freestanding multihospital cooperative that is noted for its wide-ranging diversification activities. Ms. Daniels served on the Board of Directors of the National Association for Home Care and the Hospice Association of America. She has made numerous national and international presentations on home and hospice care.

D. Michael Elliott, M.B.A., is president of SelectCare, a preferred provider organization serving southeast Michigan, and Group Health Plan of Michigan, a health maintenance organization, in Troy, Michigan. Prior to his current position, Mr. Elliott was executive vice-president of St. Joseph Health System in Flint, Michigan; president of Kensington Ambulatory Health Services; and president of Kensington Health Enterprises, a for-profit corporation with a durable medical equipment company located in Flint, Michigan. He has held a series of progressively responsible financial and administrative positions in health care in the state of Michigan and has worked in large and small hospitals as well as participated in the organization and development of health system arrangements since 1973. Mr. Elliott has an undergraduate degree in business administration from Michigan State University and a master's degree in business administration from Eastern Michigan University.

Cathy Frasca, R.N., executive director of the South Hills Health System/ Home Health Agency of Pittsburgh, Pennsylvania, is a recognized leader in the home care industry. The agency she runs is the largest multihospital-based home health agency of its kind in the nation. Ms. Frasca is a registered nurse, a licensed nursing home administrator, and a Fellow in the American College of Healthcare Executives. She is widely published and has been a presentor at many state, national, and international educational conferences. Among her numerous prestigious appointments, Ms. Frasca has chaired the AHA Governing Council of the Assembly of Ambulatory and Home Care Services.

Steven L. Griff, M.B.A., has been in hospital management since 1968 and in home health services since 1972. He is president of Home Care Information Systems, Inc., a data processing group providing software for the home health industry, and president of Home Health Associates, a multidisciplinary consulting practice. As a consultant, he has worked with health care organizations in the areas of strategic planning, marketing, management and operational systems. Mr. Griff has earned a master of business administration in health care administration from The George Washington University and a master of public administration in health policy and planning from New York University. He is a member of the American College of Healthcare Executives.

Dan Lerman, M.H.S.A., is manager of home care and hospice services in the Division of Ambulatory Care of the American Hospital Association, Chicago, Illinois. In that capacity, he is responsible for home care product development, representation and advocacy, educational programming, and technical assistance. Mr. Lerman has strong training and experience in the hospital, ambulatory care, home care, nursing home, and retirement housing fields. He holds a master's degree in health services administration from the University of Michigan School of Public Health and has a Specialist in Aging Certificate from the University of Michigan Institute of Gerontology. He is a licensed nursing home administrator and a certified public housing manager specializing in elderly housing. Prior to joining AHA, Mr. Lerman worked in a number of administrative positions in the home care and aging arena. He serves on a number of home care advisory boards and has made national and international presentations on hospital home care diversification activity.

Teri L. Louden is president and founder of Louden & Company, a firm specializing in the provision of strategic planning and marketing information and analysis for the health care industry. Louden & Company has developed a national reputation for its work in home health care, older adult markets, and health care sales and marketing. Prior to starting her own firm, Ms. Louden worked at American Hospital Supply Corporation as manager of corporate planning; Booz, Allen & Hamilton as a hospital consultant; and Baxter Travenol in both marketing and sales. She has published numerous books and articles on leading-edge health care issues and has spoken extensively at national meetings of health care associations, companies, and hospital systems.

Lawrence A. Manson, J.D., is a partner in the law firm of Wood, Lucksinger & Epstein and is responsible for the general health care practice in the firm's Chicago office. Before joining Wood, Lucksinger & Epstein, Mr. Manson was general counsel in the Office of Federal Law and Regulation of the American Hospital Association. His division was responsible for developing AHA positions on all proposed federal regulations affecting the hospital industry. Mr. Manson was president of the Illinois Association of Hospital Attorneys from 1983 to 1984 and now serves on the Board of Directors. He received his bachelor's degree from Vanderbilt University and his law degree from Columbia University.

Barbara A. McCann is director of the Accreditation Program for Hospice Care and Home Care Development of the Joint Commission on Accreditation of Hospitals in Chicago, Illinois. McCann developed and manages the first national accreditation program for hospice services in all health care settings. She is currently directing the development of a comprehensive home care accreditation program, which is targeted for implementation in 1988.

Eileen A. O'Neil, J.D., is a health law attorney practicing in Boston. She is also an assistant professor of health administration and planning at the University of New Hampshire. Ms. O'Neil has lectured and written extensively in the field of home care. Presentations include seminars given for the American Hospital Association and the National Association for Home Care as well as numerous state home health associations. She is the author of a monograph entitled *Legal Aspects of Home Health Administration,* which was funded by the W. K. Kellogg Foundation.

Patricia A. Peters, R.N., B.S.N., has been involved in home care since 1977 as a discharge planner, visiting nurse, supervisor, and administrator. She is the director of home health services for Premier Hospital Alliance in Westchester, Illinois. Ms. Peters has served as a member of the panel on managing risks and quality in hospital-sponsored home care for the Institute on Quality of Care and Patterns of Practice of the Hospital Research and Educational Trust, Chicago, Illinois. She received her bachelor of science degree in nursing from Alverno College and is working toward completion of her master's degree in hospital administration at the University of Minnesota.

Katherine Pfeifle, R.N., has over nine years' experience in the home care industry. She owns and operates a consulting firm located in Grand Forks, North Dakota. Ms. Pfeifle specializes in the provision of consultation, management, and billing services for rural home care providers throughout the United States. She is currently working on completing her master's degree in public health.

Anne L. Rooney, R.N., M.S., serves as associate director of the Accreditation Program on Hospice Care at the Joint Commission on Accreditation of Hospitals in Chicago, Illinois. Ms. Rooney's responsibilities include the management of the JCAH's hospice accreditation program. Her previous experience includes managing a home health agency's hospice program.

William J. Simione, Jr., C.P.A., is a partner at Simione and Simione, a firm of certified public accountants in Hamden, Connecticut; Boston, Massachusetts; Ft. Lauderdale, Florida; and Cleveland, Ohio. Mr. Simione has more than 20 years' experience in home care financial management and consulting. He serves on the National Association for Home Care Reimbursement Committee and Task Force on Prospective Payment/Alternative Reimbursement. He has conducted workshops on cost reporting, management information systems, fiscal management, diversification and reorganization, and budgeting and cash-flow requirements for numerous state and national hospital and home care associations.

Marion M. Torchia, Ph.D., is associate director for federal agency affairs in the Washington, DC, office of the American Hospital Association. She monitors Medicare regulatory issues, especially those relating to ambulatory care, home care, hospice, and long-term care. Prior to joining AHA in 1982, Ms. Torchia was employed by Capital System Group, a Washington-based consulting firm that provides information and research services to the federal government. While there, she managed the PSRO Information Clearinghouse for the Health Care Financing Administration. Ms. Torchia holds a doctorate in history and taught European and American History on the college level from 1967-77.

Judith Walden, R.N., is the president and executive director of Hospital HomeCare, Inc., in Albuquerque, New Mexico. She has had primary responsibility for program development, implementation, and administration of this multihospital-affiliated home health agency since its inception in 1973. Ms. Walden has delivered numerous papers and presentations at educational conferences on various home care administrative topics. She is a graduate of the University of Washington and is currently a candidate for a master of science in health administration from Trinity University.

Foreword

I am delighted to have an opportunity to recommend a most exciting publication: *Home Care: Positioning the Hospital for the Future.* Although in a more generic sense home care has been in existence for many years, hospital home care as it is today is new, exciting, challenging, and constantly changing.

I began working in home care about 20 years ago as director of the home care department of a small medical-surgical, not-for-profit, community hospital in the Steel Valley of Pittsburgh, Pennsylvania. At that time, I never envisioned that this home care program would eventually become one of the largest multihospital-based home health agencies of its kind in the nation. As the agency grew, I realized that I needed to acquire a more in-depth knowledge of program planning and development and legal and financial management as well as additional expertise in the management, operation, and marketing of a successful home health agency in a constantly changing legislative and regulatory environment. Acquiring the specialized skills required to manage any home health agency was difficult enough, but adapting that knowledge so that I could function within a highly complex hospital system appeared to be an insurmountable task. My feelings were not unique. Over the years, I have heard many other home care administrators express similar concerns.

Home health agencies are atypical health care entities that provide a complex and unique speciality: community health services. The home care industry is envisioned to become the primary focus of health care in the future. As a result of the Medicare prospective pricing system for hospitals, patients are leaving hospitals during a more intense phase of their illness and so require a multiplicity of specialized services that can be provided at home by qualified, experienced home care personnel. This pattern is expected to continue to an even greater degree in the future; and as a result, a wider scope of home care products and services, ranging from basic supportive and personal care services to highly sophisticated technology, will be provided in the home.

Hospitals have long been identified as the central core of health care services in the community and will continue to be the vital link between institutional and home care services. Hospital resources and the expertise of hospital personnel and physicians will be used by home health agencies to ensure a comprehensive, coordinated continuum of care and to appropriately provide a complete package of health care and health-related services to the community.

The value of a home care program lies in the extended care and services provided to the hospital's patients and the support given to patients as they move from one level of care to another, including readmission to the hospital. Home care patients may also require services, such as pharmaceuticals, durable medical equipment, skilled nursing care, and help from homemakers, that can be provided by many varied hospital subsidiary organizations. A hospital-sponsored home care program is an ideal resource for a hospital to use in extending and expanding its services to the community and in further enhancing already established relationships and promoting new relationships. Unlimited opportunities exist for a home care program to increase the hospital's visibility in the community and to serve as a vehicle for providing patients to the hospital and its related business ventures.

Because of the instability of federal and state funding, the private sector is anticipated to become a primary funding source for home care of the future. For example, increasing numbers of HMOs and other private insurance carriers are already including home care products and services in their benefit structure.

The American Hospital Association recognizes home care, both the Medicare-regulated and nonregulated business segments, as an integral component of the total health care spectrum. As a result of this recognition, the AHA has responded to the needs of the rapidly growing home care industry and, in particular, to the needs of hospital-based home care administrators by selecting experienced, highly accomplished, and nationally acclaimed home care experts to share their expertise as authors of this unique book.

This book is a substantive document encompassing topics ranging from global perspectives, such as fiscal and legal issues and corporate reorganization, to more finite operational issues, such as staffing and productivity. It is a timeless publication as the information presented will be as useful several years from now as it is today.

I recommend this book to anyone who is currently operating a home care organization or considering entering into any type of home care business venture. Take time to read this book in its entirety and recommend it to friends and colleagues, but possibly not to your competitors, as this book provides key information on how the hospital and the home care organization may best position themselves for ensuring their fair share of the marketplace in the future.

I have been privileged and honored to participate in this valuable book, and I know it will assist hospital CEOs, administrators of home care organizations, boards of directors, planners, fiscal officers, physicians, utilization review coordinators, and other key health care personnel in their short-term and long-range strategic home care planning endeavors.

Every success and happy reading!

Cathy Frasca
Executive Director
South Hills Health System/Home Health Agency
Pittsburgh, Pennsylvania

Chapter 1

The Home Care Opportunity

Dan Lerman

Although interest in the home care field has expanded rapidly in recent years, home care has been around for a long time and has a rich tradition. One hundred years ago visiting nurse agencies were established to care for immigrants, poor persons, and the elderly. Community support, philanthropy, and fees from patients supported these programs.

In 1947, the first hospital-based home care program was established at Montefiore Hospital in the Bronx, New York. This program was developed to serve the needs of patients just released from hospitals. It expanded the traditional home nursing role and focused on an interdisciplinary team concept that coordinated the work of physicians, nurses, therapists, aides, and social workers.

In the years since the Montefiore model was established, the home care industry has changed dramatically. A Medicare home care benefit was implemented in 1966. In 1981, the benefit was liberalized to eliminate the three-day prior hospitalization requirement and the 100-visit home care nursing limit and remove the restrictions on participation by proprietary agencies. In 1982, separate cost limits for hospital-based and freestanding home care agencies were eliminated and replaced with single cost limits based on the cost experience of freestanding home care agencies. Hospital-based agencies were permitted an add-on to the cost limits to reflect the higher administrative and general costs associated with hospital-based home care delivery. Since the introduction of the prospective pricing system in 1983, the home care program has been the fastest growing segment of the entire Medicare program and the top hospital growth area.

Dan Lerman is the manager of home care and hospice services, Division of Ambulatory Care, American Hospital Association, Chicago, Illinois.

Home Care and Home Health Care

The term *home care* refers to the wide array of products and services now offered in the home. It no longer refers narrowly to simply the provision of skilled care services alone. The service side of the home care business accounts for approximately two-thirds of industry revenue, and the product side accounts for one-third. Chapter 2 discusses these home care segments in detail. Typical home care products and services are listed in figure 1-1, below.

Another term frequently heard in the home care industry is *home health care*. This term generally refers to the Medicare and third-party-reimbursed skilled care side of the home care market. Skilled care includes the provision of nurses; speech, physical and occupational therapists; home health aides; medical social work services; and necessary durable medical equipment (DME) and supplies. The Medicare Part A home care benefit is a restrictive, highly regulated, intermittent benefit that provides, at least through 1986, cost-based reimbursement for these skilled care services and equipment when they are deemed medically necessary by a physician for a home-bound patient. Under Part A, a patient must first qualify for one of the primary services — nursing, speech therapy, or physical therapy — before being eligible for other benefits. The Medicare Part B supply benefit provides for

Figure 1-1. Typical Home Care Products and Services

Services	Products
Skilled nursing	Oxygen-Respiratory
Physical therapy	Durable medical equipment (DME)
Home health aides	Rehabilitation equipment
Social service	Daily living aids
Occupational therapy	Medical and surgical supplies
Personal care	Drug therapy
Private-duty nurses	Pharmacy
Senior sitters	Nutrition
"Tuck-in" service	Intravenous (IV) equipment
Pet and plant sitters	Dialysis
Education	Self-treatment aids
Data processing	Communications (emergency response systems)
Health promotion	Exercise equipment
Claims processing	Self-diagnostic devices
Speech therapy	Hearing aids
	Home telemetry

Adapted from presentations by David Tanner and Kaye Daniels at an AHA home care conference, *Home Care: A Key Hospital Diversification Strategy,* in San Diego, CA. 1986 Feb.

reasonable charge reimbursement versus Part A, which provides reasonable cost reimbursement.

Home care implies a much broader focus. In addition to skilled care services, home care covers such services as DME, infusion therapies, private-duty or demand care, medical-surgical supplies, self-diagnostic devices, and exercise products and equipment. Because of its broader focus, the term *home care* is the one used throughout this book except where specific reference is made to skilled care services only.

A Profitable Growth Industry

In the 1980s, the home care market has become the fastest growing segment of the hospital industry. More than 75 percent of hospitals nationwide planned to add or expand this service in 1986.[1] By contrast, less than 13 percent of hospitals offered a home care program in 1982.[2] The number of Medicare-certified, hospital-based home care agencies, which are just one segment of the broad and expanding home care market, increased 137 percent from December 1983 to October 1986 (figure 1-2, below), making hospitals the fastest growing segment of the home care industry.[3] The National Association for Home Care recently projected a 37 percent increase in Medicare home care utilization from 1984 to 1986.[4]

Figure 1-2. Medicare-Certified Home Care Agencies

Provider Type	Dec. 1983	Oct. 1986	Growth Rate (%)
Visiting nurse assns	520	502	(4)
Government	58	62	7
Official	1,230	1,176	(4)
Rehab-based	19	16	(16)
Hospital-based	579	1,370	137
SNF-based	136	109	(20)
Proprietary	997	1,899	90
Private not-for-profit	674	813	21
Other	45	2	(96)
Total	4,258	5,949	40

Source: Health Care Financing Administration

A current $3 to $5 billion home care market is projected to reach $8 to $19 billion by 1990, with an expected average annual growth of from 13 percent to 17 percent.[5] Although these projections are viewed as high by a number of industry observers, they indicate potential growth opportunities in the home care market.

The home care products and services that have high-profit potential are DME, infusion therapy, and private-duty or demand care. Skilled care, on the other hand, is generally a low-margin but high-volume service. Profitability generally varies from breakeven on the Medicare skilled service side to from 8 to 16 percent for private-duty care and from 10 to 25 percent on the DME and infusion therapy side of the market.[6] Variables such as competition, case mix, physician practice patterns, and management efficiency affect the profitability of a home care program.

According to preliminary results from a 1986 AHA hospital home care survey, 95 percent of the hospitals that provide home care have a Medicare-certified skilled care program.[7] Fifty-two percent provide private-duty or demand care, 86 percent provide home intravenous (IV) therapy, 57 percent provide DME, and 20 percent have a retail home care pharmacy or center. The new standards of the Joint Commission on Accreditation of Hospitals (JCAH), to be implemented in 1988, discuss these multiple home care product lines. Hospital-based home care programs must comply with the JCAH standards. Freestanding home care programs may voluntarily seek JCAH accreditation.

Factors contributing to this tremendous growth in home care include:

- *An increasingly aging population.* The elderly population is the highest utilizer of home care services. It is also the population that has multiple disabilities and chronic illness. From 1980 to 1990, the population of persons 75 to 84 years of age is projected to grow 27 percent; and the population of persons 85 years and over, 20 percent.[8] Such growth will place new demands on the home care industry.
- *Sophisticated technology.* Because of sophisticated technology, treatments such as home IV antibiotic therapy and total parenteral nutrition therapy permit shorter inpatient stays and increase the number of treatments that can be given in the home.
- *Strong public demand.* Strong public demand for home care is evident after 87 percent of consumers surveyed stated that they want to be treated at home rather than in institutions.[9]
- *Changing reimbursement.* The percentage of hospital outpatient revenues is expected to double by 1995 and to account for 25 percent of total hospital revenues as insurers encourage less costly outpatient care.[10] Home care will most likely account for a sizable chunk of that revenue. In addition, private insurers have greatly expanded home care benefits in recent years. More than 90 percent of Blue Cross plans and 50 percent of other commercial insurance plans now offer a home care benefit, compared to only 45 and 5 percent, respectively, in 1971.[11]

Hospital Interest

In their continued search for ways to continue providing high-quality patient care and to increase revenues, hospitals have turned to home care. Hospitals are interested in developing a home care program for four main reasons:[12]

- To satisfy patient care needs
- To provide a continuum of care and achieve internal control over the cost, quality, and access to this service
- To help manage inpatient length of stay more effectively
- To increase revenue or profitability

Home care can serve as a springboard for further hospital diversification, especially in the aging-related market. It can also keep clients within the hospital orbit, serve as a referral source for hospital product-related businesses, provide a competitive edge in marketing for hospitals trying to secure contracts with health maintenance organizations (HMOs) and preferred provider organizations (PPOs), and serve as a key component of a vertically integrated health care system.

Hospitals see home care as an inviting prospect because of the positive patient care and business impact it may have and because of the phenomenal growth in the industry. However, hospitals must exercise caution. A recent study indicated that only 1 out of 30 investor-owned home care companies that held a public stock offering in 1984 was profitable.[13] Also, such high-profit areas as home infusion therapy can be a risky business because of high capital investment, volatility of the patient base, and the limited number of these types of clients nationwide.[14]

Hospitals that are considering the home care business should look carefully at the following important issues: competition, client base, market entry strategies, referral sources, and barriers to success.

Competition

The composition of the Medicare home care market has changed dramatically in recent years: hospitals and for-profit agencies registered the fastest growth while visiting nurse associations, which once dominated the market and still provide a disproportionately large share of Medicare home care visits, showed no growth. Proprietary home care agencies now represent 32 percent of the Medicare-certified agencies; hospitals, 23 percent; state and county programs (official), 20 percent; private not-for-profit, 14 percent; visiting nurse associations, 8 percent; and all others, 3 percent. From April to October 1986, the number of Medicare-certified home health agencies declined from 6,012 to 5,949.[15] This first-time-ever decline in the number of Medicare-certified agencies reflects consolidations, mergers, and closures that resulted from competition and cash-flow problems.

Besides Medicare-certified home care agencies, major competitors in the home care market include large health care manufacturers and providers, such as Travenol, Inc.; dealers in DME and surgical supplies; staffing agencies; HMOs; chain pharmacies; independent drugstores; retail home care centers; department stores; physicians; independent practitioners; and mail-order houses. This entrepreneurial industry is extremely fragmented, competitive, and changing daily.

The average home care agency had 10 new competitors in its service area in 1985.[16] In addition, a survey conducted in 1985 indicates that 17 percent of HMO and PPO plans own their own home care businesses, and another 60 percent are interested in directly providing, rather than contracting for, home care products and services.[17] According to the preliminary results from a 1986 AHA survey, 18 percent of hospital home care programs have responded to this changing marketplace and secured active contracts with HMOs to provide their enrollees with home care products and services.[18] In addition, 10 percent of the hospitals responding to the survey report that some physicians on their medical staffs have established their own home care program. However, this competitive market has not affected 10 percent of the hospitals who serve as sole community providers of home care service.

Client Base

Nationally, 75 percent of the clients in a Medicare-certified home care agency are over the age of 65.[19] The conditions most commonly treated by home care agencies include diabetes, high blood pressure, heart and circulatory problems, carcinoma, stroke, arthritis or joint problems, respiratory ailments, bowel or bladder problems, and skin problems. In Maryland the top four Medicare hospital discharge diagnoses referred to home care programs by rank and percent are shown in figure 1-3, below.[20]

Discharge planning and analysis of case-mix management are important ways for hospitals to reduce inpatient lengths of stay and refer appropriate

Figure 1-3. Top Four Medicare Hospital Discharge Diagnoses

Diagnoses	Percent of Discharge to home care
1. Heart failure and shock	7.7
2. Cerebrovascular disorders	5.6
3. Chronic obstructive pulmonary disease	3.8
4. Atherosclerosis—over age 70	3.6

Source: National Center for Health Services Research

clients to home care programs in a timely manner. A 1986 AHA survey found that 7.7 percent of hospital discharges nationally are referred to home care programs, and of these, 61 percent are referred to the hospitals' own home care program.[21] The survey also indicated that 52 percent of Medicare home care visits are for skilled care nursing, 28 percent for home health aides, 15 percent for physical therapy, 2 percent for speech therapy, 2 percent for occupational therapy, and 1 percent for medical social services.

This survey also found that 3 percent of hospital home care clients are from birth to 20 years of age, 17 percent are 21 to 64 years of age, 64 percent are 65 to 84 years of age, and 16 percent are 85 and over.[22] The survey also shows that 17 percent of hospitals provided home care service to AIDS patients.

A study reported in the *Wall Street Journal* indicated that the average inpatient cost to treat an AIDS patient was $140,000.[23] In the coming years home care services for AIDS patients will surely skyrocket for patient care and cost containment reasons.

Significant home care growth has also occurred in the following areas for patients under age 65:[24]

- Pediatric, including patients who are dependent on a ventilator because of severe respiratory problems; are in need of phototherapy, which is used to care for jaundiced babies; require an apnea monitor; or are acutely ill, chronically ill, and terminally ill
- Psychiatric patients
- Ambulatory surgery follow-up
- Early maternity patients
- Well newborn care
- Clients with industrial and occupational illnesses
- Patients with AIDS

A study by the Illinois Hospital Association identified the three most common diagnosis-related groups (DRGs) for non-Medicare patients discharged to home care: psychoses, vaginal delivery without complications, and care for normal newborns.[25] This information would indicate that hospitals should place more emphasis on home care market opportunities in the under-65 age group. The under-65 population should account for a more sizable and profitable segment of the home care market in years ahead.

Revenue Sources

According to a 1986 AHA survey, Medicare accounts for 78 percent of the revenue from typical home care programs; Medicaid, 7 percent; Blue Cross and Blue Shield, 4 percent; commercial insurance, 5 percent; HMOs, 1 percent; self-pay, 3 percent; and other revenue, 1 percent. Hospitals must continue their commitment to serve the Medicare and Medicaid population while augmenting their payer mix with more HMO, private insurance, and self-pay clients.[26]

Market Entry Strategies

Competition and cooperation characterize the home care field. This situation is shown in the many entry strategies that can be used by a hospital that wants to become involved in home care. Hospitals have:

- Informally referred patients to a home care agency
- Formally contracted with a home care agency for service
- Formally affiliated with an existing home care agency
- Acquired home care programs
- Started their own hospital-based or freestanding subsidiary program
- Developed joint ventures with a wide variety of partners

The first four of these strategies require the hospital to become involved, either formally or otherwise, with an already established home care agency. The last two strategies involve the hospital beginning a new business on its own or in conjunction with partners who may or may not be providers of health care. These last two market-entry strategies require some additional discussion.

How have hospitals initially developed home care programs? Figure 1-4, below, identifies hospital responses to start-up, acquisition, joint venture, and contract or agreement strategies for the five major home care market segments. Hospitals have generally started up skilled care, private-duty or demand, IV therapy, and retail home care pharmacy services. Less than half of the hospitals started their own DME business. Acquisition has not been a major home care development strategy for hospitals. Less than 1 percent have acquired DME businesses and only 6 percent have acquired skilled care programs. The most prominent home care joint ventures are in the DME

Figure 1-4.   Initial Development of Home Care Programs by Type of Service

Service	Method of Initial Development (%)			
	Start-up	Acquisition	Joint Venture	Contract or Agreement
Skilled care	80%	6%	4%	10%
Private duty	70	6	11	13
IV therapy	70	3	7	20
DME	47	1	16	36
Health care pharmacy or center	83	3	0	14

Source: Preliminary results, AHA's *Hospital Home Care Survey—1986*

and private-duty or demand segments. The most common contract or agreement arrangements are with DME and IV therapy businesses.

Eighty-three percent of hospital-sponsored retail home care pharmacies or centers have been started up by hospitals.[27] Pharmacy is an extremely important product line; research at Yale-New Haven Hospital found that 85 percent of all persons discharged from hospitals require prescription drugs and 95 percent of the persons referred to home care need prescription drugs.[28]

Hospital-Based or Freestanding Program

A hospital deciding to enter into home care must decide whether the home care agency should be hospital-based or freestanding. To effectively make such a decision, hospitals must understand the distinction between hospital-based and freestanding home care agencies. Under the Medicare program, a hospital-based home care agency is a department of the hospital and so files under the hospital's cost report and has the same governing body as the hospital. A freestanding agency files a separate cost report and has a separate governing body. Freestanding agencies submit the cost report to a regional home care fiscal intermediary. Through 1986 at least, hospital-based programs file with the hospital's fiscal intermediary. The Health Care Financing Administration (HCFA) is studying the merits of having hospital-based programs file with a regional home care fiscal intermediary.

Hospital-based home care programs receive an add-on to the single freestanding-agency Medicare cost limits to cover the higher administrative and general costs that hospital-based agencies incur. Overhead allocations can also be shifted from the hospital to the home care department. The advantages of a hospital-based home care agency are the tremendous access to patients, physicians, and hospital resources, such as finance, planning, health records, data processing, and infection control. However, a hospital-based program is highly regulated and much less flexible than a freestanding program. Through 1986, Medicare-certified home care agencies were reimbursed on a cost basis. The federal government is studying alternate home care payment methods, such as prospective pricing, competitive bidding, and capitation.

After hospitals decide on whether the home care agency should be hospital-based or freestanding, they must decide whether the agency should be for-profit or not-for-profit. A 1986 AHA survey indicates that with the exception of retail pharmacy, most of the services provided by a home care agency—that is, skilled nursing, private-duty care, IV therapy, and DME—are provided on a not-for-profit basis (figure 1-5, next page).[29] In addition, 89 percent of those responding expect to organize as a hospital-based program; and 11 percent, as a freestanding program.[30]

On the basis of these results, an inference can be made that hospitals are not yet maximizing home care business opportunities if the private-duty or demand, DME, and IV therapy programs are not being managed with

Figure 1-5. Not-for-Profit versus For-Profit Services for Home Care

Home Care Service	Not-for-Profit	For-Profit
Skilled nursing	89%	11%
Private duty	62%	38%
IV therapy	81%	19%
DME	60%	40%
Retail pharmacy	49%	51%

Source: Preliminary results, AHA's *Hospital Home Care Survey—1986*

the market and entrepreneurial orientation necessary to be successful in these product lines. In addition, Medicare step-down cost report methodology limits the ability to maximize private-duty or demand services provided within a Medicare-certified home care program. Also, hospital-based DME and IV therapy programs receive reasonable-cost reimbursement under Part A of Medicare, but freestanding businesses can receive Part B reasonable-charge reimbursement, which is a more attractive payment arrangement. Hospitals must consider these points when evaluating hospital-based or freestanding development.

Hospital Partners

Figure 1-6, next page, identifies how hospitals in a 1986 AHA survey responded to questions on their preferences for joint venture partners. For skilled care services, the most preferred joint venture partners for the development of a home care business are not-for-profit home care programs and other hospitals. For-profit home care programs are clearly the most preferred joint venture partner for private-duty or demand services. National product companies ranked as the top joint venture partner for IV therapy, and local product companies are the preferred joint venture partner for the provision of DME services.[31]

Hospitals often formally contract or informally refer patients to home care programs if the hospital does not directly provide a particular service. Figure 1-7, page 12, shows the percentage of hospitals who formally contract or informally refer patients to the five major home care services when the hospital does not directly provide the service. Results indicate that the vast majority of patients are informally referred to other providers.[32] Hospitals that informally refer patients must consider such issues as the safety, quality assurance, and risk management procedures of the organization to which they are referring patients. These organizations must be evaluated;

Figure 1-6. Choices of Joint Venture Partners by Type of Home Care Service

Service	Home Care Agency		Other Hospitals	National Product Co.	Local Product Co.	Nursing Home	Physicians	Other
	For-Profit	Not-for-Profit						
Skilled care	21%	37%	32%	0%	0%	5%	0%	5%
Private duty	47	13	13	0	0	7	7	13
IV therapy	20	5	20	40	0	5	0	10
DME	12	0	16	20	32	4	0	16
Retail pharmacy	0	0	0	0	0	0	0	100*

Preferred Joint Venture Partners (%)

*Retail pharmacies will most likely engage in joint ventures with community pharmacies.

Source: Preliminary results, AHA's *Hospital Home Care Survey—1986*

**Figure 1-7.   Forms of Home Care Referral by Type
of Home Care Service**

Service	Formal Contract	Informal Referral
Skilled care	38%	62%
Private duty	16%	84%
IV therapy	28%	72%
DME	20%	80%
Retail pharmacy	9%	91%

Source: Preliminary results, AHA's *Hospital Home Care Survey—1986*

and responsibilities, liabilities, continuity of care, and the patient transfer process must be clearly understood and delineated between the hospital and the organization to which informal referrals are made.

Hospitals that develop their own programs and directly provide all services have greater control over cost, quality, and patient access to home care but also incur greater risk and liability. As an example, 27 percent of hospitals formally follow up home care discharges once the home care illness episode has ended, according to the results of a 1986 AHA survey.[33] More follow-up phone calls, mailed questionnaires, or visits may be required to best serve patients and limit the hospital's liability.

Hospitals must think creatively and in an entrepreneurial vein when establishing home care venture arrangements. A leading freestanding home care agency in Hawaii is structuring a joint venture that has as venture partners a hospital, a physicians' group, an HMO and PPO plan, and an insurance company.[34]

Referral Sources

However the hospital structures its own home care program, it must develop a strong internal and external referral base. Emergency departments, ambulatory surgical centers, rehabilitation programs, long-term-care facilities, birthing centers, medical office buildings, and geriatric assessment clinics, as well as physicians, nurses, therapists, discharge planners, and pastoral care providers, are key internal referral sources.

Hospital internal referral bases are strong but must be strengthened. Results of a 1986 AHA survey indicate that for hospitals that offer these services:[35]

- 14 percent do not refer from the emergency department to the home care program

- 18 percent do not refer from the ambulatory surgery center to home care
- 11 percent do not refer from the rehabilitation facility to home care
- 14 percent do not refer from the long-term-care facility to home care
- 8 percent do not refer from medical office buildings to home care
- 45 percent do not refer from birthing centers to home care

External referral sources are HMO and PPO plans, employers, insurers, community physicians, pharmacists, persons living at elderly housing sites, staff and attendees at senior centers, staff from community health and aging agencies, and consumers and their families. Freestanding cancer centers and high-tech medical parks are also emerging as referral bases.

Barriers to Success

The following list includes key barriers to the success of a hospital-sponsored home care agency:

- Commitment by executive management of the hospital
- Lack of authority and resources
- Home care administrator reporting relationships
- Market competition
- Adequate reimbursement, especially if more professional intensive services have to be offered at home
- Regulatory atmosphere
- Management expertise, which is often hard to find
- Quality control management
  - Prevention, avoidance, and minimization of risk
  - Staff skills and retention
  - Poor customer and clinical service
- Capital investment requirements
- Lack of interest by physicians
- Poor data-base development: limited clinical and fiscal data to make timely management decisions and slow transition from manual to computerized record systems

Reporting relationships, in particular, play a key role in the ultimate success or failure of a hospital home care program. A 1986 AHA survey found that 28 percent of directors of hospital-sponsored home care agencies report directly to hospital vice-presidents, 24 percent to hospital chief executive officers, 17 percent to assistant administrators, 14 percent to directors of nursing, 4 percent to system corporate officers, 3 percent to a governing board, and 10 percent to others.[36]

Hospital home care experts claim that home care development or expansion may be hindered when the home care director does not report directly to executive management. Quick decisions and a market and business orientation are essential to take advantage of new markets, clients, products, and services in the rapidly changing home care field. Layers of bureaucracy and inappropriate reporting relationships may stifle entrepreneurial initiatives and opportunities.

Overview of the Book

Hospitals that look to home care as a means to satisfy patient care needs, provide a continuum of care, manage inpatient length of stay more effectively, and increase revenue are faced with a challenge and an opportunity. Diversifying into home care is not simple or easy. Special clinical and business management skills are required.

A successful home care business requires a strong business and market orientation, a skilled and caring staff, and person-oriented high-quality service. Home care is a *people* business, and the caring component is crucial to success.

This book provides hospitals interested in diversifying into home care and those already involved in home care with an overview of all aspects of the home care business: market segmentation, strategic planning, corporate structures, legal issues, operational considerations, financial management, quality assurance, risk management, marketing and promotion, HMO contracting, and regulatory affairs. A collection of patient case histories provides examples of the various types of patients who can benefit from home care. Six home care program models provide structural and operational details on the various types of home care agencies that a hospital can sponsor.

The home care market is market driven, entrepreneurial, and consumer oriented. It is composed of a wide array of service and product lines. This book helps hospitals determine how home care can affect their futures and how to maximize client service and business opportunities.

Notes

1. Barry Moore, "CEOs Plan Resource Shift for 1986," *Hospitals* (1985 Dec. 16. 59(24):69-72).

2. American Hospital Association, *Hospital Statistics, 1983 edition* (Chicago: AHA, 1984).

3. Personal communication from Diane Milstead, Health Care Financing Administration, 1986 Nov. 5.

4. Presentation by Val J. Halamandaris, president of the National Association for Home Care, on the AHA home care teleconference, *Winning Ventures: There's No Place like Home,* in Chicago, 1986 Mar. 20.

5. Teri Louden, "Home Health Care Opportunities in Market on the Rise," *Modern Healthcare* (1983 Dec. 13(12):109-112).

6. Presentation by Dan Lerman at the International Health and Economic Institute, St. Thomas, Virgin Islands, 1986 Apr. 19.

7. American Hospital Association, *Hospital Home Care Survey—1986,* unpublished preliminary results.

8. Susan Van Gelder and Jill Bernstein, "Home Health Care in the Era of Hospital Prospective Payment: Some Early Evidence and Thoughts about the Future," *Pride Institute Journal of Long-Term Care* (1986 Winter. 5(1):3-11).

9. Teri Louden, *Home Care Market Outlook* (Chicago: SMG-Louden Ventures, 1985).

10. Arthur A. Andersen & Co., and American College of Hospital Administrators, *Health Care in the 1990s: Trends and Strategies* (Chicago: Arthur Anderson & Co. and American College Hospital Administrators, 1984).

11. Personal communication from Neal Hollander, vice-president, provider affairs, Blue Cross of Western Pennsylvania, Pittsburgh, 1986 Nov. 13.

12. Presentation by David Tanner on the AHA home care teleconference *Winning Ventures: There's No Place like Home* in Chicago. 1986 Mar. 20.

13. "Rummaging for Med Tech Bargains," *Venture.* (1985 Apr. 7(4):29).

14. Presentation by David Tanner at the AHA conference *Home Care: A Key Diversification Strategy* in New Orleans, 1986 May 16.

15. Health Care Financing Administration, "Providers and Suppliers of Services" (file maintained by HCFA's Office of Survey and Certification), 1986 Nov. 7.

16. Presentation by Teri Louden on the AHA home care teleconference, *Winning Ventures: There's No Place like Home,* in Chicago, 1986 Mar. 20.

17. Teri Louden, *Home Care-HMO/PPO Perspectives* (Chicago: Louden & Co., Mar. 1986).

18. *Hospital Home Care Survey—1986.*

19. *Building a Long-Term Care System: Home Care Data and Implications* (Washington, DC: U.S. House Select Committee on Aging. 1984 Oct. Pub. No. 98-484).

20. M. Meiners and R. Coffey, *Hospital DRGs and the Need for Long Term Care Services: An Empirical Analysis.* (Rockville, MD: National Center for Health Services Research, 1984 July).

21. *Hospital Home Care Survey—1986.*

22. *Hospital Home Care Survey—1986.*

23. "AIDS Costs: Employers and Insurers Have Reasons to Fear Expensive Epidemic, *Wall Street Journal* (1985 Oct. 18. 18:1, 21).

24. "Non-Medicare Home Care Clients Provide Market Opportunities," *Outreach.* (1986 Jan.-Feb. 7(1):5)

25. "Potential Home Health Expansion Identified," *Discovery,* newsletter of the Illinois Hospital Association (1985 Sept).

26. *Hospital Home Care Survey—1986.*

27. *Hospital Home Care Survey—1986.*

28. Presentation by David Tanner at the AHA conference *Home Care: A Key Hospital Diversification Strategy* in New Orleans, 1986 May 16.

29. *Hospital Home Care Survey—1986.*

30. *Hospital Home Care Survey—1986.*

31. *Hospital Home Care Survey—1986.*

32. *Hospital Home Care Survey—1986.*

33. *Hospital Home Care Survey—1986.*

34. Presentation by Kaye Daniels on the AHA home care teleconference, *Winning Ventures: There's No Place like Home,* in Chicago. 1986 Mar. 20.

35. *Hospital Home Care Survey—1986.*

36. *Hospital Home Care Survey—1986.*

Chapter 2

Market Segments

Steven L. Griff

Home care has consistently led the list of alternative delivery services that hospitals report they have in operation or are planning to offer. What these hospitals seek to build on is the logical flow of patient referrals from the inpatient and outpatient settings and the extension of their role to the delivery of care at home. Before a hospital decides to enter the home care market, it must understand that this market is not a single homogeneous one. Rather, it is a diverse collection of products and services that, for this discussion, is segmented into *skilled care; private-duty or demand service;* and *durable medical equipment (DME).* Skilled care and private duty or demand are both service businesses; DME is a product business.

Hospitals planning to enter the home care market need to recognize that the market segments differ in the types of service to be provided, the specific client population being served, the regulatory environments, and the financial risks and opportunities each segment offers. This chapter discusses these differences for each segment of the home care market.

Skilled Care Segment

Skilled care is sometimes referred to as the medical model of home care because skilled care services are closest in character, level, and intensity to the services provided on an acute care basis. Generally, physicians are required

Steven L. Griff, M.B.A., is president of both Home Health Associates and Home Care Information Systems, Inc., Totowa, New Jersey. All statistics in this chapter are based on the experience of these firms.

to certify that skilled care services are medically necessary. Skilled care is the largest segment of the home care market, and it is the segment most directly affected by the pressures to reduce the lengths of hospital stays.

Services Provided

The services generally encompassed by a skilled care program include the *primary* services of nursing, physical therapy, and speech therapy and the *secondary* services of occupational therapy, social service, home health aides, supplies, and equipment. The terms *primary* and *secondary* are a reflection of the reimbursement rules of the major payer, the Medicare program, and reflect the fact that a client qualifying for coverage and receiving one of the primary services also becomes eligible to receive the secondary services and to have that care financed by Medicare.

Client Description

The client in the skilled care segment is often receiving care that is part of a program of treatment begun during an inpatient stay. Care may also be provided preparatory to hospital admission or may be a continuation of the care that was begun in another alternative care setting.

In the past, home care patients have been predominantly elderly and have included individuals who were recovering from strokes or from such procedures as cataract surgery or hip replacement and patients with onco-logic diagnoses. As home care has moved more into the mainstream of med-ical practice, the client population for home care has begun to include younger individuals, including those receiving nutritional support (either enteral or parenteral) and intravenous antibiotic therapy. Also receiving home care are the premature neonate and children with severe respiratory-related illnesses.

Referral Mechanism

The client in the skilled care segment is referred directly by or with the con-currence of the attending physician. This referral is often through the hospital discharge planning mechanisms. The hospital nurse or social worker may be the party to originally identify the need for skilled care services and may assist the physician with the referral.

Referral may also be by the clients themselves or the clients' family. In either instance, the policies of the agency and third-party payers generally require that the attending physician concur.

Approximately two-thirds of the persons referred to skilled care come directly from hospitals. Therein lies the concern of the freestanding providers as to the potential for hospital domination of the market.

Physician's Role

Skilled care is provided under the direction of the attending physician. Orders for all services must be in writing and must be renewed at 60-day intervals. This procedure reflects the requirements of the major payer, the Medicare program, and therefore tends to be applied to all clients registered with the agency.

Requirements for Coverage

Certain requirements must be met if patients are to qualify for skilled care. The majority of the providers use the Medicare eligibility guidelines because generally 60 percent to 100 percent of their clients are Medicare-reimbursable beneficiaries. These guidelines are frequently adopted in whole or in part by other payers, such as Blue Cross or commercial insurers.

The Medicare guidelines state that an individual must require skilled care to qualify for coverage. These guidelines also specify that such care can only be provided by a licensed professional. Before therapy can qualify as skilled care, it must result in improvement and progress toward a goal; maintenance therapy is not considered skilled care in terms of coverage qualification under the Medicare program.

The Medicare guidelines also require that the individual receiving skilled care be *essentially homebound*. Through the years, this requirement has been the subject of varying interpretations. In some instances, the fiscal intermediary has ruled that to be considered homebound, the individual must never leave his or her residence, not even to go onto the front porch or to be taken to a physician's office or medical facility for diagnostic work. At other times, the interpretation has been more liberal, with *essentially homebound* interpreted as being unable to leave a residence easily or on a regular basis. The manner in which the homebound requirement is applied has also had a significant impact on the volume of services that are delivered.

Duration and Intensity of Services

The care provided by the skilled care provider is generally categorized as *intermittent;* that is, it is not continuous service. The professionals employed by the agency visit the client to provide services as needed. Generally clients are not visited daily. The typical professional visit is less than one hour. Home health aides spend approximately two hours per visit, two to three times a week. The average duration of a case is approximately 60 days and typically includes 16 to 18 visits. With increasing utilization review, the number of visits has declined drastically to approximately half in some areas.

However, the actual duration and intensity of service reflects regional usage patterns that differ according to professionals and consumers, geographic conditions, intermediary influence, and the types of client that the provider serves.

Financing and Reimbursement

Medicare is the major third-party payer providing coverage for patients of home care programs. Medicare pays the home care agency an interim rate per visit. A year-end settlement is based on the agency's filing of a Medicare Cost Report to adjust the total payment to actual cost. Cost is limited to those costs that the Medicare program recognizes as reimbursable and to a maximum allowable cost per visit.

The maximum allowable cost per visit is calculated independently for each type of visit and applies for the agency's entire fiscal year. The rate is uniform for all agencies, with adjustments based on the wage index for the geographic area in which the agency provides service, an inflation factor to reflect wage rates in the area, and for hospital-based agencies, an adjustment to reflect the higher administrative and general costs that the agency incurs as a result of being hospital based.

Medicaid coverage varies from state to state. In some states, reimbursement is *cost based* and is calculated in the same manner as are Medicare costs. In other states, a rate is set periodically by the administering body. Medicaid may function like Medicare and provide unlimited coverage that is dependent on medical need or may impose limits on the amount of care that is provided. Prior approval may also be required. Some states have provided expanded levels of supportive care under their home care benefit, and others have provided less care than does the Medicare program.

Coverage with respect to Blue Cross and commercial insurance plans is derived directly from the stipulations of the insured's insurance policy. For the most part, commercial coverage is charge based and may be subject to deductibles and coinsurance. For Blue Cross plans, coverage may be based on costs or charges or may be based on a negotiated rate.

Another type of coverage that is becoming increasingly prevalent is negotiated reimbursement contracts, in which the rate of payment to the home care provider is made on the basis of a preestablished, mutually agreeable fee. These contracts may be with preferred provider organizations (PPOs), health maintenance organizations (HMOs), or major insurance carriers. Such contracts reflect the changing nature of health care reimbursement and the emergence of the need to be price competitive to negotiate contracts for the provision of service to the membership of organized groups.

Certification, Licensure, and Certificate of Need

To provide service to Medicare beneficiaries, the home care agency must be certified by the Medicare program. Such certification requires that the agency comply with the standards that have been set by the federal government and pass an inspection conducted to determine compliance with these *Conditions of Participation*. The inspection process is generally carried out for the Medicare program by a unit of the state government. During the inspection, the organization must demonstrate compliance with the requirements of various other governmental programs, such as those programs designed to protect against discrimination, and must establish that the agency is fiscally competent.

In some states, such as Massachusetts, New Hampshire, New York, New Jersey, and California, the home care agency must also be licensed and may require a certificate of need. The requirements for licensure and certificate of need vary from state to state. However, for the most part, state requirements parallel the Medicare program and add special concerns of the individual state.

Competition

Hospital-based home care programs compete with other established home care providers. A hospital planning to deliver skilled care must assess the effect such competition may have and the community's potential reaction to that competition. An existing agency may have deep community roots and a positive public image as a result of a long history of community-oriented service.

The role of the physician is extremely important in any discussion of competition. Some physicians may see the referral of patients to skilled care in the home as taking revenue from their practices. Also, the home care program may offer services that physicians provide in their offices, for example, blood pressure monitoring or laboratory services. If physicians view home care as infringing on their prerogatives, they will not make referrals. Such action is disastrous for home care agencies because they especially depend on physicians when working with clients in need of skilled care. To be successful, the home care agencies must complement the physician's practice.

Special Considerations

Because the majority of third-party payers reimburse skilled care in the home on a cost basis, home care agencies have little opportunity for profit. A surplus can be generated only on the charge-based commercial insurance and demand-service clients. Depending on the extent of free care that must be provided, the program may operate at minimal gain or loss.

Hospital-based programs may find that the greatest direct financial incentive home care offers the parent organization lies in the ability to shift overhead from the acute care facility to an area that is cost reimbursed. With this in mind, many home care agencies have elected to be hospital based to benefit from overhead allocations from the hospital to the home care program.

This attitude obviously ignores the other benefits of operating a home care program: shortening length of stay, maintaining contact with the patient, and providing a full range of services to the hospital's medical staff. These benefits are positive public relations aspects of home care as is the advantage of a position in the home services market as a link to other home-based services, such as demand services and DME.

Factors Critical to Success

The factors critical to success in the operation of a skilled care program in the home include having access to an appropriate-size referral base, having the ability to market effectively to that referral base, and most important, having the acumen to manage the program efficiently and effectively.

Private-Duty or Demand Service

Private-duty or demand service caters to the discretionary needs of the client. The orientation and behavior of a private-duty program more closely approach that of a business selling a product than a health care agency performing in a regulated environment. The private-duty market is similar to temporary office services and so is often referred to as the staffing model of home care.

Services Provided

The private-duty home care agency frequently has a full range of services available. This kind of agency employs registered nurses, licensed practical nurses, physical therapists, occupational therapists, homemakers, companions, household assistants, and household aides. In practice, the major portion of the business lies in providing home health aides and companions. Generally, the call for the other services is more limited.

The services provided by the homemaker or companion in the private-duty segment of home care and the services provided by a home health aide in the skilled care agency are quite similar. The major distinction is that the duties of the aide in the skilled care agency are generally restricted to the immediate personal health care needs of the individual while the homemaker goes beyond this care to become involved with general housekeeping activities.

Agencies in the private-duty business are commonly under contract to certified home care agencies. Private-duty agencies may also provide home health aide or other services to individuals who are clients of skilled care agencies. In this instance, the billing is to the certified provider, who, in turn, bills the third party. Other sources of business for the private-duty agency are individuals who qualify under public assistance or government programs for the aging.

Client Description

The client generally requires assistance because of a disability, illness, or the infirmities of age. The client generally does not meet the skilled care criteria that clients of a Medicare-certified provider must meet. Care is desired instead of required.

Many of the clients are elderly. However, a significant number of clients may require assistance when a newborn comes home or when one spouse is recuperating from an illness and the other needs to work full time.

Referral Mechanism

Clients receiving care in the private-duty segment of the home care market have generally made contact with the provider directly, or the contact has been initiated by a member of the immediate family unit. Advertising in Yellow Pages directories and print media are the principal vehicles used to make the public aware of sources of assistance. Referrals through friends who previously used the agency are also important.

Physicians, hospitals, and community agencies generally do not directly make referrals. However, they play a role by providing information about sources of service to prospective clients, who may then investigate the options and make their own purchase decisions.

Additional sources of referral include parties who are responsible for the care and well-being of others. Examples of such persons are trust officers and attorneys who are acting as executors for estates and have broad responsibility to provide for the beneficiaries.

Physician's Role

The physician's role in the private-duty market segment is limited. Agencies generally keep physicians informed about the services being rendered to their patients more as a way to create physician awareness than as an operational requirement. Orders from a physician are required only when state law or professional practice acts dictate that the professional providing service may render the care only under medical orders.

Requirements for Coverage

Private-duty home care services are provided on a discretionary basis because the client desires the assistance. As a result, few regulations limit the client's access. The only significant barrier is an economic one: the client must have the ability to pay.

Other requirements reflect the reasonable standards of safety and propriety in the delivery of any service. The services requested may not exceed limits imposed through state professional practice acts or licensure standards for the business or individual practitioner. The service must also meet reasonable safety standards for both the client and employee.

Duration and Intensity of Service

The duration and intensity of private-duty services are based on the desires and finances of the individual. For example, care may consist of support for a few hours a day and a few days a week or the services of a live-in employee who is available around the clock or someone who comes in just overnight so that the family may sleep.

In some cases, such as when a baby nurse moves in with the family for a few days after the mother and child come home from the hospital, services are required for only a short time. In other cases, service may continue for an indefinite period; for example, assistance may be provided to enable a family to keep an elderly, invalid parent at home rather than in an institution.

Financing and Reimbursement

In the private-duty environment, the prevalent pattern of payment is direct payment of charges by the client. However, many agencies will fill out insurance forms so that the client can be reimbursed. Other agencies will bill third-party payers directly. The third parties are generally major medical carriers or supplemental insurers.

Careful procedures are generally required to ensure that the client can pay the charges. Weekly billing cycles and rapid follow-up tend to control accounts receivable. The dependency of the client on the agency and the desire that services be maintained encourages a surprisingly low bad-debt experience.

Contracts with medical assistance programs or other providers tend to be highly competitive. Government contract awards are made almost solely on the basis of price. Organizations that engage in this portion of the private-duty business generally earn low margins on a high volume. Cash flow on these contracts is often a problem.

Certification, Licensure, and Certificate of Need

Standard commercial licenses commonly apply to the private-duty business, and health agency licensure is generally not applicable. Some states are moving toward licensure because of the health care orientation of the services provided by many of these companies. However, the common pattern is for the organization to operate in the same way that personnel and temporary employment agencies do.

Certificate of need is a state option but generally does not apply. Florida had certificate of need until 1984 but then discontinued it. In Maine, licensure and certificate of need apply to both skilled care and private-duty services. Other states are investigating if they should regulate private-duty programs.

Competition

The makeup of the private-duty market is diverse. Several large chain and franchise organizations are attempting to establish national name recognition by offering their units shared support services and assistance with training and organization. The industry also includes a substantial number of independent operators, small agencies that are locally controlled, and individuals who contract directly with the patient.

Special Considerations

Private-duty home care is almost totally a labor-intensive business. The labor is most frequently managed as an on-call pool. The usual arrangement is for staff to be paid only for billable hours worked.

Staff turnover tends to be high, and so recruitment and training becomes an ongoing effort. Training programs are offered frequently to attract potential employees. Participants are not generally compensated for attending these programs. Satisfactory completion of the prescribed program qualifies the individual to be on the agency's roster and to be called for assignment.

Personnel are often on the roster of several companies and work whenever they can get an assignment. Some agencies offer fringe benefits based on actual time worked as a means of creating loyalty and encouraging the availability of personnel.

Factors Critical to Success

Critical factors for success in the private-duty business are marketing and the organization's responsiveness to requests for service. The ability to develop an adequate labor pool is key to the organization's ability to establish a reputation of high quality and reliability. Competitive pricing must also be maintained.

Durable Medical Equipment and Supply

A durable medical equipment (DME) and supply business is predominantly a product business. The emphasis is on distributing material of a medical nature. The business problems are similar to those encountered in the management of any retail enterprise: materials handling, scheduling, and distribution. In addition, a DME business must consider the issues related to rental equipment: tracking of stock, durability, and maintenance.

Services Provided

By definition, *durable medical equipment* (DME) is equipment designed to assist injured or ill patients in their homes. The term is often used broadly to refer to all of the items of supply and equipment that are financed by third-party payers or sold directly to clients. Typical products include ambulatory and comfort aids, such as wheelchairs, canes, commodes, and hospital beds; home oxygen therapy, including respirators, ventilators, and other inhalation therapy equipment; prosthetic devices; nutritional support equipment, including pumps, solutions, and tubing; ostomy supplies and devices; medical supplies; and health-related items, such as bandages, pads, and personal assistance and convenience items that help the debilitated individual to manage more independently.

Client Description

Individuals use these services either because they are prescribed as part of a planned program of care or because the individual desires them as a discretionary convenience item. Thus, this market may be either third-party financed or self-directed.

The client for DME uses items that have been prescribed because of the individual's medical condition or need. Individuals with chronic obstructive pulmonary disease require oxygen and respiratory equipment. Individuals recuperating from corrective surgery or an accident may need wheelchairs and other ambulation devices.

The self-referred client may desire an almost endless array of products. The elderly may purchase bathroom assistance devices to make personal hygiene more comfortable. Younger individuals may purchase exercise equipment. Persons of any age who are concerned about their health may purchase blood pressure monitoring devices.

Referral Mechanism

Referrals come from a number of professional sources including physicians and such ancillary personnel as physical therapists, occupational therapists, rehabilitation therapists, and ostomy nurses. In some cases, the order is placed directly with the dealer. In other instances, clients are instructed on their needs and the potential sources of supply and left to acquire the item by themselves.

Home care agencies are major referral sources. The necessary supportive supplies and equipment are often identified by the home care staff when they are providing care to individuals in their homes.

In addition to the clients who are professionally referred, some clients are self-referred. Because of the existence of this discretionary market, many companies choose to maintain stores in retail locations so that various products can be displayed.

Physician's Role

Because DME is both a professional-referred and self-referred market, the physician's role depends on the particular item required. The physician must generally write orders for those items that are going to be reimbursed by third parties but may only advise the client on the purchase of discretionary products. The physician sometimes defers specification (and actual ordering) to another party, such as a physical therapist or a home care program.

Requirements for Coverage

When a third party finances the acquisition of DME, a physician's order is generally required, and the recipient is subject to guidelines that determine qualification for DME services.

The Medicare program often imposes specific criteria for services that it believes may have been abused. An example of this is requiring the documentation of blood gas levels to determine if oxygen services are needed. Guidelines have also been issued on when different modes of oxygen delivery (cylinder, liquid, or concentrator) are to used. Commercial carriers frequently follow the same criteria set by the government.

The market for individually prescribed items for the self-pay market is growing. Among the items being purchased with increasing frequency are blood pressure devices; home emergency dental kits; and self-diagnostic laboratory test kits, the best known of which is the home pregnancy test kit.

Duration and Intensity of Service

Because of the wide mix of conditions under which DME is acquired and the diversity of products, no uniformity in utilization exists. Supply items, which are usually suitable for only one-time use, are often required on an ongoing basis. Equipment rentals can be for many months or for a few days. For example a patient who has chronic obstructive pulmonary disease or who requires nutritional support may need oxygen or medical supplies for an indefinite period.

Financing and Reimbursement

Medicare coverage for DME services is predominantly under Part B, with the rate based on customary and prevailing charges. Part B covers 80 percent of the charge. Claims are subject to an annual deductible. Reimbursement under Medicare Part A is 80 percent of reasonable cost.

For Medicare, the charge is prospective, and so the difference between the cost of service and the Medicare rate can represent profit to the provider. This situation is different from that of skilled care services, which is reimbursed on a cost basis.

The preponderance of all DME is acquired under third-party reimbursement, with Medicare the major third-party payer. The coverage for commercial carriers is dependent on the client's individual policy, with the dollar amount calculated as some portion of the dealer's charge.

Certification, Licensure, and Certificate of Need

Certificate of need and certification do not apply to the DME market segment. Dealers must apply to Medicare program for approval to participate. However, this application is basically a process of establishing a billing identity. Standard mercantile permits are all that is required to enter the DME market.

Competition

A large number of DME businesses are owner operated, are not affiliated with any central source or franchising agent, and are limited in their number of locations. Owners of DME businesses may also be wholesale distributors to doctors and hospitals. Other segments of the dealer base include drugstores; department stores, such as Sears & Roebuck; and catalog and mail order dealers.

Major companies are significantly increasing their involvement in the DME market. These companies have built their networks through a combination of business start-ups and acquisitions.

Current DME dealers are concerned about the entry of hospitals into the DME market. After all, hospitals have an extremely close relationship with the most critical element in a DME business's success: the consumer of service.

Factors Critical to Success

The DME market has matured significantly during the past few years. Although it was once an easy business to run and one whose success was virtually assured, today significantly greater management acumen is required. Margins have been reduced so that efficiency of operation is essential for the business to be financially viable. A thorough knowledge of billing requirements is critical if the dealer is to appropriately cope with the more stringent regulatory limitations. This implies quality business systems and automation. To operate as efficiently as possible, dealers are installing sophisticated software systems to track clinical and fiscal data.

In almost any geographic area, a competitive environment can be assumed. To be successful, the dealer must provide a full range of services and at competitive prices. Clients want the convenience of one-stop shopping that fills all their needs reliably and at competitive prices. Responsiveness, complete product lines, timely delivery, availability of clinical consultants, and good service are all factors that the purchaser considers when deciding with whom to establish a business relationship. A new dealer who starts out with a limited product line and reduced service capacity but with the intent of expanding as the business develops has little chance of succeeding.

Integrated Care

One of the incentives for providing home care services is being able to care for patients as they progress through the various stages of their illness. Home care is the next step along a continuum that may begin in the acute care hospital and progress to the home care agency. Home care is not a single market, but rather several markets that are intertwined. Patients may receive different types of care — skilled care, private pay, DME — with one type following the other or in combination and with care provided by one or a combination of providers.

Involvement in the multiplicity of home care service areas represents an opportunity for integration, that is, the provision of various components of the services used by the homebound individual regardless of the level of acuity. The total revenue generated is maximized if a full spectrum of services is offered.

The condition of home care patients does not necessarily improve. Some patients, for example, the patient who needs a ventilator, receive subacute-level services for extended periods. The condition of other patients may worsen, and they then have to return to the more intense acute or inpatient level of care. Involvement by a particular institution in the provision of services at home helps retain contact with the patients and reduces the risk of losing them to another provider.

Home care is different from the services that most acute care facilities are accustomed to delivering. Home care is unique because its practitioners work without direct supervision to provide services at many individual sites. This situation necessitates specialized mechanisms for organizing staff and ensuring the quality of care. Added to this is that home care is subject to a complete, separate set of reimbursement and regulatory constraints.

The various segments of the home care business are complementary, and all can be integrated with hospital services. Skilled home care patients may have laboratory work provided through the acute care facility or a related laboratory. They may also need DME or medical supplies, or they may purchase supplementary services because they desire a level of support beyond that which is available through third-party financing. Private-pay clients may receive active treatment at outpatient facilities or may purchase items at their discretion from a DME company.

The home care market is maturing, and major opportunities in the development of home care programs still exist. Entry requires that the provider select the service it wishes to develop based on its individual strengths and corporate objectives and then develop and implement these services with excellence.

Chapter 3

A Strategic Plan

Teri L. Louden

Strategic planning is critical to the long-term success of any business. The purpose of planning is to routinely assess market and internal conditions and develop strategies that ensure a strong market position. The planning process also integrates new venture plans with existing business strategies.

Home care planning efforts should consist of both short-range and long-range strategies. In addition to developing an overall strategic plan, each of the many home care product or market segments should have its own unique plan because of the wide differences in reimbursement, success factors, and customer base for each segment.

Planning is particularly important in the home care market because of the rapidity with which change is occurring. The variety of both positive and negative forces affecting the industry also make planning particularly difficult. The use of home care is being affected positively by such underlying forces as the aging population, pressures for more cost-effective health care, and consumer demand. However, negative forces are causing a decrease in revenues and profits. Some of these negative forces are changes in Medicare home care reimbursement, bidding by health maintenance organizations (HMOs) for home care products and services, and increased competition.

With all the changes on the home care horizon, many hospitals may argue that planning is impossible. On the contrary, understanding the market and developing a plan is imperative precisely because of the environment of change and uncertainty. Indeed, rapid change represents an opportunity for those organizations that are positioned for the future through effective long-term planning.

Teri L. Louden is president of Louden & Company, Chicago, Illinois.

Developing a home care strategic plan should yield these concrete results:

- Clear decision on which products and services should be included in the hospital's home care product and service portfolio
- Definition of target markets and a marketing strategy for reaching key decision makers
- Specific expectations for the home care business that will serve as a tool for measuring future performance
- Background data and analysis necessary to obtain approval and funding from both internal and external sources and to track performance

The Strategic Planning Process

The strategic plan consists of four main elements:

- *Formulation of goals and objectives.* At the heart of a successful strategy is a clear understanding of what the hospital wants from its home care business (its goal) and the steps it must take to get what it wants (its objectives). Identifying these goals and objectives in the initial planning stages ensures the coordination of the home care strategy with overall hospital objectives.
- *Environmental assessment.* The home care business is affected by a large number of external factors, such as market dynamics, competitive actions, and regulatory issues. Data on how these factors affect the hospital's opportunities in the various home care market segments must be collected and analyzed.
- *Internal assessment.* A strategy should incorporate an internal review of the hospital. This analysis requires taking an organizational inventory, evaluating capabilities and weaknesses as they relate to requirements for a successful home care venture, and assessing internal resources.
- *Strategy development.* On the basis of the environmental and internal assessment, strategies are developed to meet the goals and objectives. The strategies cover the key areas of product and service development, marketing, finance, and organizational issues.

This chapter outlines a five-step approach for initiating a home care strategic plan (figure 3-1, next page):

- Task force selection
- Formulation of goals and objectives
- Data collection
- Data analysis and issue formulation
- Strategy development

Figure 3-1 also shows that strategic planning is an ongoing effort. Organizational goals and objectives must be continually refined in light of the new

Figure 3-1.   Strategic Planning Flow Chart

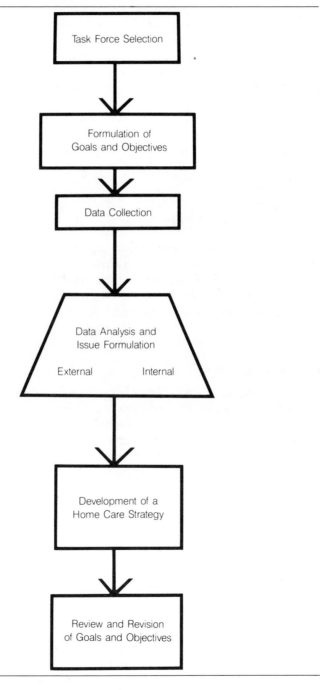

issues and opportunities that are identified through data analysis. Persons responsible for the hospital's home care strategic planning cycle must be concerned with how to ensure that the process goes beyond a one-time analysis of market opportunities. The best way to institute regular review of the developed strategy is to integrate the initial home care strategic plan into the hospital's general planning cycle. If this integration is not possible, then at least the general planning requirements of the hospital should be considered when the format for the home care plan is developed.

The general framework for planning described in this chapter should be tailored to the specific organization. The scope of the strategic plan should reflect the organization's specific needs, management requirements, and available resources.

Task Force Selection

A home care task force is responsible for collecting and analyzing data, identifying issues and opportunities, and advising on home care strategy. It is both a means of accessing information and a tool for sharing the work load. After the implementation of a home care program, a task force can also serve as an ongoing mechanism for ensuring the smooth, high-quality operations of home care businesses and ventures.

Why a Task Force

A task force approach works particularly well in the development of a home care strategy because information must be collected and analyzed from many areas, both inside and outside the hospital. Home care information is particularly scattered, reflecting the decentralized discharge process found in most hospitals. Further, interest in home care crosses departmental lines and so requires knowledge from many functional areas.

Using a task force alleviates the risk of planning in a vacuum. The end product of these cooperative efforts is a stronger plan: with better, more accurate information available, the organization faces fewer surprises in the implementation phases. Issues are more likely to be identified and discussed during the planning process rather than after the strategy has been formalized. Also, the strategy developed by the group may represent a more creative approach than could have been devised by any one individual.

Sound political reasons exist for using the task force approach. A task force with members from key areas enables everyone to participate. Enthusiastic members of the task force help sell the program to colleagues throughout the hospital. Further, the setting up of a task force draws attention from all levels of staff and is an indication that management views the project as a priority. Finally, the program may be easier to implement because task force members act as facilitators out of a sense of ownership.

Recruitment of Task Force Members

Task force members should represent the various areas of the hospital that refer patients to home care. A team of six to eight members works well. Larger teams can become unwieldy.

The core group shown in figure 3-2, below, should definitely be represented on the team. Additional members can be recruited from the list of all other areas that make referrals to home care.

Individuals from departments with relatively large home care referrals must be included on the task force so that the task force is ensured access to data on the volume of referrals. Also, the task force must include at least one key member of the medical staff who is a strong supporter of home care.

The persons selected for the task force should be interested in and committed to seeing the project through to completion. Prospective members must be willing to devote time and energy to the team.

The goal of the recruiting process is to assemble a team that inspires enthusiasm and creates momentum to complete the project. Therefore, several aspects of the overall group composition must be considered:

- *Visibility.* The credibility of the task force is greatly enhanced if a few high-ranking staff members are recruited. Having members who can use political clout to secure needed resources may be especially helpful. Credibility is also enhanced if the task force has the overt support of a respected and influential physician.
- *Organization within the task force.* To function effectively, any group needs a combination of skills and abilities. The task force should have a balance of leaders and workers. Collecting and analyzing data requires a certain skill level, and the task force should include some members who are able and willing to do this work.
- *Group dynamics.* The person who is selecting task force members must consider how prospective team members may interact in a group

Figure 3-2. Task Force Members

Core Group	Other Areas Involved in Home Care Referral Process
Administration	Pharmacy
Discharge planning/social service	Nutrition
Physicians	Outpatient clinics
Nursing	Occupational therapy
Respiratory therapy	Speech therapy
Physical therapy	

Source: Louden & Company

setting. Checking on how prospective members have worked together in the past may help avoid potential conflicts.

The last ingredient for a successful task force is management support. Even the best task force cannot succeed without the support of hospital management. Members of the task force need to devote significant time to the development of a home care strategic plan, and this requirement can create problems unless top management makes a conscious investment decision to support the task force's activities.

Formulation of Goals and Objectives

Hospital's Goals and Objectives

A home care strategy is effective only if it satisfies the goals of the hospital. Therefore, understanding these goals at the outset is essential if the evaluation of home care opportunities is to be meaningful.

A hospital may want to enter the home care market for a variety of reasons (see figure 3-3, below). For instance, a hospital may have financial motives for considering the development of a durable medical equipment

Figure 3-3. Objectives for Hospital Home Care Programs

Marketing
- Continuum of care
- Broad range of products and services (full-service model)
- Application to groups (HMOs, insurance companies, employers)
- Joint ventures with physicians

Financial
- Additional revenues and profit
- Readmission of patients
- Reduced length of stay
- Leverage of existing resources, such as financial resources, image, facilities

Home Care

Community Service Image
- Enhancement of community image
- Public relations
- Fulfillment of mission

Patient Concern
- Involvement in discharge planning process
- Home care quality-control measures
- Patient satisfaction

Source: Louden & Co.

(DME) business. Another hospital may have marketing reasons for developing a home care business. For this hospital, the actual bottom-line profits may be seen as less important than the reduction of length of patient stays through the provision of home care.

The hospital's goals will determine which home care businesses and markets should be targeted and will provide guidance in making such operational decisions as whether to own the operation or seek a joint venture relationship, what specific products and services to include on the home care menu, and how to relate the home care operations to existing hospital businesses. For example, if a hospital is considering home care to appeal to HMOs and to increase referrals to home care by physicians, it should plan to offer a full range of products and services at a competitive price. To accomplish this goal, this hospital may consider participating in a joint venture, particularly with physician groups, rather than totally owning the home care business.

In determining goals, the hospital must assess its risk profile. Some home care businesses are riskier than others, particularly those businesses that require heavy capital investment. One way of participating in home care while minimizing the risk is to enter a joint venture relationship with a current home care provider. During the initial planning stages of the venture, the hospital should make sure that the other venture partner understands how much risk the hospital is prepared to take. If the hospital understands how much risk it can afford to take, it will be better able to tailor its home care strategies to avoid unnecessary risk.

Different types of organizations will necessarily have different goals. A regional or national chain or affiliated hospital group is more likely to participate in joint ventures with a national home care provider that can service the needs of all of its hospitals. A local hospital may prefer to join forces with a small, local vendor that it has worked with over the years.

Rural and urban hospitals may also differ in their home care goals. With more providers in their market, urban hospitals spend more time trying to identify unmet consumer needs and assessing their ability to compete effectively. Rural hospitals may have an obligation to provide home care if no alternative providers are available in their service area. However, rural hospitals must carefully consider the high cost of providing home care when staff members must travel long distances between visits to patients.

Role of the Task Force

The role of the task force in formulating goals and objectives for home care varies depending on management. Task force members may be asked to identify possible goals and objectives or to refine goals and objectives that have already been established by management. Objectives can be identified through interviews with management and discussions among task force members.

In any event, management and the task force must be in agreement on what the goals and objectives for the home care program will be. Both groups must also agree on the exact wording of the objectives. One method of deciding on specific home care objectives is to ask management and task force members to rank order those objectives they think are best for the hospital's home care program. These rankings can then be used to establish the priorities of various home care objectives.

Data Collection

Data collection provides information needed to analyze the market and assess the organization's capabilities. The data collection process should be organized in advance to save time and money, avoid duplication of effort, and ensure that all necessary information is gathered.

Top management must be committed to the data-gathering effort because it takes a significant amount of time and crosses departmental lines. Management support is essential to secure cooperation from all areas and to avoid delays in the process.

Sources of Home Care Data

Home care information is abundant and comes from a variety of sources, both inside and outside the hospital. Figure 3-4, next page, lists possible sources of home care data and examples of the kinds of information that can be obtained from internal and external sources.

Hospital staff members can provide a wealth of knowledge about the health care industry as well as a perspective on the internal environment. The task force should make use of this resource whenever possible. However, one problem with obtaining information from in-house sources is that much of it is decentralized and thus difficult to find and time-consuming to collect. The task force will save time if it can identify key persons in the hospital who are knowledgeable about home care and who understand the flow of information across departments.

The task force may want to examine patient health records to see how many patients are discharged into a home care program. Past referrals to home care are good indicators of potential opportunities. Patients discharged from the hospital are the major market for hospitals who do not anticipate referrals from their competitors. Patients' health records are a possible source of information on discharges. Unfortunately, however, the health records may not provide any follow-up information on the provision of home care services after the patient has been discharged. To get such information, the task force may have to collect detailed discharge data on each patient for a period of several months.

Many outside groups are also good sources of information. For example, vendors of home care products can project the hospital's volume by

Figure 3-4. Sources of Information and Examples of the Kinds of Information to Be Obtained

Internal Sources: Physicians and Hospital Personnel	Examples of Information
• Physicians:	• Knowledge of home care
— Key medical staff leaders	• Referral volumes—past and present
— Major home care referrers	• Characteristics of patients referred
— Physicians who do not refer to home care	• Criteria for referral
• Discharge planners	• Referral process
• Social workers	• Agencies or companies referred to and why
• Nursing staff	• Support of hospital program
• Physical therapists	• Interest in financial participation (physicians)
• Occupational therapists	
• Respiratory therapists	
• Pharmacists	

External Sources	Examples of Information
• Home care agencies and companies frequently used by the hospital	• Volume of referrals received from the hospital by referral department
• HMOs and PPOs	• Type of services or products provided by home care providers
• Third-party payers: Medicare, Medicaid, private insurance companies	• Geographic coverage
	• Criteria used by HMOs and PPOs to evaluate home care companies
	• Reimbursement coverage and rates
	• Filing requirements, processing time
	• Denial rates, appeals process

Source: Louden & Company

reviewing their records and determining what volume of home care referrals they obtain from the hospital,. Vendors are also good sources of market and competitive information. Customer groups, such as local employers and HMOs, can provide information on their specialized needs and on their criteria for selecting home care providers. Government demographic data is available and can be analyzed for a local market to help predict potential demand for home care. Also, with the recent growth in home care, much information is being published by associations, trade magazines, and business publications.

Data Collection Methods

Two general methods are used in data collection. *Primary research* involves performing basic market research, usually to understand customer-based issues. *Secondary research* consists of sifting through existing research to locate information pertinent to the hospital's market.

Primary Research

Primary research can be structured to address specific home care questions that cannot be answered by searching through available data or literature. It is particularly useful in gaining an understanding of the home care referral process, market needs, home care political issues, and internal capabilities. Three approaches for collecting primary data are:

- *Interviews.* Interviews can be conducted in person or over the telephone. The interview format allows the interviewer to probe responses or clarify questions. Interviews of key hospital staff members should provide the task force with a clear understanding of the discharge planning process.
- *Focus groups.* Focus groups allow the hospital to obtain information in an informal atmosphere that promotes interaction between participants. Usually focus groups consist of 5 to 10 persons and one moderator who loosely guides the discussion; a focus group does not usually have a formal structure. This type of discussion is helpful in identifying customer needs and developing new ideas. However, the task force should avoid drawing specific conclusions from focus-group discussions because the small size of the groups limits the validity of the conclusions. The suggestions, ideas, or recommendations from a focus group often serve as a good basis for conducting more extensive and more formal research.
- *Written surveys.* Written surveys can be used to collect many types of market and internal information. For home care strategy development, the task force can use a survey to monitor the hospital's discharges to home care. Because hospitals do not routinely collect this data, the task force will need to develop a survey that follows patient discharge activity for several months at least. Figure 3-5, next page, shows examples of information that should be collected.
  Before performing this research, the task force must fully understand the discharge planning process so that it can collect all the information it requires. Information on the discharge planning process in the hospital can be obtained by interviewing appropriate staff members.
  Once an effective instrument for collecting home care discharge data is developed, it should be used as an ongoing measurement of

Figure 3-5.   Home Care Patient Discharge Tracking Information

Home Care Patient Characteristics	Method of Payment
• Age	• Medicare
• Sex	• Medicaid
• Geographic location	• HMO
• Living alone or with relatives or friends	• Private insurance
	• Self-pay
Services or Products Required	**Department Referring**
• Detailed breakdown of home care services needed	• Discharge planning
	• Respiratory therapy
• Detailed breakdown of equipment need	• Physical therapy
	• Other
Physician Information	**Home Care Company Referred to**
• Name of physician referrer	• Agency
• Specialty	• DME company
• Age of physician	

Source: Louden & Company

the hospital's home care activity. Summarizing this information on a monthly basis will help the task force and hospital management to understand the hospital's home care referral base.

Secondary Research

Secondary research often turns up useful, low-cost data and is worth the time required to identify and secure information. Secondary research provides a good knowledge base for designing and conducting primary research.

The methods for gathering data are straightforward: literature searches, reading, and phone calls to secondary sources. Because a lot of information is currently available on home care, the task force must use a disciplined approach to avoid spending too much time on this effort.

Comparison of Research Methods

Figure 3-6, next page, compares the advantages and disadvantages of primary and secondary research. In sum, primary research is superior because it is

Figure 3-6. Comparison of Research Methods

Research Method	Advantages	Disadvantages
Primary research	• Timely data • Situation specific • Identifies customer needs and unmet market opportunities	• Expensive • Time Intensive
Secondary research	• Low cost • Fast and easy to collect	• Outdated information • Not situation specific • Information may not be available

Source: Louden & Company

specific to the hospital's situation, provides more timely data, and gives the hospital a clearer idea of what the customer wants.

However, the cost of primary research is high, in both time and money. The task force will need to develop an appropriate research plan by weighing financial and timing constraints against research needs and internal research capabilities.

Costs for primary research can be controlled by using members of the home care task force, as well as students or part-time researchers, for selective interviewing. Despite the costs, the benefits of primary research justify its use, and hospitals should not neglect this kind of research.

Data Analysis and Issue Formulation

At this point, the task force must analyze the data to identify key strategic issues and opportunities. This process involves looking at two broad areas:

- Environmental factors: marketplace, competition, reimbursement, legal issues, technology
- Internal factors: human resources, physical resources, financial resources, hospital politics, hospital organizational and structural issues, physician preferences

In this section, each of these areas is discussed and the factors to consider within each area are outlined.

Environmental Factors

Data on environmental factors should include information on the marketplace, competition, reimbursement, legal and regulatory issues, and technology.

Marketplace

The assessment of opportunity by market segment should begin with an evaluation of the hospital's customer base. This type of assessment enables the hospital to predict the demand in its service area for home care products and services. Forecasting the demand for home care is at best an inexact science, requiring a creative meshing of several approaches:

- *Macro formula-based forecasting models.* Various agencies and organizations have published models that forecast overall home care demand on the basis of population in a given area. Figure 3-7, below, shows examples of commonly used home care planning formulas. The forecasts that result from these formulas vary widely, as these forecasts are for a particular organization in a specific geographic location. Home care is a rapidly changing industry and is highly dependent on local attitudes and the reimbursement climate. Consequently, wide geographic variations in market potential exist. Further, these macro models predict *overall* demand for home care, rather than the demand for individual lines of business. Also, because these models are historically based, they do not reflect the recent changes

Figure 3-7. Macro Formula-Based Home Care Demand Forecasting Models

Author	Formula
Department of Health, Education and Welfare	.067 x population over age 65
Kaiser-Permanete System	.07 x hospital discharges
Southwestern Pennsylvania HSA	.04 x hospital discharges x 2
Piedmont HSA	(.07 x population over age 65) + (.005 x population under age 65)
National League for Nursing	(.026 x population over age 65) + (.013 x population under age 65)
Ohio Department of Health	(.002 x population under age 14) + (.0115 x population age 15-64) + (.118 x population age 65 and over)
Georgia Department of Human Resources	(.14 x population 65-74) + (.25 x population age 75 and over)
New Jersey/Pennsylvania HSA	(.06 x population age 65 and over) + (.08 x hospital med/surg discharges) + (.5 x nursing home discharges)
University of California	(.118 to .160 x population over age 65) + (.15 to .30 x nursing home population) + (.03 to .09 x hospital discharges)

Reprinted with permission of the National Association for Home Care, from *Caring* magazine, July 1984, p. 18.

in the market, such as the impact of Medicare prospective pricing. In spite of these shortcomings, these models provide a quick and easy starting point for estimating market potential.

- *Hospital-based projections.* The relevant market for most hospitals is their home care discharges. The data from the task force's survey of patient discharge activity provides recent, situation-specific data from which the task force can forecast demand. This forecast must be annualized and augmented by any anticipated nonhospital referrals, such as those from physicians and nursing homes. Again, although the information from this source is recent, it is still historical, and therefore, its use is limited in developing forecasts for a rapidly changing market.
- *Customer need-based forecasting.* An understanding of customer needs can be the basis for a meaningful prospective forecast of the demand for home care. Using primary and secondary data, the task force should analyze the following questions:
  - What are the key customer-targeted market segment options?
  - For each segment, what are the relevant demographics and psychographics, and what implications do they have for home-care-related needs?
  - How do the needs of customer groups translate to demand for home care products and services?

  Customer need-based forcasting can be difficult to quantify, and the cost to do so may be prohibitive for some hospitals. However, the need-based method is powerful because it correctly establishes the customer as the focus for planning, and it can result in creative new ways of meeting customer needs.

Using a combination of the three types of forecasting and tailoring the analysis to the particular organization should result in a good understanding of the marketplace. The external and internal factors provide tools for analyzing the attractiveness of the market and the hospital's potential for success in the various segments.

Competition

The growth in home care has attracted many new competitors to a market traditionally served by small local providers. Home care represents a diversification opportunity for many of these new providers, who may be hospitals, local pharmacies, national medical products companies, DME manufacturers and suppliers, consumer package goods companies, drugstore chains, and private entrepreneurs.

Hospitals must perform an extensive review of the competition that does the following:

- Identifies major competitors and assesses their strengths and weaknesses
- Predicts potential competitive reaction
- Plans a counter response for the hospital
- Refines the forecast of patient demand in light of the review of the competition

Competition even exists inside the hospital. The hospital cannot afford to forget that physicians have home care preferences and the power to refer patients to outside providers.

Reimbursement

Changes in the reimbursement structure have a massive effect on the utilization of health care. Prospective pricing has fueled the growth of home care as hospitals try to control costs by reducing average length of stay. Although diagnosis-related groups (DRGs), the basis for prospective pricing, have not yet been applied to home care, the reimbursement climate is changing as government attempts to control spending. Examples of changes in home care reimbursement include the 1985 Medicare rental and sale guidelines for low-cost DME and Medicare caps on home care agency charges. Given the rapidly changing climate for the home care scene and the wide variations in reimbursement practices across the country, the home care task force must carefully assess the effect of changes in reimbursement policies on the hospital's ability to do business.

Customer groups — HMOs, insurance companies, and employee groups — are emerging as major forces in the reimbursement picture. These large customers control huge numbers of patients and are increasingly concerned with the cost of health care. One innovation being marketed to provide consumers with protection from the high costs of extended home care use and nursing home stays is insurance for long-term care. If this kind of insurance becomes widespread, it could have a significant positive impact on the future demand for home care.

Legal Issues

Home care is a heavily regulated industry, and a major source of patient-oriented regulations is Medicare. These regulations are designed to protect the consumer and third-party payers.

Because of these many regulations, the task force should be aware that entering into or expanding a home care business, both for start-up operations or joint ventures, can raise complex legal questions. These legal questions need to be evaluated with respect to their effect on the hospital's potential home care business. Five major legal issues have special implications for home care providers:

- *Kickbacks.* The Medicare-Medicaid Antifraud and Abuse Amendments of the Social Security Act prohibit seeking or receiving remuneration for patient referrals.
- *Patient's rights.* Medicare requires freedom of choice, which means that patients must not be coerced or compelled to use a particular provider. Hospital personnel may only *recommend* providers.
- *Corporate structure and tax issues.* Hospitals must ensure that their organizational structure is appropriate for a home care operation. Hospitals planning joint ventures need to be especially aware that such ventures may affect their tax status. They also need to understand the advantages and disadvantages of a partnership versus a corporate structure for the home care business..
- *Liabilities.* Hospitals entering the home care market must consider both insurance and malpractice issues. The hospital must understand the effect that a home care program will have on its insurance rates.
- *Licensing.* Hospitals must comply with state certificate-of-need (CON) requirements.

Chapters 4 and 8 discuss organizational structure and legal issues, respectively, in more detail.

Technology

Advances in disease treatments and product technology have resulted in more home care therapies and a greater number of patients with conditions amenable to home treatment. For example, the increased portability of pump devices allows cancer patients to receive continuous chemotherapy infusion while carrying on their normal daily routine. Computer technology, through the use of in-home patient monitoring and control systems, is also expected to have a major impact on home care in the future. The task force needs to assess technological developments as they relate to home care opportunities under consideration. The task force also needs to be aware of future advances in technology and the impact of these advances on the home care business.

Internal Factors

An analysis of internal factors requires an assessment of how well the organization is positioned for participation in the home care market. This assessment includes taking an inventory of the resources necessary for success in home care as well as an evaluation of how readily the hospital can make the transition to providing home care.

Human Resources

Does the hospital possess, or have access to, the staff required for home care? The home care organization may require specialized staff, and so a decision on whether to transfer personnel from the hospital must be made. If this action must be taken, employee willingness, pay scales, benefits, and special home care training must be considered. If internal staff is not available or if transferring staff is not feasible, the task force must look to the local labor supply. Top management of the hospital will need to dedicate time to the home care effort, particularly in the early phases before a home care manager is added to the staff.

Physical Resources

The various home care business segments have different physical resource requirements, which correspond to the level of total investment required and the risk or return relationship of the business. For example, a DME operation has relatively high capital requirements, such as the need for warehouse facilities, delivery vehicles, equipment inventory, maintenance equipment, and perhaps retail showroom space for walk-in business. Investors are rewarded with higher rates of return on a DME business relative to home care service businesses. At the other end of the spectrum is a home care agency, which is essentially a people business that has a less favorable average return on investment.

Hospitals must evaluate their available physical resources in light of the requirements for operating the home care businesses under consideration. The hospital may have facility space or equipment that can be devoted to home care operations, or it may need to use existing vendors because of the lack of available facilities and the high cost of investing in new facilities and equipment.

Financial Resources

The task force needs to determine the financial investment required for home care opportunities in terms of initial capital investment and working capital needs. Does the organization have the necessary capital, or does it have access to the necessary funds? Is management willing to make the level of investment required to succeed in the home care business? Is it willing to take any potential downside financial risks?

Members of the financial staff of the hospital should be asked to do a financial analysis. Outside accountants with home care expertise can also be used as necessary. Projections on investment, income and expenses, and cash flow should be detailed for each home care option that the task force is considering.

Hospital Politics

Does the organization have an entrepreneurial environment that promotes innovation? This question is a difficult one to answer because it is subjective in nature. However, the answer is critical to the overall success of any potential home care venture. The task force should make some effort to evaluate the entrepreneurial spirit of the organization by looking at several areas:

- Are the personalities of management and staff flexible and able to deal with change?
- Do key constituents, particularly in the physician group, support the idea of home care?
- Does the hospital enjoy a track record of successful new ventures, or would this venture into home care be the first such venture?

Hospital Organizational and Structural Issues

The organizational structure of the home care business is ultimately determined by the home care strategy. The task force members should consider various options for structuring the home care business by answering questions such as the following:

- What type of corporate identity should the home care business have?
- To what extent should the home care operation be coordinated with other outpatient areas?
- How should the home care business relate to the main business of the hospital?
- Who will have home care management accountability, and what reporting relationships will be appropriate?

Answers to such questions depend on the particular home care businesses being considered, the existing corporate structure, and management philosophy. Expert legal counsel should be consulted with regard to for-profit and not-for-profit issues and the placement of home care in the organizational structure of the hospital. Chapter 4 discusses some of these issues.

Physician Preferences

The success or failure of a home care program depends on the reaction of the hospital's physician group. The hospital must recognize that the physician is a key player in this relationship because physicians can specify a provider along with their prescription for home care products and services.

In the data-gathering phase of the planning process, physicians were interviewed. How did they define quality for home care providers? What were the key preferences of physicians for any home care program? By integrating these findings into the home care strategy, the hospital has a greater chance of gaining physician support for its home care operation.

Another area to consider is whether staff physicians are involved in any other home care business. Through affiliation agreements, many physicians have interests in these businesses, and these arrangements can have a negative impact on the hospital's chance for success in specific home care market segments.

Strategy Development

The result of strategy development is a thoughtful, cohesive plan for the hospital's future in home care. This plan will become the blueprint for implementing the hospital's participation in a home care business. The task force must develop a home care plan that is based on the hospital's goals and objectives, its risk profile, and the issues that were identified in the analysis of external and internal factors.

The resulting strategy statement should cover the following areas:

- *Customer target markets.* On the basis of the customer survey, who is the customer target market for home care products and services? Once the needs of this target group are identified, the home care program and other new venture strategies can be tailored to serve these customers.
- *Quality control procedures and evaluation systems.* Measuring and monitoring the quality of home care is particularly difficult because the nature of care given in the home requires independent judgment and limited direct supervision. Nonetheless, problems relating to quality must be considered, and mechanisms must be put into place to ensure ongoing monitoring of patient care and satisfaction.
- *Financial projections.* Such projections should include forecasts of revenue and expenses, cash flow, ratio analysis, and breakeven expectation for the strategy the team has developed.
- *Marketing plan.* Although the details of a marketing plan can be determined during the implementation stages, the task force should first identify the image that the home care business should project. General strategies can be outlined for communicating the image to target customers, decision makers, and referral resources. Because home care is still a relatively new concept, education is the primary key to a successful marketing program.
- *Selection of home care businesses and identification of products and support services to be offered.* Product-line decisions are heavily influenced by the hospital's goals. Consideration should be given to what segments of the home care business the hospital wants to develop. The task force should address whether the hospital or the home care operation will have responsibility for the major areas of support services listed in figure 3-8, next page.

Figure 3-8. Form for Indicating Responsibility for Support Services

	Responsibility	
Service Components	Hospital	Home Care Provider
• Physician and staff education		
• Patient and family education		
• Discharge planning coordination		
• Reimbursement management—billing and collections		
• Patient care visits		
— Nursing		
— Therapies		
— Other		
• Quality control		
• Buying and inventory of supplies		
• Delivery of supplies and equipment		
• Patient support services		
— 24-hour coverage		
— Family support		
• IV Pharmacy Compounding		

Source: Louden & Company

- *Alternative home care entry vehicles.* Given the hospital's goals, should the hospital achieve its home care goals by starting its own business, acquiring an existing provider, or entering into a joint venture relationship? The start-up and acquisition options require more capital and have a higher level of risk but allow the hospital the greatest degrees of control.

  The joint venture option is the fastest, least capital-intensive way to get into the business, but the ongoing relationships involved can be complex to manage. A joint venture can be arranged in many ways, from a complex corporate partnership structure to a simple fee-for-service arrangement. The decision depends largely on whether appropriate joint venture candidates are available in the hospital's service area and on how much time and effort hospital management wants to devote to starting up a home care business. Timing is also a consideration, as start-ups and acquisitions can greatly extend market entry time.

Finally, the task force should plan a time line for the implementation of its home care strategic plan. Management needs to know when they can expect to have an operating business. The specific lead times required vary tremendously depending on the segment of the home care business the hospital is developing, and a workable timetable is necessary to coordinate all the implementation steps.

The task force should establish a number of checkpoints during the start-up phase so that it can evaluate the implementation of the plan. One particularly critical point to identify is when to hire a manager whose sole job is to direct the home care efforts.

A Reminder

Three keys to a productive planning process are:

- The strategic planning process should be ongoing, with the results and findings from this effort used to refine home care goals and objectives.
- Management commitment and involvement are critical to the success of a home care program. Management's input is needed at several stages, and its enthusiasm and influence should be used to smooth any resistance encountered along the way.
- The task-force approach works well for developing a home care strategic plan. Assembling an enthusiastic, action-oriented group from appropriate departments of the hospital gives the home care program the best possible start.

Chapter 4

Organizational Structure

Lawrence A. Manson

A hospital that is attempting to choose the optimal organizational structure for a new home care venture must consider several issues:

- Should the home care project be operated as a hospital department, or should it be a freestanding unit?
- Should the hospital develop the project on its own, or should it participate in the project with other hospitals, physicians, existing home care agencies, or other organizations?
- Should the home care organization be operated on a not-for-profit or a for-profit basis?
- What is the organizational form best suited to the home care venture?
- How does the proposed home care venture fit in with the existing structure of the hospital and its related organizations?

The decisions that hospital managers make with regard to each of these issues influences the range of options available to them. Figure 4-1, next page, uses a decision tree to show the possible paths a hospital may take in determining the organizational structure for its home care program. This chapter discusses each of the decisions that hospital managers must make as they plan a home care venture.

Lawrence A. Manson, J.D., is a partner in the law firm of Wood, Lucksinger & Epstein, Chicago, Illinois.

Figure 4-1. Decisions That Must Be Made in Determining the Appropriate Organizational Structure for Home Care

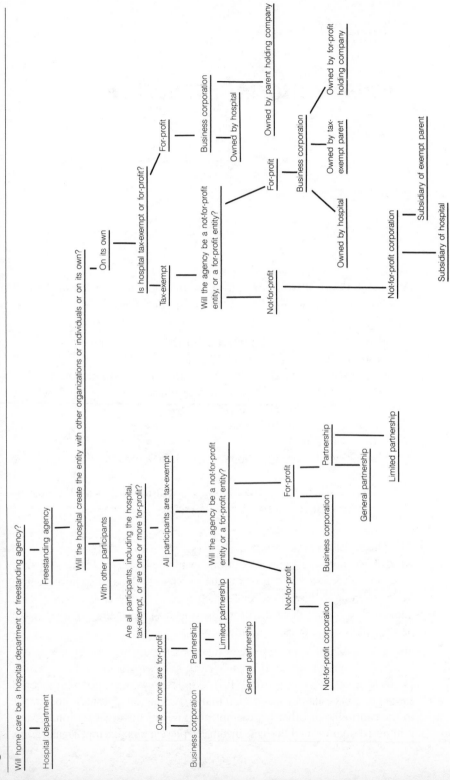

Hospital-Based Program or Freestanding Agency

The hospital that plans to offer home care services must first decide whether this service is to be offered in a hospital-based program or in a new, separate entity. For Medicare purposes, a home care agency is hospital based when it is:[1]

- Operated under the hospital's license
- Financially integrated with the hospital
- Operated under common professional supervision with the hospital
- Subject to the bylaws and operating decisions of the hospital's governing board

A hospital-based home care agency does not file a separate Medicare cost report but is included in the hospital's cost report. One possible advantage to the hospital of having a hospital-based home care program is that the hospital can allocate a portion of its total overhead to the home care program.

In addition to the potential reimbursement advantage, a hospital-based program also offers other advantages. A hospital-based program does not require separate licensure and accreditation. The hospital's control over a hospital-based home care program is more direct, and the organizational structure of such a program is usually simpler. Also, the hospital can assign its employees to the home care program or switch home care employees to another hospital department.

If the home care agency is a freestanding, independent agency, it must have a separate employer identification number and separate payroll system. Depending on the organizational relationship between the hospital and the agency, the agency can be viewed as a joint employer with the hospital for purposes of calculating overtime hours.[2] If employees are shared between the hospital and a freestanding home care agency, each facility must keep careful records on the calculation of overtime pay to avoid inadvertent violations of the Fair Labor Standards Act.

Unrelated Business Income

A hospital-based home care program does have one problem to worry about that a freestanding agency does not. If the hospital is tax-exempt and the home care program is not separately incorporated, revenue from some activities of the home care program can be considered *unrelated business income* by the Internal Revenue Service (IRS). Unrelated business income is income earned by a tax-exempt organization that is carrying on a business not related to the charitable or other tax-exempt purposes of the organization.[3] A tax is imposed on unrelated business income to prevent a tax-exempt organization from having an unfair advantage over taxable entities engaged in the same business.

For hospitals, one issue in determining if an activity is considered related is whether the activity enhances the hospital's primary role of providing health care to its patients. Activities of the hospital that are carried out for the convenience of the hospital's patients do not give rise to unrelated business income.[4] For example, hospital laboratory services performed for hospital inpatients and outpatients are part of the hospital's tax-exempt activities. However, the provision of laboratory services for private physicians or other laboratories is considered in most cases to be unrelated to the hospital's tax-exempt purpose, because the hospital is not serving its patients but is competing with other referral laboratories.[5]

For home care services, the IRS has ruled that a person receiving medical services at home is considered a patient of the hospital for purposes of the unrelated business income provisions as long as the services are provided by, and are under the supervision of, the professional staff of the hospital as an extension of its inpatient and outpatient care.[6] Under this interpretation, many activities of a hospital-based home care service are not classed as unrelated business income. However, activities, such as the provision of durable medical equipment (DME), that compete with non-tax-exempt businesses and that are removed from the hospital's general patient care activities and so do not require the professional services of hospital staff can cause the hospital to realize unrelated business income, which is taxable.

To estimate the potential tax liability of the operation of unrelated businesses, the hospital must take into account expenses as well as gross income. Expenses solely attributable to the unrelated business are deductible according to the general rules governing business deductions.[7] Furthermore, when personnel and facilities are used both for tax-exempt activities and for the unrelated activities, expenses related to the facilities (including overhead) and salary and benefit costs are allocated between the tax-exempt and unrelated activities.[8] A deduction may be claimed for the amounts allocated to the unrelated business.

If unrelated business income seems to be a serious problem, the hospital can set up a separate corporation to operate the home care service. If the governance standard and other criteria for hospital-based status described in the beginning of this chapter are met, such a program can be considered a hospital-based program for Medicare purposes even though it is separately incorporated.

If the hospital organizes its freestanding home care program as a partnership, it may not escape taxation of unrelated business income resulting from partnership operations (see the section "Organizational Forms of For-Profit Entities" later in this chapter). For federal income tax purposes, a partnership is treated as conduit through which income flows to the partners. When the partnership's business is unrelated to the tax-exempt purpose, the tax-exempt organization receives unrelated business income from partnership operations.[9] However, if the partnership furthers the organization's tax-exempt purpose, the partnership is not deemed an unrelated business, and so the income from the partnership is not considered unrelated.[10]

Rate Review and Certificate of Need

Two issues that must be considered in determining whether the home care program should be hospital-based or freestanding are rate-review and certificate-of-need laws. A hospital-based program that is not separately incorporated is generally considered to be a part of the hospital for rate-review purposes and consequently is taken into account in determining the hospital's cost base and rates. A separately incorporated home care agency may or may not be subject to rate-review laws, depending on the agency's relationship to the hospital and the laws in a particular state. State rate-setting statutes vary widely. Depending on the specific requirements of state law, a rate-review agency may or may not look to related organizations in determining the costs and revenues to be attributed to the hospital.

Hospital-based and freestanding home care agencies may also be treated differently for certificate-of-need (CON) purposes. Under the federal Section 1122 program, a review of certain capital expenditures is required, including expenditures that substantially change the services of a health care facility.[11] The addition of a hospital-based home care program is considered a substantial change in the hospital's services because it involves the addition of a new clinically related service.[12] Therefore, the initiation of the hospital-based home care program requires Section 1122 review, regardless of the amount of capital expenditure.

The treatment of home care programs varies under state CON laws. In some states, home care agencies are included in the definition of health care facilities, and in such states the establishment of a home care program requires CON review whether the program is hospital-based or freestanding. In many states, the offering of home care services by a hospital is considered a new institutional service that requires review.

A CON review is also required for expenditures by or on behalf of a hospital for the purchase of medical equipment. Whether capital expenditures for a freestanding home care agency are considered to be on behalf of the hospital depends on the degree of common control and operational involvement between the hospital and the agency.

Hospital-Funded Project or Joint Venture

If the hospital decides to create a freestanding home care organization, it must next decide whether it should finance and operate the project entirely on its own or whether it should seek the participation of other parties in a joint venture. A *joint venture* is technically an association between two or more legally independent parties to create a new enterprise and to share in the rewards and economic risks of this new entity. The term is used in this chapter to refer to any cooperative venture.

Potential participants in a joint venture may be existing home care agencies, other hospitals, or equipment suppliers. The joint venture can be structured either as a corporation or as a general partnership or as a limited partnership if the venture is to be a for-profit one (see the section "Organizational Forms of For-Profit Entities" later in this chapter).

Tax-Exempt Status

A tax-exempt hospital must carefully structure any for-profit venture so that it does not endanger its tax-exempt status. An organization that is exempt from taxation under Section 501(c)(3) of the Internal Revenue Code (I.R.C.) may not have any portion of its income inure to private individuals and may not engage in nonexempt activities unless these activities represent an insubstantial part of its operations. (These requirements are discussed in the section "Organizational Forms of For-Profit Entities" later in this chapter.)

Generally, a hospital may participate as a shareholder in a business corporation without endangering its tax-exempt status because the shares may be viewed as an investment. Even if the hospital owns 100 percent of the stock in the for-profit subsidiary, its exemption is not endangered so long as the for-profit business is formed for a bona fide business purpose and the hospital, as a tax-exempt shareholder, does not actively participate in the day-to-day business of the subsidiary.[13] The participation by the hospital as a general partner in a joint venture is more problematic, because general partners usually participate in the management of the business and are therefore responsible for its liabilities.

Joint venture activities that are related to the hospital's tax-exempt function of providing care to the hospital's patients neither endanger the hospital's tax exemption nor result in the realization of unrelated business income. Examples of joint ventures that are related to a hospital's tax-exempt purpose include the construction of a medical office building by a partnership formed with a hospital as general partner[14] and participation by the hospital in a joint venture with a partnership of physicians to purchase a CAT scanner.[15] When the proposed activity is not related to the hospital's tax-exempt purpose and involves the sharing of earnings with for-profit organizations and individuals, the hospital's tax-exempt status can be endangered.[16]

Conflict of Interest

An additional problem that must be avoided in any joint venture involving physicians is a conflict of interest on the part of a physician who certifies that a patient needs home care services. Medicare does not pay for home care services unless the physician who established the home care plan certifies, and periodically recertifies, that the home care services are required.[17]

A physician who has a "significant ownership interest in, or a significant financial or contractual relationship with" the home care agency providing the services has such a conflict of interest.[18] A *significant financial or contractual relationship* is defined as a relationship involving contracts, leases, or other business transactions that amount to more than the lesser of $25,000 or 5 percent of the agency's operating expenses in any fiscal year. A *significant ownership interest* exists if the physician owns more than a 5 percent interest in the capital, stock, or profits of the agency or in any mortgage or obligation that is secured by the agency and that represents 5 percent or more of the agency's assets. A significant ownership interest also exists if the physician is an officer, director, or partner in the agency. However, these restrictions do not apply to a sole community home care agency or to a physician who is an uncompensated officer or director.[19]

Tax-Exempt Organization or For-Profit Business

Once a tax-exempt hospital decides that the home care venture is to be organized as a freestanding entity, it must first determine how the project is to be financed and then decide whether the home care entity is to be a tax-exempt, not-for-profit organization or a taxable, for-profit organization. An organization can be not-for-profit without being tax-exempt.

Whether a corporation is for-profit or not-for-profit depends on the purposes of the corporation, as expressed in its articles of incorporation. State corporation acts generally define the purposes for which a not-for-profit corporation may be organized. To qualify for exemption from federal income taxes, a corporation must not only be a not-for-profit corporation under state law, but it must also meet the requirements for tax-exempt status set forth in the I.R.C. and the Treasury Regulations.

Although organizations other than corporations, such as trusts and unincorporated associations, can also qualify for tax-exempt status, these organizational forms are not generally appropriate for home care ventures. Also, partnerships are not typically organized on a not-for-profit basis; the Uniform Partnership Act describes a partnership as "an association of two or more persons to carry on as co-owners a business for profit."[20] Therefore, this discussion of tax-exempt entities assumes that the entity is organized as a corporation.

Qualifications for Tax-Exempt Status

To qualify for federal tax-exempt status, a not-for-profit corporation must serve a religious, charitable, or educational purpose or other purposes that are recognized as tax-exempt.[21] The determining consideration for a home care program is whether the provision of services is a charitable activity. The IRS says that the provision of home care services may be viewed as a charitable activity because the promotion of health is generally considered to be a charitable purpose.[22] Therefore, an organization that provides home care services on a not-for-profit basis may be tax-exempt if its services are available to the general public and if any excess of income over expenses is used to provide care for patients who cannot pay or to expand the organization's services.[23]

A tax-exempt organization must be both organized and operated exclusively for a tax-exempt purpose.[24] The *organizational test* is met if the articles of incorporation of the home care entity limit its activities to the provision of home care services and other charitable purposes and does not empower the corporation to engage in nonexempt activities except as an insubstantial part of its operations.[25] The *operational test* is met if the home care entity engages primarily in tax-exempt activities.[26] An entity is not operated exclusively for tax-exempt purposes if it engages in lobbying activity[27] or if any part of its earnings inure to the benefit of any private shareholder or individual.[28]

Inurement

The prohibition on inurement of earnings to private individuals is a factor that should be given particular attention in the planning of tax-exempt home care ventures. Clearly, this provision prevents a tax-exempt organization from being organized as a business, or for-profit, corporation, which pays dividends to its shareholders. Private inurement can also take less obvious forms, such as providing compensation to officers, managers, physicians, or others that exceeds normal and customary compensation for the services provided. Also, an incentive compensation plan can result in private inurement.[29]

Private inurement is absolutely prohibited for organizations that are exempt under 501(c)(3) of the I.R.C., even if the amount of earnings that inure to private individuals is negligible in comparison with the total earnings of the organization. This treatment contrasts with the treatment of unrelated business income. An organization may retain its tax-exempt status even if it realizes unrelated business income as long as the unrelated business activity is not a substantial part of the organization's total operations.

Private Foundation

In addition to qualifying for federal tax-exempt status, a not-for-profit organization should also apply for a determination by the IRS that it is not a private foundation. A private foundation is organized and operated for a tax-exempt purpose and does not receive support from the general public or provide funds to a publicly supported organization. The criteria for recognition that the organization is not a private foundation are too detailed to be fully described here.[30] Generally, however, the following types of organizations are not considered to be private foundations:

- Organizations, such as hospitals or medical research facilities, that qualify for the maximum charitable contribution limit[31]
- Organizations that receive more than one-third of their support from specified sources and less than one-third of their support from investment and from unrelated business income (less the tax on such income)[32]
- Organizations that provide funds to a publicly supported organization and that have an organizational relationship with the publicly supported organization[33]

Organizations that are tax-exempt by virtue of Section 501(c)(3) of the I.R.C. are presumed to be private foundations unless they notify the IRS to the contrary.[34] Private foundations are subject to a tax based on the tax benefit derived from their tax-exempt status.[35] Therefore, as part of the planning for a new not-for-profit home care organization, the hospital should examine its sources of funding and its projected operating and capital budgets to determine whether the organization can qualify for non-private-foundation status on the basis of its source of support or whether another basis for this classification must be sought.

State Taxes

Finally, an organization that is exempt from federal income taxation may not be exempt from state income, sales, and other taxes. The corporation must examine the laws of each state in which the corporation operates to determine whether it is exempt from state taxes.

Choice between Tax-Exempt and For-Profit Status

Choosing between tax-exempt and for-profit status for the home care entity that is being created by a tax-exempt hospital is a crucial decision in the planning process. In some cases, the organizational objectives of a planned home care entity clearly indicate that the entity does not qualify for tax-exempt status. In other cases, the hospital must explicitly weigh the advantages and disadvantages of tax-exempt status to decide whether its objectives can best be served by a not-for-profit business.

The principal advantage of tax-exempt status is, of course, the exemption itself. A tax exemption decreases the organization's expenses and permits the organization's managers to make decisions without regard to tax implications (unless unrelated business income is involved). A second major advantage of tax-exempt status is being able to deduct contributions made to the tax-exempt organization.[36] Also, the tax-exempt organization may have access to tax-exempt financing, providing that bonds issued by the organization are *qualified 501(c)(3) bonds* under the Tax Reform Act of 1986.[37]

A major disadvantage of tax-exempt status concerns the prohibition against private inurement that was discussed earlier in this chapter. This restriction limits the financing sources available to the organization, because no return of earnings to participants is permitted. Also, this restriction limits the organization's ability to structure compensation packages for its managers that are competitive with compensation offered by for-profit businesses. Another important disadvantage is that the assets of a tax-exempt corporation may not be distributed to a nonexempt entity even if the tax-exempt corporation is dissolved.[38] This prohibition restricts the organization's flexibility to adapt to changes in the competitive environment. Another disadvantage may be the expense involved in applying for tax-exempt status.

The choice between tax-exempt and for-profit status frequently comes down to a choice between lower tax liability and greater organizational flexibility. In addition, the hospital must give consideration to the organization's place in the overall corporate structure of the hospital and its related organizations.

Organizational Forms of For-Profit Entities

After the hospital reaches a decision on whether the freestanding home care agency is to be entirely financed by the hospital or financed with the participation of other investors, it must then select an appropriate organizational form for the home care venture. Both the corporate form and partnership form have special advantages and disadvantages.

The basic difference between a corporation and a partnership is that a corporation is an independent entity that has an existence entirely separate from its shareholders. In a partnership, the interests of the partners are not fused to create an independent entity but instead remain identifiable. Because of this basic difference, corporations and partnerships are treated differently under the law.

Liability

Perhaps the most significant difference concerns the liability of the owners of the enterprise. Shareholders of a corporation are not liable for the debts and obligations of the corporation, but general partners of a partnership are liable for the partnership's obligations. Therefore, if a claim cannot be satisfied out of the partnership's assets, the claimant can collect from one or more of the general partners. (Limited partners have limited liability, like shareholders of a corporation. This feature of limited partnerships is discussed later in this section.)

The limited-liability attribute of the corporate form can be an advantage in home care ventures. The extent of agency exposure to potential liability for patient injury depends on the kinds of services that the home care agency provides and the types of patients it serves. For example, an agency that provides DME can be liable to a patient who was injured because the equipment was defective in design, improperly manufactured, or negligently maintained. In another example, a home care agency that employs registered nurses, licensed practical nurses, or other health care personnel can be held liable if a patient is injured because the agency's employees were negligent in the performance of their duties, were performing tasks for which they were not qualified, or were inadequately supervised. As the number and complexity of the furnished services increase, so does the potential liability of the home care agency.

If the home care agency is organized as a corporation, the shareholders, that is, the sponsoring hospital or its related corporation and other participants, are not liable in most circumstances for the obligations of the agency. This factor can be significant if the agency's exposure to potential liability is substantial. However, if adequate commercial insurance to cover the activities of the agency is available at a reasonable cost, the agency can purchase insurance to protect itself against reasonably foreseeable losses and thereby minimize the secondary liability of its sponsors. In this case, the limited-liability feature of the corporate form is less significant.

Federal Taxes

Another major difference between corporations and partnerships is the treatment accorded them for federal income tax purposes. A corporation is a taxpayer and is required to report and pay income tax on its taxable income. Furthermore, if a corporation distributes income to its shareholders, the distribution is, in almost all cases, treated as a dividend that must be included in the shareholder's taxable income. For an individual shareholder, this situation results in what is called the *double taxation of corporate income:* corporate income is taxed once through the income tax paid by the corporation and again through the taxation of the individual shareholder's income.

Double taxation may not be a problem, however, if all the shareholders are corporations. A business corporation is entitled to a deduction of 80 percent or 100 percent of the dividends it receives, depending on its relationship to the distributing corporation.[39] If the shareholder is a not-for-profit corporation, the dividends are usually viewed as passive investment income that is not taxed as unrelated business income.[40] (The section "Hospital-Funded Project or Joint Venture" earlier in this chapter discusses the issues involved in a tax-exempt corporation's ownership of a for-profit business.)

A partnership is not a taxpaying entity, although it is required to report partnership income.[41] For federal tax purposes, a partnership is treated as a conduit: income flows through the partnership to the partners and is taxed as part of the partners' income. Because income is not taxed at the partnership level, the income of the partners is not subject to double taxation as is the case with corporate income. Therefore, one advantage enjoyed by partnerships is the avoidance of double taxation. However, the most significant tax advantage enjoyed by partnerships is the availability to the partners of income tax deductions and credits arising from partnership activity.

The partnership is treated as a conduit not only for the purpose of attributing income and gain, but also for the purpose of attributing losses, deductions, and credits to the partners.[42] Therefore, accelerated cost recovery system (ACRS) deductions, depreciation, and other deductions and credits are attributed to each partner according to the partner's distributive share. For general partners, the losses, deductions, and credits of the partnership can generally be offset against the partner's income from other sources.

However, if the partner is a tax-exempt organization, the availability of these deductions and credits is not an advantage. For this reason, the individual partners in a partnership venture between a tax-exempt corporation and individual investors should contribute the largest percentage of the capitalization and should receive the largest distributive share of partnership income and losses.

Organizational Requirements

Another difference between corporations and partnerships are organizational requirements. A corporation is created when the state in which it is incorporated grants it a corporate franchise. To maintain its existence, a business corporation must file annual reports (customarily with the Secretary of State for the state of its incorporation) and must pay state franchise taxes. In addition, the corporation must observe the formalities required by the state's corporation act, such as the requirements for annual meetings of the shareholders and the directors.

One organizational advantage of the corporate form is the ease with which ownership interests can be transferred. Although a corporation may restrict the transferability of its shares by imposing restrictions in its articles of incorporation,[43] corporate shares are generally freely transferable. The only formal requirement imposed is the recording of the transfer on the records of the corporation. This feature may make investment in a corporation more attractive to some individuals. Of course, the significance of this feature depends on whether shares of the particular corporation are generally traded in an organized market.

A partnership is usually created through the execution of a partnership agreement.[44] An interest in a partnership is not freely transferable as are shares of a corporation. The Uniform Partnership Act provides that no person can become a member of a general partnership without the consent of all the partners.[45] The partnership must keep records of the capital contribution of each partner and must determine the distribution of partnership income, gains, losses, deductions, and credits according to the terms of the partnership agreement. Consequently, partnership accounting can be a complex undertaking. Finally, the Uniform Partnership Act contains detailed provisions governing the dissolution of a partnership and the winding up of its affairs.[46]

One organizational form that contains elements of both the corporate form and the general partnership form and that is suitable for a hospital-sponsored home care venture is the *limited partnership.* The limited partnership must have at least one general partner, who is liable for the partnership's obligations.[47] Like shareholders of a corporation, limited partners are not liable for the partnership's obligations so long as they do not participate in the control of the business.[48] Although this limited-liability feature is similar to a corporation, the limited partnership continues to be treated as a conduit for tax purposes. However, because the limited partners cannot participate in the management of the enterprise, the ability of limited partners to use tax deductions and credits of the partnership is limited by the passive-activity provisions of the Tax Reform Act of 1986.[49]

The advantages and disadvantages of the corporation and partnership and limited partnership forms must be evaluated on an individual basis by hospitals seeking to sponsor home care ventures. For example, two not-for-profit hospitals that plan to jointly establish a freestanding home care agency may find it most advantageous to use the corporate form. Because both hospitals are tax-exempt, neither can benefit from the tax advantages of the partnership form, but they may gain some benefit from the limited-liability feature of a corporation. In contrast, two for-profit hospitals that are generating income from their other operations can benefit from the tax advantages of the partnership. Therefore, they may choose to organize as a partnership if the partnership business can generate tax credits and deductions during the early years of its operation. Such an arrangement may be suitable for a DME supplier. For a home care venture that is organized by a hospital and that obtains most of its capitalization from individual investors, the limited partnership form may be the most attractive. In many cases, the individual investors benefit from the tax treatment accorded to partnerships but do not want to assume the liability associated with general partner status.

Integrating with the Hospital's Corporate Structure

After hospital management decides to create a new organization to operate the home care venture and delineates the general characteristics of the new organization, it must then integrate the home care entity into the overall organization of the hospital and its related corporations.

When the only existing corporation is the hospital itself, the options are limited. If the hospital is tax-exempt and the home care entity is also to be tax-exempt, the home care venture can be organized as a not-for-profit corporation. The hospital can maintain control over the home care corporation through provisions in the articles of incorporation and in the bylaws that designate the hospital as a member of the corporation, give the hospital authority over the selection of directors and officers, and require the approval of the hospital for certain corporate actions. If the home care organization is a joint endeavor of a tax-exempt hospital and one or more tax-exempt entities, control of the home care corporation can be shared by the participants. A for-profit home care venture can be organized as a business corporation, with stock owned by the hospital alone or by the hospital and other venture participants. If the home care venture is to be organized as a partnership, the hospital can be a general partner or a limited partner if its interest is solely that of an investor. However, if the hospital is tax-exempt, special consideration should be given to the issues concerning the participation of tax-exempt organizations in business partnerships.

In a reorganized corporate system, several organizational options are available. A multicorporate structure is frequently designed to separate for-profit activities from tax-exempt activities and to separate health care provider activities from nonprovider activities. By selecting the appropriate organizational framework, some of the problems identified in earlier sections of this chapter may be minimized. A not-for-profit hospital can endanger its tax-exempt status by acquiring a partnership interest in certain partnerships whose activities are unrelated to the hospital's exempt purpose. This problem is avoided if a for-profit holding company or for-profit subsidiary in the hospital's corporate structure participates in the partnership.

A hospital-based home care program is treated for certificate-of-need and rate-review purposes as part of the hospital, and this factor must be taken into consideration in deciding between a hospital-based program and a freestanding home care agency. However, a separately incorporated home care agency may still be integrated with the hospital for certificate-of-need and rate-review purposes, depending on the agency's organizational relationship to the hospital and on the requirements of individual state laws. Placing the control of the home care agency with a not-for-profit holding company or a for-profit subsidiary of the hospital's parent corporation may help to avoid this problem. Nevertheless, in some states the home care agency is still regarded as related to the hospital even if control of the agency rests with another corporation.

A hospital planning to launch a home care venture must ensure that the organization and operation of the home care entity is consistent with the overall objectives and management style of the hospital. A successful planning process takes into account not only the specific issues identified in this chapter but also the more intangible elements of organizational philosophy.

Notes

1. 46 Fed. Reg. 38014 (June 5, 1980).

2. 29 C.F.R. § 791.2(b)(3).

3. I.R.C. §§ 511-513.

4. I.R.C. § 513(a)(2).

5. See, for example, Carle Foundation v. United States, 611 F.2d 1192 (7th Cir. 1979) (pharmacy sales); Rev. Rul. 85-110 (laboratory services).

6. Rev. Rul. 68-376, 1968-2 C.B. 245.

7. Treas. Reg. § 1.512(a)-1(b).

8. Treas. Reg. § 1.512(a)-1(c).

9. I.R.C. § 512(c). This applies even if the tax-exempt organization is a limited partner. Rev. Rul. 79-222, 1979-2 C.B. 236.

10. GCM 39005, Dec. 17, 1982 (Exempt Organization Reporter [CCH], New Developments ¶6740).

11. 42 C.F.R. § 123.404(a).

12. 42 C.F.R. § 123.404(a)(3)(ii).

13. GCM 39326, Aug. 31, 1984 (Exempt Organization Reporter [CCH], New Developments ¶6925).

14. See, for example, Ltr. Rul. 780058.

15. Ltr. Rul. 8201072.

16. Ltr. Rul. 8206093, ¶54,823 P-H Fed. 1982. (A tax-exempt organization was a general partner in a limited partnership in which for-profit entities were also general partners.)

17. 42 C.F.R. § 405.1633.

18. 42 C.F.R. § 405.1633(d).

19. *Medicare and Medicaid Guide* (CCH) ¶11,455.

20. Uniform Partnership Act, § 7; Ill. Rev. Stat. ch. 106½, § 7 (1985).

21. I.R.C. § 501(c)(3).

22. Rev. Rul. 72-209, 1972-1 C.B. 148.

23. Rev. Rul. 72-209, 1972-1 C.B. 148.

24. Treas. Reg. § 1.501(c)(3)-1(a)(1).

25. Treas. Reg. § 1.501(c)(3)-1(b)(1)(i).

26. Treas. Reg. § 1.501(c)(3)-1(c)(1).

27. Treas. Reg. § 1.501(c)(3)-1(c)(3).

28. Treas. Reg. § 1.501(c)(3)-1(c)(2).

29. However, see Rev. Rul. 69-383, 1969-2C.B. 113, which provides that a hospital's tax-exempt status is not endangered when the hospital compensates a radiologist on the basis of a percentage of department income.

30. The requirements are described in Treas. Reg. §§ 1.509(a)-1 through 1.509(a)-6. See also I.R.S. publication 557, *Tax Exempt Status for Your Organization.*

31. I.R.C. § 509(a)(1). Organizations that qualify for the maximum charitable contribution limit are listed in I.R.C. § 170(b)(1)(A). (This section also includes private foundations and organizations that are not private foundations by virtue of § 509(a)(2) and § 509(a)(3) of the I.R.C.; such organization do not, however, qualify under § 509(a)(1) for designation as an exempt organization that is not a private foundation.) In § 170(b)(1)(A), certain organizations, such as hospitals, are described by function; also included are organizations that normally receive a substantial part of their support from governmental sources or from direct or indirect government support. Home care agencies, according to an IRS ruling, are not hospitals for purposes of § 170(b)(1)(A). Rev. Rul. 76-452. Therefore, a home care agency that wants to qualify as a nonprivate foundation under § 509(a)(1) must receive a substantial part of its support directly or indirectly from the public or from the government.

32. I.R.C. § 509(a)(2).

33. I.R.C. § 509(a)(3).

34. I.R.C. § 508(b).

35. I.R.C. § 507(c).

36. I.R.C. § 170. As noted in note 31, home care agencies are not hospitals, and therefore contributions to a home care agency do not qualify for the maximum percentage limitation on charitable contributions unless the home care agency qualifies under § 170(b)(1)(A)(vi). Corporations as well as individuals may claim a deduction for charitable contributions, but a business corporation that is related through corporate affiliation to the home care agency may not be entitled to a deduction for a contribution to a related tax-exempt corporation. For example, if the business corporation is owned by a tax-exempt parent company that controls the home care agency, the contribution may be viewed as a disguised dividend.

37. Pub. L. 99-514, § 1301; I.R.C. §§ 103, 141 *et seq.*

38. Treas. Reg. § 1.501(c)(3)-1(b)(4).

39. I.R.C. § 243, as modified by Pub. L. 99-514, § 611.

40. Treas. Reg. § 1.512(b)-1(a).

41. I.R.C. § 701.

42. I.R.C. § 702.

43. A corporation that restricts the transferability of its shares is a close corporation. See Ill. Rev. Stat. ch. 32, §§ 1201, *et seg.*

44. The Uniform Partnership Act does not require the execution of a written agreement in order to create a partnership. Ill. Rev. Stat. ch. 106½, § 7 (1985).

45. Ill. Rev. Stat. ch. 106½, § 181(g) (1985). However, a partner can assign his right to partnership income. Ill. Rev. Stat. ch. 106½, § 27 (1985).

46. Ill. Rev. Stat. ch. 106½, §§ 29-43 (1985).

47. Uniform Limited Partnership Act, § 1; Ill. Rev. Stat. ch. 106½, § 44 (1985).

48. Ill. Rev. Stat. ch. 106½, § 50 (1985).

49. Pub. L. 99-514, § 501.

Chapter 5

Operational Considerations

Cathy Frasca

One of the keys to the success of a home care organization, or any business venture for that matter, is the effective delivery of its products or services. Indeed, the effectiveness of agency operations largely determines the image that patients, families, survey teams, physicians, insurance carriers, and the overall community have of the home care organization.

In general, the operational aspects of a home care organization can be divided into two critical components: patient care management and staffing. This chapter describes specific elements of these components that affect and enhance a home care organization's effectiveness. Examples used in this chapter are based on the experiences of South Hills Health System/Home Health Agency (SHHS/HHA). Although these examples are based on the experiences of a large multihospital-based home health agency, they illustrate general principles that have wide applications.

At the outset, however, the special operational concerns that apply to hospital-based agencies need to be discussed. A hospital-based agency, which is more commonly referred to by the Health Care Financing Administration (HCFA) and Medicare as *provider-based,* functions as an integral component of a hospital system. In contrast, a *freestanding agency,* in the broadest sense, is any home health agency not defined as hospital-based

---

Cathy Frasca is the executive director of South Hills Health System/Home Health Agency, Pittsburgh, Pennsylvania. Also contributing to this chapter are Meg Wise Christy, director of research and development; Dolores Deegan, staffing coordinator, James Graeca, director of finance; Mary Ann Miller, director of staff development; JoAnn Parzick, director of patient care; Mary Ann Schmidt, director of program and operations; Helen Triebsch, home care department director; and Donna College, consultant.

by HCFA and Medicare. The operating principles of a freestanding agency may not necessarily apply to a hospital-based agency, but some operating principles of a hospital-based agency can apply to a freestanding agency.

A hospital-based agency is unique in several respects. It operates under more restrictions than does a freestanding agency. It shares the same board of directors as its parent hospital system. Because the hospital-based agency is considered a department of the hospital, Medicare regulations require the hospital to allocate a portion of its indirect costs to the agency just as it does for any other hospital department. Medicare regulations recognize these allocations by allowing hospital-based agencies to receive an add-on to the freestanding agency's cost limits. (For a discussion of the federally mandated Medicare step-down cost methodology, see chapter 7.)

A hospital-based agency must comply with all requirements for a home health agency and a hospital department. For example, the state of Pennsylvania has more than 200 surveying organizations and regulations that cover hospitals. In addition to either being directly or indirectly affected by these hospital regulations and surveying organizations, a hospital-based agency must also meet Medicare certification, JCAH accreditation, and state licensure requirements.

Administering a patient care management system for home care within a full-service hospital is often difficult because many policies and procedures of the parent hospital may not be compatible with those of the home health agency. For example, home care policies relating to on-call status and inclement weather may be a low priority for the hospital but are a high priority for a home health agency. Hospital policies relating to occupational health and safety may not include how to cope with wild dogs, broken stairs, potential rapists, or firearms, but these issues are important ones for personnel in a home health agency. Unnecessary delays in filling vacant positions present certain elements of risk in a hospital setting. However, similar delays in filling vacant positions in a home health agency not only reflect these same risks relating to patient care, but also generate negative budgetary variances because referrals cannot be efficiently processed and home visits cannot be made. The resulting reduction in revenues is inescapable. In addition, agency credibility may also be threatened if the agency is perceived as being consistently unable to respond to referrals in an efficient and effective manner..

For any home care program, the key element for success is flexibility in policies and procedures. The provision of home care services outside the institutional setting presents a unique challenge because of the unpredictable nature of the community setting and the variables inherent in each home environment. These challenges, as well as those that are present in a continually changing home care industry, require that a home health agency employ seasoned, highly qualified, and experienced community health care specialists.[1]

In addition, the agency's policies and procedures must conform to the situations encountered in the home care environment. On-call policies that require the employee to remain on the hospital premises and respond to calls within 10 minutes are overly restrictive and expensive for the home care setting. A more appropriate home care on-call policy is one that allows the employee to be available by telephone and to respond to calls within 30 minutes. This less restrictive on-call policy is also more cost-effective because the employee is compensated only for the time actually spent interacting with patients.

As with any home care organization, the manager of a hospital-based home health agency must be concerned with the personal safety of each employee. Because the home care environment is the whole community, a wide variety of safety risks may be encountered. Staff members must understand that their personal safety is a high priority. Operational policies that encourage the use of vacation days when snow and ice make roads unnegotiable are inclined to reduce job-related injuries from falls and automobile accidents. Those few patients who absolutely must be visited on an icy day can be seen by one nurse in an all-terrain vehicle.

Patient Care Management

The patient is the focus of all home care services. Patient needs arise not only from the health situation itself, but also from sociopsychological factors. Focusing on the patient's needs, expressed or unexpressed, leads to specific, measurable, and achievable goals for patient care. Developing and carrying out a plan for home care based on these goals is a dynamic, ongoing process.

This section discusses aspects of patient care management. It covers the care of the patient from discharge from the hospital through discharge from the home care program and focuses on the skilled care segment.

Hospital Discharge

Planning for a patient's discharge from the hospital to a home health agency is a process that may begin at the time of admission to the hospital or even before the patient is admitted to the hospital. Early planning allows the patient to receive hospital care that is managed in the most appropriate, expedient, and cost-effective manner and helps the health care provider respond to the total needs of the individual patient.[2]

Discharge planning is a systematic process of assessing the patient's abilities and limitations while the patient is still hospitalized, planning for the care initiated in the hospital to be continued at home, and coordinating resources to facilitate this care. Joint discharge planning with staff members from both the hospital and the home health agency ensures a comprehensive, coordinated continuum of patient care. The process of facilitating the patient's transition from one health care setting to another involves the patient, the patient's family, and a team of health care professionals.

Perhaps the most effective model for facilitating discharge planning is the adoption of *grand rounds*. The grand-rounds format for discharge planning requires the regular participation of each head nurse as well as a social work staff member, discharge planner, and home care staff member assigned to each nursing department. These individuals comprise the discharge planning team. The function of this discharge planning team is to regularly review each patient's condition and make judgments about the probable level of care that will be required for that patient at discharge. Members of the team should use grand rounds as an opportunity to project what available resources the patient is likely to require so that the referral process is begun as early as is appropriate. In some hospitals, the diagnosis-related-group (DRG) or utilization review (UR) coordinators may wish to attend these rounds to obtain information regarding each patient's progress.

The home health agency's involvement in the hospital's discharge planning process is vital. Staff members from the agency function as the link between the hospital and the community and promote the patient's continued integration into all appropriate, available services. The participation of the agency in discharge planning benefits the home care department serving that hospital in three major areas:

- The agency has direct access to the information and services needed to best plan and meet the needs of the home care patient.
- The agency is ideally positioned to be able to quickly respond to the changing needs and demands of its hospital and the patients it serves.
- The agency's active involvement in the hospital's discharge planning process ensures the true continuity of patient care, a major characteristic of a high-quality home care program.

The team concept is the only workable basis for any discharge planning model, and the key to its success is *communication*. The communication that takes place as the hospital and the home health agency work together in the discharge planning process facilitates the successful coordination of the services that each party provides.

Discharge planning rounds provide a number of benefits for the hospital as well as for the home health agency. These rounds allow personnel from the agency to give feedback to the hospital staff about the progress of recently discharged patients who are being visited by the home care staff. Rounds also provide an opportunity for the home care staff member to give a report on how well each currently hospitalized patient who has had home care in the past has been able to cope at home. This report helps the discharge planning team project how well individual patients may be able to manage following their current hospitalization. The report must have enough detail to allow the discharge planning team to make some predictions about the patient's strength, determination, and level of independence. It should also indicate resources that can be tapped to help make home care a successful experience for the patient.

Referral

The patient's attending physician must be involved in the decision to refer a particular patient to skilled home health services. If the initial skilled care referral comes from any team member other than the physician, the head nurse or another member of the discharge planning team must secure the physician's approval before proceeding through the referral and coordination process. This approval must be verified, with the physician's signature either on the patient's health record or on the home health agency's treatment plan.[3] The home care staff involved in the referral must discuss the patient's needs with the attending or referring physician. Such contact between the home care staff and the physician is essential throughout the time the patient is receiving home care. The physician's approval is generally not required if the patient is going to receive private-duty or demand services and is paying for services personally rather than through Medicare or other insurance.

The coordination process at SHHS/HHA includes an assessment of the appropriateness of the referral. The patient must meet the following SHHS/HHA eligibility criteria:

- The patient must need intermittent skilled care services.
- The patient must have a physician to supervise care.
- The patient should have a care giver in the home to assist with the implementation of the care plan.
- The patient must be essentially homebound.

Inevitably, inappropriate referrals occur. Such referrals may include patients who do not meet the eligibility criteria or who have demonstrated through past experience with the agency that they are inappropriate candidates for home care services for such reasons as previous noncompliance with agency policies or an unsuitable home environment. If a referral is inappropriate, the discharge planning team must look for appropriate alternatives for the patient. Occurrences of inappropriate referrals emphasize the need for early discharge planning so that sufficient time is available to pursue available alternatives.

The early involvement of the patient and family in the referral process is essential. Such involvement enables the patient to establish a rapport with home care team members at an early stage. This early contact facilitates communication after the patient has been discharged and seems to promote improved compliance with the discharge plan of care. Early patient and family involvement also assists in the prompt identification of inappropriate referrals, especially of those patients who should really be referred to a skilled nursing facility.

Intake

The home care intake process, which is a vital function of a home health agency, includes all those activities performed by the agency during its involvement in the hospital discharge planning process, in the home care referral process, and in the coordination of the referral before the patient is actually admitted to home care. This process requires agency staff to be keenly aware of supplemental services available in the community, such as home-delivered meals, transportation, and available persons to provide respite for caretakers.

During the intake process, the agency's staff are actually performing a pre-home-care planning function that is multifaceted and includes:

- Identifying the care needs of the patient and the support needs of the family
- Determining the availability of appropriate home care staff to provide care to the patient
- Processing the patient's health insurance to determine coverage for home care services and discussing this information with the patient and family
- Identifying and obtaining the appropriate ancillary services, such as equipment, supplies, and community services

In addition to participating in the discharge planning process and in the home care referral, the intake staff uses all available hospital resources to obtain as much information as possible about the patient requiring home care. Often the information needs of the home health agency differ from those of the hospital. The agency needs information on the home environment and the availability of a care giver in the home situation. For example, a patient who experiences acute episodes of dyspnea (difficult or labored breathing) should eliminate multiple trips up and down stairs and should have a care giver available to assist with the normal activities of daily living.

Developing a specific form for gathering this information provides consistency in the type of information secured. Home care intake staff use the patient's health record, communication with hospital staff and the physician, and interactions with the patient and the family to complete the intake form. Figure 5-1, next page, shows the intake form used by SHHS/HHA.

Ongoing documentation of the agency's discharge planning activities is reflected on the patient's health record. This documentation assists the hospital in meeting its regulatory requirements and also aids communication among the professionals involved in the discharge planning process.

Agency intake staff should be able to work well as team members and have a high level of communication skills and rapport with and respect from hospital staff members. At least daily, the intake staff report to department managers within the agency to ensure that the home care staff is ready to meet the needs of the patient and family at the time of the patient's discharge from the hospital.

Figure 5-1. Example of an Intake Information Sheet

```
                        INTAKE INFORMATION SHEET

Name: _____ Room No.: _____  Intake Person: _____

Referred to: _____ By: _____ Date: _____

Plan of Treatment: Signed [ ]  On Chart [ ]  Send [ ]  To Come [ ]

Insurance: To be Checked [ ] Has Home Care Coverage: Yes [ ] No [ ] Partial [ ]

Payment Responsibility Discussed with Patient/Family: Yes [ ]  No [ ]

Discharged Discussed with: _____

Equipment: _____ Supplier: _____

Home Environment: _____
                                                    Telephone
Responsible Caretaker: _____ Relationship: _____ No.: _____

S.S. Involved: Yes [ ]  No [ ]  Social Worker: _____

Past Medical History: _____

Reason for Admission to Hospital: _____

Course during Stay (include therapy reports): _____
_____
_____
_____
```

LAB TESTS	VITAL SIGNS	CATHETER
	Blood	Size _____
	Pressure _____	Date _____
	Pulse _____	Inserted _____
	Respiration _____	Irrigation ___
	Weight _____	
EKG: _____	Diet _____	
X Rays: _____	Allergies _____	

```
Treatment or Dressing: _____
Surgery: _____
```

Diagnosis – Principal:	
	M.D. Appointment: _____
	Specific Orders or Instructions: _____
Additional:	_____
	_____
Medications:	Activities: _____
	_____

Admission

When the intake process is completed, the patient is ready to be admitted to the home health agency. At that time, a folder containing appropriate clinical and insurance forms, intake information, and any special instructions regarding the patient is turned over to the agency and becomes part of the home care patient's health record. The patient is then considered admitted to the home care program.

Once the patient has been admitted, the management staff of the agency must identify the most appropriate staff person to function as the patient's home care coordinator. Theoretically, any health care professional could assume this role. To minimize duplication of effort and streamline the agency's operation, SHHS/HHA designates the service provider who makes the first visit as the coordinator. The identification of the service provider who makes this first visit is determined on the basis of the patient's condition and the physician's orders. Social workers, occupational therapists, respiratory therapists, and nutritionists are usually not named as home care coordinators because the services they provide are not considered by Medicare to be *core services*. Consequently, an initial evaluation visit by one of these providers is not reimbursable under the Medicare program. As a result, the home care coordinator is most often a registered nurse.

The home care coordinator is responsible for:

- Initial patient assessment that occurs after the patient is admitted to home care
- Ongoing evaluation of the patient
- Identification of any potential problems

A miniconference between the intake person, who has been actively involved with the patient prior to discharge from the hospital, and the selected home care coordinator is held to review and clarify the physician's orders and to determine the special needs of the patient.

After being assigned to a new patient, the home care coordinator performs the initial home and patient-family assessment. Ideally, this assessment should be completed within 48 working hours of the patient's hospital discharge to ensure the continuity of care and the early identification of additional patient needs, complications, or noncompliance with the care plan.

During the admission process, the home care coordinator must establish an initial care plan that implements the physician-approved plan of treatment. This care plan includes:

- Identification of the patient's principal and secondary needs
- Goal setting relative to those needs and appropriate time frames to facilitate case management
- Identification of the appropriate skilled and unskilled services required to best meet the goals set
- Incorporation of the physician's initial orders into the care plan

The establishment of the patient's initial care plan requires the home care coordinator's involvement with the patient, the family, and the physician. Initially, the physician's approval for home care intervention and agreement regarding the services to be provided are essential. The identification of specific needs and goals is most effective when the patient and family can perceive these needs and goals as their own, not merely as ones identified by a professional for them. Therefore, the home care coordinator meets with the patient and family and explains the proposed care plan. After the plan has been discussed, the patient and family enter into a verbal agreement with the home care coordinator to do their part to implement the plan. This verbal agreement is important because the goals expressed in the care plan can only be achieved with the full commitment of the patient and family.

After identifying the patient's needs and goals and noting which home care services are needed to implement the physician's treatment plan, the home care coordinator confers by telephone or in person with the physician to secure approval of the specific details of the care plan. This conference should be accomplished within 24 hours of the patient's initial assessment to facilitate early action on the patient's care plan. The home care coordinator should confirm in writing the subjects and key points discussed with the physician.

Thus, the establishment of a care plan by the physician and the home care coordinator creates the patient care team, which includes appropriate members of the home care professional and paraprofessional staff, the patient and family, and the physician. Through the interdependent and collaborative efforts of this team, the highest quality of care possible under the agreed-upon and prescribed treatment plan can be provided.

The patient's home care health record, with appropriate patient identification data, insurance information, and intake and referral forms, is routed to those professional staff members who are assigned to the patient care team. The design of the referral form is multidisciplinary to reflect all of the services provided for any given patient. The routing of referral forms does not replace the informal patient care conferences among the care givers but does facilitate the rapid, smooth, and accurate implementation of the patient's care plan. The referral form used by SHHS/HHA is shown in figure 5-2, next page.

Schedule for Home Visits

After all members of the patient care team have had an opportunity to assess the needs of the patient that are specific to their area of expertise, the home care coordinator can develop the patient's home care visit schedule. The frequency of visits is directly related to the identified needs of the patient and the goals and time frames specifically set for meeting these needs. Visits should be scheduled to best facilitate the goals of the care plan and to avoid overstressing the patient (for example, multiple visits by various care givers should not be clustered in one day).

Figure 5-2. Example of Referral Form

```
                          HOME HEALTH AGENCY      [ ]  Nursing
Unit _____    REFERRAL FORM         [ ]  Mental Health
Patient's Name _____[ ]  Speech Pathology
Age _____ D.O.B. _____ Telephone No. _____[ ]  Physical Therapy
Address _____[ ]  Occupational Therapy
Directions to Home _____[ ]  Respiratory Therapy
         _____[ ]  Social Work

Caretaker _____ Relationship _____ Telephone No. _____
Hospital _____ Adm. Date _____ Disch. Date _____
Diagnosis _____
Date of Onset/Surgery _____ Mental Status _____
Precautions and/or Limitations _____
Physician _____ Signature _____
```

NURSING Referral Date _____	OCCUPATIONAL THERAPY Referral Date ____

NURSING   Referral Date _____
Specific physician's orders:

Comments:

MENTAL HEALTH   Referral Date _____
Current frequency of nursing visits:
Mon. ___ Tues. ___ Wed. ___ Thurs. ___ Fri. ____
Attending psychiatrist? _____
Reason for referral:

SPEECH PATHOLOGY   Referral Date _____
Reason for referral:
Word finding problems _____
Problem understanding your speech _____
Slurred speech _____
Harsh or hoarse voice _____
No voice _____
Swallowing problems _____
No speech _____
Specific orders _____

Previous Speech Therapy: Yes ___ No ___
Where _____ When _____
Comments:

PHYSICAL THERAPY   Referral Date _____
P.T. Orders:

Plan of Treatment
Sent | | | | | | | | |
Ret. | | | | | | | | |

OCCUPATIONAL THERAPY Referral Date ____
Secondary problems affecting rehabilitation:

O.T. Orders: Eval/training/exercise in
( ) Range of motion
( ) Muscle strengthening
( ) Coordination
( ) Hemiplegic program
( ) Activities of daily living
( ) Transfers
( ) Homemaking
( ) Work simplification/energy conservation
( ) Joint protection
( ) Perceptual
( ) Prosthetic/orthotic
( ) Adaptive equipment
( ) Architectural barrier assessment
( ) Others
Comments:

RESPIRATORY THERAPY   Referral Date ____
R.T. Orders:

SOCIAL WORK   Referral Date ____
Patient's Soc. Sec. No. _____
Was hospital Social Work involved? Yes [ ] No [ ]
Name of worker _____
Reason for referral:

The cost-effectiveness of the visitation pattern must also be considered. A cost-effective visitation pattern permits service providers to make visits in each sector of their assigned geographic areas at regular intervals. This practice allows each service provider to systematically and effectively visit each patient residing in that sector. The primary benefit of this systematic visitation pattern is that it does not require the service providers to drive back and forth across their assigned geographic area in the course of a day's work. Consequently, they can spend the maximum amount of time with patients and the minimum amount of time traveling. The major drawback in strictly adhering to this policy is that the unique needs of individual patients may be sacrificed in the name of efficiency. At SHHS/HHA, the general practice of using geographic visitation patterns while routinely making exceptions based on specific individualized needs of patients provides excellent results.

As team members conduct their individual assessments of the patient's needs and review the orders on the initial treatment plan, they may spot discrepancies between the orders that were written while the patient was still hospitalized and the most effective treatment modality for the patient at home. Either the home care coordinator or the direct service provider must discuss these discrepancies with the attending physician. The advantage of having the home care coordinator contact the physician is that the physician need relate to only one home care professional for the care of each patient. The advantage of having the direct service provider contact the physician is that the details of the assessment and evaluation, with all the appropriate supporting data, are related to the physician in the taxonomy of that direct service provider's discipline. If the physician has any questions, they are more likely to be answered concisely by the direct service provider. Perhaps the best plan is to look at each individual case and then decide who will contact the physician.

The home care coordinator is responsible for monitoring the overall visitation pattern and for maintaining open communication among team members. Team members must share any changes in their visit patterns with others in the group so that they can adjust their schedules as needed. Any changes in the visit schedule, especially those altering the frequency of visits, must be verified in writing by the physician before being instituted.

The patient's and the family's role in the home care visit is vital. They must be able to communicate their needs and their ability to handle schedule and treatment regimens to the home care coordinator. The home care coordinator is the conduit for the flow of information from the patient and family to appropriate members of the home care team. This essential communication link begins with the verbal agreement that is developed during the home care coordinator's initial contacts with the patient and family and continues until the patient is discharged from home care.

Careful documentation in the home care patient's health record of all services provided during home visits is vital. This record serves as a communication tool as well as a verification of patient care and regulatory compliance. Team members keep only the most recent documentation with them as a working tool. All previous documentation is centrally filed for total team accessibility. The patient's health record includes, in addition to visit documentation, all physician-signed treatment plans, all team members' progress summaries, and other multidisciplinary communications to the physician regarding the patient. The health record should reflect a total profile of each patient receiving home care services.

Team Conferences

Team conferences on patient care range from the most informal discussions to highly sophisticated, management-level conferences to discuss case management problems. At SHHS/HHA, each home care coordinator maintains a binder of case conference forms for each active patient. Whenever a case conference occurs, the personnel involved record the following information on the case conference form: the date, the initials of those attending, and comments regarding the nature of the conference. This form becomes a part of the patient's permanent health record when the patient is discharged from the home health agency.[4]

There are five levels of team conferences:

- *Mini case conference.* The purpose of a mini case conference is to allow individual staff members the opportunity to discuss and coordinate patient services. This conference is called a mini conference because it usually involves only two or three providers, who discuss issues relating only to their specific services. The meeting is face-to-face whenever possible; however, telephone contact is also acceptable. During the conference, the providers may realize that they cannot solve the problem under discussion. In such a situation, the quick involvement of management staff is essential.[5]
- *Monthly case conference.* In a monthly case conference, direct service providers review all of their current patients with the clinical supervisor in their discipline. This monthly review allows the clinical supervisor to review each patient's treatment program, care plan, and progress and to record the results of the discussions on each patient's conference form. Unresolved problems are reported immediately to the appropriate level of management.[6] This conference is also helpful in supervising staff members as it clearly reflects each direct service provider's clinical skills and style of case management.
- *All-services case conference.* An all-services case conference, which is held monthly, provides the structure for interdisciplinary communication on the care of all patients who are receiving more than one professional service from the agency. One particular patient is chosen as the focus for the meeting. All staff providing care for that particular

patient must be present. The discussion is recorded on a case conference form that becomes a permanent part of the patient's health
record. This conference is also used for problem solving so that professionals who are not currently assigned to that patient can provide
input, which may or may not result in their direct involvement with
the patient at some later time.[7] Because this conference is similar in
nature to grand rounds in a teaching hospital, it is also a useful
mechanism for providing in-service instruction to staff members.
* *Interdisciplinary patient care review.* A quarterly interdisciplinary
patient care review is conducted to ensure that established policies
and procedures are followed in providing patient services, to ascertain that patient care is being maintained at an optimal level, to identify gaps in services, and to evaluate the quality of agency
documentation. This review is conducted by a standing agency committee made up of nurse representatives from each department in the
agency, a representative from each allied health care discipline, and
a representative from management. The committee reviews a random
sampling of records of discharged patients from each home care
department and professional discipline. The evaluative results are
recorded on a form and forwarded to the quarterly utilization review
committee.[8]
* *Quarterly utilization review conference.* The quarterly utilization
review conference represents the highest level of review within the
agency. It is used to promote high-quality patient care, increase the
effective use of services by providing a concurrent review of active
patient records, monitor patient care, and interface the agency's utilization review with the parent hospital's quality assurance program.[9]
To achieve these goals, the conference regularly evaluates the
following:
  − Quality and appropriateness of care being provided, including
    accessibility, timeliness, and need for services
  − Proper utilization and coordination of the various home care
    disciplines
  − Effective resolution of problems relating to patients with complex
    needs or patients who are not responding to treatment
  − Review of patient situations that require termination of care because
    of unresolvable patient situations

  The persons involved in a utilization review conference include
professional representatives from the entire scope of home care services offered by the agency. In addition, a physician and an administrative representative of the agency should be present. The group's
overall goal is to ensure appropriate case management and high-
quality patient care. Any decisions on patient care policies and procedures that come out of this conference must be communicated to all
agency staff members.

Patient Recertification

The home care coordinator is responsible for initiating a patient care recertification every 60 days. In the recertification process, each patient's care plan is reviewed and evaluated to determine the adequacy and the appropriateness of continued care.

In the course of caring for the patient, each person providing care adds documentation on the patient's progress to the patient's health record. These notes also include recommendations for any changes in services provided by the team.

During the recertification process, the treatment plan is resubmitted to the patient's attending physician for review and approval. Any changes must be authorized by the physician in writing before the expiration of the current orders. After the new treatment plan is received from the physician, the home care coordinator is responsible for communicating to other team members any new or additional orders that the physician may have documented.

Discharge from Home Care

From the time home care services are initiated, the patient and family should be prepared for the patient's ultimate discharge from the home health agency. The discharge plan is developed as a joint effort by the patient care team in conjunction with the patient, the family, and the physician to help the patient improve or maintain current level of functioning. The physician's written approval is needed before the patient can be discharged.

Before the actual discharge date, the patient and family must have a clear understanding of what is expected of them after the home care team is no longer visiting. Each professional on the patient care team reviews with the patient the portion of the plan for postdischarge care that concerns that professional's particular discipline.

In addition, the home care coordinator prepares a home care discharge summary. This summary compares the initial assessment data on the patient with the patient's status at the time of discharge from the agency. It states the goals of the patient care plan and how those goals have been met. It also lists ongoing patient care needs and outlines how they will be met after the patient is no longer receiving home care services. The discharge summary becomes part of the patient's permanent health record.

The patient's home care coordinator usually makes the final home visit. During this visit, instructions from all members of the patient care team are reviewed and reinforced. The patient's follow-up with the physician is discussed (for example, the patient is reminded of the date of the next appointment), and the importance of this follow-up is emphasized. Available and appropriate community-based support services are identified for the patient and family. When the patient does not have a family member or caretaker present at the time of the final visit, the home care coordinator attempts to communicate the discharge information to the patient and then by telephone to the family member or caretaker indicated by the patient.

When the patient is being discharged to another health care facility, the home care coordinator and the other members of the patient care team may communicate with the facility on significant patient needs and the care plan used in the home setting. This communication is followed up by sending a copy of the home care discharge summary to the receiving facility.

Once the discharge documentation has been added to the patient's home care health record, the record is closed. At this point, final invoices are submitted, along with any necessary clinical documentation, to the insurance carrier. In addition, a copy of the patient's home care discharge summary is sent to the referring hospital or skilled nursing facility so that the circle of care has been completed and regulatory requirements have been met. Discharge summaries are also sent to referring physicians for their office records.

Most home health agency discharges are routine: that is, the patient no longer requires home care services, and so, with the physician's approval, the patient is discharged. However, the agency may terminate services to a patient, after notifying the physician and following appropriate administrative policy, for other reasons, such as:

- The patient is no longer homebound.
- The patient's condition changes so that the patient now requires care or services other than those that the agency can provide.
- No one is available in the home to give the required care to the patient between visits from the patient care team.
- The patient or family refuses to cooperate in working toward treatment goals.
- The patient moves out of the agency's visiting area.
- The patient changes physicians, and the new physician does not order home care services.
- The patient dies.

The decision to discontinue home care services can also be made at any time and for any reason by the physician, the patient, or the family on the patient's behalf if the patient cannot make the decision.

Staffing

The importance of adequate staffing cannot be overemphasized. Over time, the patient load of most home health agencies increases as the agency becomes known in the community. Having a sufficient number of well-trained, experienced staff to handle this volume is essential. However, maintaining a sufficient number of experienced staff for each discipline is often more complicated than it appears to be.

Management Philosophy and Practice

Meeting the personnel needs of a home health agency is an important part of providing services in a professional and fiscally sound environment. Each one of the departments at SHHS/HHA maintains a full staff of registered professional nurses and other care givers in numbers sufficient to meet the direct care needs of its patient population. Each care giver is assigned a caseload of patients for whom he or she retains primary responsibility. Department managers assign patients to staff members on the basis of the geographic locations of the patients. This practice reduces the amount of travel time and allows the home care staff members to become familiar with the demographic characteristics of and the resources available in their territory. It is also a cost-effective and cost-efficient way of managing the department's resources.

The agency must also have additional trained and qualified nurses and other care givers available to meet the needs of patients whose care giver is ill or on vacation or unable to handle an unusually high volume of visits. The agency can meet the fluctuating volume of service requests in three ways:

- Assign part-time care givers to each department
- Assign part-time care givers to a centralized staffing pool
- Use a staffing agency

No matter which method is used, budgetary flexibility is essential to ensure financial success. One way to ensure flexibility is to use a variable as opposed to a fixed budget. The variable budget provides a mechanism for adjusting and monitoring expenses that are truly volume related while holding other overhead expenses constant. In a variable budget, expenses are calculated relative to the number of units of service (visits) provided. The variable budget allows the department manager to expand and contract the pool of workers as needed to meet the volume of service required on any given day.

Experience and judgment are required to determine how many care givers should be assigned to a department in the home health agency, how many should be assigned to the centralized staffing pool, and how many will be needed from a staffing agency. Factors that affect these numbers include the size of the agency, the relative number of new patients visited daily, the health and safety of individual staff members, and the availability of appropriately prepared part-time personnel.

The SHHS/HHA has found that all three methods of staffing are required to meet a large agency's staffing needs. The best procedure is for each department in the agency to first cover unassigned visits with the department's regularly assigned nurses. If more help is required, the department calls on its part-time nurses or requests additional coverage from the agency's centralized staffing pool. If all of the nurses in the centralized staffing pool are assigned and a significant need still exists, the staffing coordinator calls a staffing agency with whom previous arrangements have been made.

Part-Timers Assigned to Department

Assigning part-time care givers to a specific department in the agency maintains continuity and consistency of care in the absence of the regularly assigned care giver and gives the department manager considerable flexibility in granting vacation requests and in allowing staff members to participate in educational opportunities. At SHHS/HHA, these part-time nurses are permanent part-time employees who receive benefits, such as holidays and vacation days. This practice tends to foster dedication and incentive. The agency also derives benefits from this arrangement because it has a permanent source of personnel that is already trained and oriented in agency procedures and policies.

This combination of staffing arrangements contributes to the health of the department as a whole by not overburdening the full-time staff, who would otherwise have to step in for their absent colleagues. Part-time employees can visit patients at the previously scheduled time in most instances, and so no patient visits need to be rescheduled. Full-time employees do not have to increase their travel time or expenses to cover for absent care givers. Additionally, this practice eliminates the need to obtain the physician's approval for altering the patient's frequency of visits and changing the appointed visit day. Departmental revenue is not lost because visits do not have to be canceled.

Assigning part-time care givers to each department of the agency has additional benefits. These care givers are also known to the attending physicians, who may have more confidence in the care being given their patients when they work with persons with whom they have developed a relationship. The part-time care givers soon learn the geographic area of the agency; and therefore, nonproductive hours as a result of getting lost or using inefficient travel routes are reduced. The full-time and part-time care givers learn to function as an efficient team. The major disadvantage of assigning part-time care givers to each home care department is that one department may not have enough volume to supply the part-time care givers with as many hours of work as they may desire.

Centralized Staffing Pool

A centralized staffing pool is used to meet needs that cannot be covered by each home care department's full-time and part-time personnel. At SHHS/HHA, part-time nurses are hired for a centralized staffing pool and assigned to various departments on a daily, weekly, or monthly basis as the need arises.

The staffing coordinator at SHHS/HHA is responsible for hiring, training, orienting, assigning, and supervising the nurses in the centralized staffing pool. These part-time nurses are not guaranteed any specific number of hours of work per week and must be willing to provide staff relief in any department of the agency. The staffing coordinator conducts regularly scheduled meetings with the nurses in the centralized staffing pool to ensure that they are informed of any changes in agency policies and procedures and to give them an opportunity to discuss problems, concerns, and ideas.

When a home care department at SHHS/HHA needs someone from the centralized staffing pool to provide relief or to handle additional volume, the department manager contacts the staffing coordinator. The staffing coordinator assigns a nurse to the requesting department for the specified time. The home care department then prepares an assignment, which includes specific directions to each patient's house and a full report of the patient's condition along with the objectives for the scheduled visit. The nurse from the staffing pool receives this report, completes the assignment, and reports back to the home care department before returning to the pool for reassignment.

Staffing Agency

Another method of dealing with increased visit volume is to use the services of a staffing agency. This step cannot be taken quickly, and so for the best results, the agency's staffing coordinator meets with representatives of several staffing agencies well in advance of any expected use. At these meetings, the staffing coordinator communicates the agency's expected standards for education and experience, the nature of assignments, and the duties expected of a nurse. The staffing coordinator is also responsible for checking the credentials and references of each staffing agency that may be used.

After ascertaining that the staffing agency will be able to appropriately fill the home health agency's needs, the staffing coordinator, in cooperation with the staffing agency, makes arrangements to provide an orientation for staffing agency personnel who may be assigned to the home health agency. Such an orientation ensures that these temporary personnel understand the requirements of the home health agency and their assigned duties and that they know how to interface with the agency staff, where to turn for assistance, and how to report problems.

Using staffing agencies has a number of significant disadvantages. Perhaps the most problematic disadvantage is the lack of continuity that arises from the rapid turnover among staffing agency personnel. The result is that the home health agency's patients, staff members, and attending physicians find it difficult to build a meaningful professional relationship with a staffing agency nurse. Additional disadvantages include the frequent need to orient new staffing agency personnel and the costliness of this means of providing personnel.

Allied Health Staffing

Each of the three methods, either singly or in combination, of achieving appropriate nurse staffing is appropriate for providing a pool of available allied health care professionals. However, in some regions of the country, allied health care professionals are a scarce commodity. If no staffing agencies offer the services of allied health care professionals and if only a limited number of professionals are willing to work part-time, the home health agency must find other ways to meet its need for these essential services.

Perhaps the most widely used method of obtaining additional allied health care staffing is to make contractural arrangements with professionals on a per visit basis. Professionals who agree to work under this type of arrangement are often called *independent contractors.* Many hospital-based agencies approach professionals who work in the hospital's rehabilitation departments to ask if they are interested in making home visits in the evenings and on weekends. These professionals are generally reimbursed on a per visit basis.

When using independent contractors from any source, the agency must be sure that they receive an appropriate orientation to the agency. Developing effective communication mechanisms to use with independent contractors, who are often unable to attend regular staff meetings, is also crucial. Supervision of independent contractors must also be individualized to meet the needs of the professional and the agency.

Staff Recruitment and Selection

Staff recruitment in the home care industry is no easy task. Because the market demand for qualified, experienced home care staff is at a peak, the competition for available professionals among home health agencies is often keen. For example, establishing an effective home care rehabilitation program is difficult, if not impossible, without a full complement of allied health care specialists, including those in physical therapy, occupational therapy, speech and language pathology, social work, psychiatric mental health nursing[10] and respiratory therapy.[11,12] Yet some of these professionals are in short supply. Establishing clear criteria for the selection, orientation, staff development, and evaluation of all home care staff is paramount to the success of any home health agency.

Selecting the appropriate prerequisite skills for home care staff members requires knowledge of the pool of available personnel in the agency's service area as well as knowledge of the home care field. The best advice that can be given on this subject is that a home health agency should not hire anyone who does not have a minimum of two years of recent clinical experience.

Nearly every specialty in nursing is needed in home care. However, a background in medical-surgical nursing is the most appropriate. Even a large home health agency is unlikely to be able to afford the luxury of assigning a nurse to an entire caseload of patients whose care requires only one specialty.

Most agencies require that home health aides have a high school diploma or equivalent. Many agencies also require some form of certification or training as a nursing assistant. The requirement of certification should be considered carefully before it is instituted. Recruiting certified aides is difficult if no educational institutions in the area offer the certification or if such certification is prohibitively expensive.

For allied health care professionals, recent clinical experience is especially crucial if the agency has no management staff in that discipline. The SHHS/HHA uses a matrix reporting system, which creates allied health care departments headed by a member of each discipline who has had extensive clinical and home care experience. The matrix arrangement requires that each allied health professional report to the director of his or her allied health department for all supervision relative to the practice of his or her profession and to the director of the department to which he or she is assigned for the care of each patient as a member of that department's team. A large agency, such as SHHS/HHA is able to use an arrangement of this type because it employs a large number of allied health staff for each professional discipline and because it covers a wide geographic area. An alternative method of providing clinical supervision and consultation may be to contract with the agency's parent hospital for this service.

Because of the requirement for a minimum of two years of clinical experience, the home care department of a hospital will probably pay higher starting salaries to its nurses than do the other clinical departments of the hospital. This higher pay is essential to attract and retain persons with the level of skills that is necessary in the home care setting, where supervision and consultation are several miles away. Some hospitals that give annual raises on the employee's anniversary date for only the first few years of the employee's tenure may need to extend the number of years for such raises in order to retain an experienced home care staff. Offering a pay differential to nurses who have a baccalaureate may be one way to attract and retain qualified individuals. When the agency is having difficulty attracting persons with a particular specialty, it may have to develop special incentive programs. One such program may be to give a bonus to any employee who is instrumental in the recruitment of someone with the desired specialty.

Home health aides may also require a salary that is higher than the salary of nursing aides in the hospital. In making such salary determinations, the agency must carefully evaluate the duties of the aides in each setting. Some home health agencies assign aides to more complex tasks than do their parent hospitals. The home health aides' salary should be commensurately higher if their usual assignments are significantly more complex or require additional training and more independent judgment than do the assignments of nursing aides in the hospital.

Before the home health agency employs any person, it must check all references. Because of the unique features of the home care setting, all employees must be extremely self-motivated and capable of autonomous decision making. Checking each applicant's references is one way of ensuring that each new employee will have these essential skills. When hiring individuals who have been employed by the parent hospital of the agency, the agency has the extra advantage of being able to use the hospital's personnel records as a source of information about the potential employee. The person evaluating the qualifications of a prospective employee should remember that teaching specific clinical skills is easier than teaching interpersonal skills. An individual who demonstrates excellent interpersonal skills but has few current clinical skills may have the potential to become a better employee than does a person with excellent clinical skills and poor interpersonal skills.

The SHHS/HHA has a low incidence of staff turnover, with 70 percent of all employees having more than five years' tenure with the agency. Nevertheless, full-time staff nurse positions as well as other direct-service positions at SHHS/HHA become available from time to time through attrition or because of increases in patient volume. When openings occur, staff members are generally recruited by postings within the agency and its parent hospital system, by newspaper advertising, and by word of mouth. Candidates for employment with the agency are often recommended by current staff members.

Determining when a new position should be added requires the development of standards to measure volume and productivity, which is discussed later in this chapter. However, these standards can be used only as guidelines because applying them requires the assessment of additional factors that affect a department's ability to function. These additional factors may include level of care of current patients; the number of admissions and discharges; and additional responsibilities, such as the increasing burden of mandatory documentation, that staff members must shoulder.

The hiring of new staff nurses at SHHS/HHA is done centrally by the staffing coordinator, who screens all applications for employment and conducts all initial interviews. The staffing coordinator has final authority in hiring nurses for the agency's centralized staffing pool. When a permanent position is to be filled in one of the home care departments, the manager of that department also interviews the applicants and then makes the final decision.

A few of the requirements for nurses at SHHS/HHA are a current registered nurse's license in the commonwealth of Pennsylvania, a current Pennsylvania driver's license, and two to four years of recent medical-surgical experience. Preference is given to applicants who have either community health experience or a bachelor's or master's degree in nursing. During the hiring interview, the staffing coordinator also considers references, a broad range of nursing experience, the ability to communicate and relate to others, patient assessment skills, independent decision-making experience, time management and organizational skills, empathy, the ability to practice in an unstructured environment, flexibility and adaptability to new situations, and a sense of humor.

At SHHS/HHA, the time during which a new nurse does not function at an optimal productivity level is reduced by offering open full-time positions to current part-time nurses. The part-time nurses already have acquired experience in the agency and have established relationships with department managers and other staff members. Thus, these nurses can be fully functional in less time. This hiring practice is also an additional incentive in recruiting part-time home care nurses for the agency.

Hiring for all allied health care services at SHHS/HHA is done by the allied health care director responsible for that particular discipline. No uniform employment requirements exist because each professional discipline is unique and has established individual employment requirements. These requirements conform to Medicare's *Conditions of Participation for Home Health Agencies* and to Pennsylvania's licensure and certification laws. Most disciplines also require employees to be graduates of a school that is accredited by a nationally recognized standard-setting group for that particular discipline. Experiential requirements vary widely and are primarily related to the supply of available professionals in that discipline. Additional skills that indicate a high probability of success for potential allied health care employees are similar to those identified for nurses: the ability to function autonomously in a remote, varied, and unstructured environment; flexibility; assessment skills; independent decision-making experience; and interpersonal skills.

Dress Code

An agency dress code serves several purposes:

- It ensures that there will be some similarity among staff members in standards of dress.
- It provides some measure of protection for staff members and for patients, who can identify agency callers from others by their appearance.
- It assists in marketing the agency by increasing its visibility.

The type of dress code to be adopted is a matter of individual agency choice. Some agencies select a certain color that all employees must wear when representing the agency. Other agencies have specially designed uniforms that are similar to those worn in the airline industry. The type of uniform is less important than the function it serves: providing a specific identity to a group of diverse individuals.

Orientation

Staff orientation in a home health agency should consist of both formal and on-the-job training. This orientation begins with the new employee's exposure to the roles and responsibilities of all members of the home care team. Because an agency's success in both qualitative and financial terms depends on the ability of its staff to manage patients and to document patient care so that it is reimbursable, an important aspect of orientation is developing professionals into responsible team members. To this end, the new employee's ability to give the required care and prepare the required documentation is assessed, and specific training is provided, as needed, during the orientation period.

The practice at SHHS/HHA is to require all new employees to complete a three-week orientation program, "Introduction to Home Care," which is held in a central location to acquaint new staff with the organization and function of the home health agency and the hospital system of which it is a part. This orientation program is derived from a general outline that is individualized for each new employee. The general orientation to the agency's policies, procedures, services, and forms is conducted as frequently as is needed to accommodate new employees. Orientation to the specific department and on-the-job training are conducted by the clinical supervisor or allied health care director at the assigned department and in the community. A skills inventory is used to assess the level of each new employee's clinical skills. In addition, detailed observations are made of the employee's ability to perform in the unstructured community setting.

Another method for orienting employees, especially when more than one new employee is hired in a department, is to assign each new employee to a preceptor, who is a staff member from the same discipline as the new employee. The preceptor's job is to work closely with the new employee under the direction of the clinical supervisor or the allied health care director.

Some departments prefer to use the preceptor method of orientation because it exposes new employees to a diversity of styles and encourages them to be creative and flexible while teaching them the framework within which they must function. Other departments prefer to assign orientation exclusively to the clinical supervisor or allied health care director because they believe that the new employee is less confused when only one individual provides the orientation.

In addition to the orientation already described, an orientation program covering all of SHHS/HHA's available services—physical therapy, occupational therapy, social work, speech and language therapy, rehabilitation nursing, and respiratory therapy—is held approximately every six months. Attendance is mandatory because these programs are helpful to new employees who may have come to the agency without an in-depth knowledge of how these services can most appropriately help their patients.

At the end of a three-week period, the new employee and the agency's director of staff development, along with the employee's supervisor, evaluate the orientation process and discuss any topics that may need further clarification. This meeting completes the three-week orientation process. A form certifying the employee's participation in the orientation process is signed by those staff members involved. This form then becomes part of the employee's personnel file. New employees have an initial probationary period of six months, with a performance evaluation required at the end of the first three months and another at the end of the first six months.

Training and Education

An important responsibility of any home health agency is the ongoing education and training of its staff members. Whereas on-the-job training and in-service education are especially well suited to internal agency training activities, continuing education appears to be accomplished best through external seminars and workshops and through formal educational programs awarding academic credit.

As new service programs are added, each staff member must be trained for the delivery of that specific service. Also, fostering the educational development of each staff member should be of concern to the agency. These objectives provide the foundation of an agency's educational program.

Staff training and education at SHHS/HHA are coordinated with other programs under the auspices of the director of staff development. The goal of the director of staff development is to provide opportunities for agency personnel to acquire the knowledge, understanding, and skills necessary to safely and effectively perform the functions specified in their job descriptions. Staff training is directed toward three specific needs:

- Training to help those persons without adequate preemployment preparation to do their jobs
- In-service training to keep the staff up-to-date on health care information and changes in agency policies or health practices
- Continuing education for administrative and supervisory personnel to maintain and upgrade their ability to do their jobs

Staff development activities at SHHS/HHA are now largely decentralized. The decision to decentralize in-service education and on-the-job training was made after the completion of an assessment of the needs of staff members in various departments and an evaluation of the ways in which a centralized program was meeting these needs. The large size of SHHS/HHA and its structure, with nine offices and nine allied health care services, dictated the need for change. Prior to decentralizing the in-service education function, the agency held regularly scheduled in-service programs in a central location. As the agency grew, accommodating an increasingly large group of staff members in a centrally located facility became difficult. As the agency's geographic area expanded, staff members providing services on the periphery of the geographic area had a more difficult time attending these centrally located programs. Also, as staff members developed increased expertise, the agency found it difficult to identify meaningful in-service programs that would benefit all employees. Scheduling in-service programs that required large blocks of time also became difficult.

Since the development at SHHS/HHA of a decentralized educational model, staff training and education is conducted by each of the nine home care departments of the agency through its own educational council. Educational councils are composed of the department director and three or four direct-service providers who represent all of the department's staff members. The director of staff development assists the councils in planning and presenting programs, developing evaluation tools, and disseminating information about in-service opportunities. The director of staff development also maintains centralized records of all in-service programs.

The decentralized training program allows each home care department to provide for the specific training needs of staff assigned to that department. It also enables a greater number of the home care staff to participate in training programs. Occasionally, centrally located programs are presented when a specific need is identified throughout the agency or when a program is costly to present.

An additional benefit that SHHS/HHA has experienced as a result of decentralizing staff development has been a reduction in the number of hours, agencywide, spent in travel, with a concurrent reduction in travel expense. During the first year of operating under the decentralized system, the number of educational programs held in each department doubled. This increase resulted primarily because of the shift in location from central to local. In addition, departments were able to hold shorter and more frequent in-service programs because of the reduced travel times involved.

The director of staff development spends time with each educational council, giving advice and assistance in planning each in-service program. This role is essential to maintaining the same level of quality at the departmental level as could be offered through centralized programs. The agency expects that decentralized training will make it easier to measure how well the training programs increase knowledge and skills and to coordinate agency training with that of corresponding departments in the parent hospital system and the participating hospitals.

Job Descriptions

The home health agency should have complete and accurate job descriptions for every position in the agency. These descriptions should clearly delineate each job's overall responsibilities to the agency and to the patient and should indicate precisely what tasks the incumbent is expected to perform. Good job descriptions cover the position and not the person currently holding the job. Therefore, a job description should not need to be changed when a new person is hired. Job descriptions should be reviewed every three to six months for new positions and at least annually for every position so that any changes in responsibilities and duties can be incorporated. Because job descriptions are central to the determination of how well each employee is functioning, and in many instances may be the foundation for determining salary increases, the agency needs to make sure that each job description is accurate and up to date.

The process of developing a job description begins with a statement of why the position was developed. From there, the person writing the job description should identify the major responsibilities or accountabilities of the job. The job description should identify the position's supervisor and any positions that report to the position being described. The job description should be sufficiently detailed to convey the nature and extent of the job and yet flexible enough to allow the incumbent to individualize his or her approach to the job.

South Hills Health System, the parent corporation of SHHS/HHA, uses a job questionnaire developed by Hay Associates, a management consulting group, as a first step in writing a job description. This job questionnaire takes the individual through the steps already described and asks additional questions to enable the human resources department of SHHS to place the position in relation to all other positions in the organization so that appropriate job classifications and salary ranges can be determined.

Sometimes a person may be hired to fill a perceived need, and in such cases, no finalized job description may exist. Often the development of a new position and program within the agency is best served by delaying the writing of a job description until a person is actually hired for that job. This new employee may be the person most qualified to complete the job description. The process of completing the job questionnaire for a position also helps the new employee to learn about the agency. The new employee is thus directly involved in the development not only of the position he or she fills but also of the program in which he or she works.

Evaluation

Staff positions are usually divided into exempt (salaried) and nonexempt (hourly) categories. Each category contains a number of levels. A staff nurse position may be exempt or nonexempt. At SHHS/HHA, staff nurses are nonexempt. Classifying nurses in this way enables them to be paid for over-time worked. Administrative staff and management personnel are exempt staff positions. Within the exempt classification, positions are classified as management or nonmanagement as defined under the U.S. Fair Labor Standards Act.

Hay Associates also worked with SHHS to develop several tools for evaluating job performance and measuring achievements against expectations for each employee. Job performance is evaluated on a scale ranging from provisional to distinguished. In considering overall job performance, achievement in each of several job responsibilities is weighted. The sum of these indicates the employee's overall rating. Salary increases for exempt employees are directly contingent on the level of job performance. Nonexempt employees receive annual salary adjustments based on areawide wage scales.

Productivity

The development of productivity standards provides the agency with a benchmark against which it can measure its day-to-day activities for efficiency. Because third-party reimbursement is based solely on a per visit basis, all staff activities centered around that visit, such as direct-care time, travel time, documentation time, conferences, meetings, and any other previsit and post-visit activities, must be built into the productivity standard. Other issues to be considered in establishing a standard are complexity of the visit and levels of care. For example, an initial visit may take more time than follow-up visits.

An important issue is the variances that can exist in travel times for different agency personnel. For example, to meet volume demands, one department may have six full-time nurses but only two home health aides or two physical therapists to cover the same geographic area. Also, a nurse may be assigned patients who live 10 or more miles from one another.

In the initial development of the agency's productivity standards, the agency may find that management engineering time studies are useful. Frequently used standards are the hour per visit or visits per day. Figure 5-3, below, shows the productivity standards used at SHHS/HHA.

Even though visit volumes are monitored daily by department directors at SHHS/HHA, the hours per visit and the visits per day are only calculated on a monthly basis. These calculations are based on total staff hours worked per department divided by the total number of visits for that same period. Calculating productivity of all the nurses by department allows the department to account for fluctuations in productivity that occur throughout the month. For example, a nurse working in an area that does not require a lot of travel time balances the productivity of a nurse in an outlying area who cannot meet the quota for that day because of the travel time involved

Figure 5-3. Productivity Standards Used at South Hills Health System/Home Health Agency

	Hours/Visit	Visits/Day
Registered nurse	1.4	5.7
Psychiatric nurse	2.3	3.4
Hospice nurse	2.7	2.9
Home health aide	1.6	5.0
Respiratory therapist	2.0	4.0
Physical therapist	1.55	5.2
Occupational therapist	2.9	2.7
Social worker	3.0	2.7
Speech-language pathologist	2.0	2.0

or the complexity of the required care. A nurse who works in an outlying area may not meet the quota one day but may balance this loss of productivity when he or she makes scheduled visits on another day to several patients located in a senior citizens' apartment complex. This practice of calculating by department also balances out visits that cannot be made because of weather conditions, meetings, or sick leave. The productivity of nursing in all departments in the agency is then combined and used to determine the overall productivity expectations for nurses. Then, the productivity of other departments, such as physical therapy or social work, are calculated according to overall agency performance. However, breakdowns of staff performance per department are available for monitoring individual staff productivity.

Several steps need to be followed in the development of productivity standards:

- Analysis of various possible productivity standards
- Analysis of the agency's past and future performance probability
- Selection of a specific standard
- Development of specific tools and procedures to enhance the agency's ability to conform to the selected standard
- Implementation of the standard
- Evaluation of the usefulness of the chosen standard

Analysis of Possible Productivity Standards

Productivity standards may take several forms, as previously discussed. Perhaps the most popular is the standard based on *hours per visit*. This standard is determined by dividing the total number of visits made during a specified period by the total number of hours that direct-service providers worked during that particular period.

Another often used productivity standard is the *number of visits made in an average working day*. This standard is determined by averaging the number of visits made in a certain period and dividing by the number of working days in that period.

Still another productivity standard is the *number of visits per admission*. This standard is calculated by dividing the number of visits made during a particular period by the number of admissions that occurred during that same period.

A myriad of other factors, such as admissions per day or week, discharges per any given period, or indirect hours per patient or time, may be used to develop productivity standards. No matter what factors are used, the agency must be certain that the standards it develops are realistic, useful, and relatively easy to calculate and that variations in their results are easy to track and explain.

In selecting a productivity measure, the agency should make use of data that it already routinely collects. If the agency routinely keeps records of the number of visits by discipline, number of admissions to the agency, and number of hours spent in direct service to patients, then using visits per day, hours per visit, and visits per admission as productivity standards may be expeditious.

Analysis of Past and Future Performance Probability

After determining which type of standards are most appropriate, the agency must study its operational data to calculate what its performance relative to these measures has been in the past. By calculating agency performance for previous periods, the agency can identify an entire range of possible performance variations. Then the agency should analyze these variations to determine what events within the agency were affecting performance to create those particular performance ratios.

Determining what has been done in the past that is reasonable and acceptable helps to develop a visit standard that will become a key management tool. If developed properly, the standard can predict staff performance in future years. Such predictions can be helpful when preparing budgets, trying to establish staff needs according to volume projections, and monitoring and balancing the budget. These predictions are particularly significant as cost ceilings are imposed for individual home care service units as well as aggregate ceilings for total agency services. Agency policies should include provisions for the continued review and analysis of each standard on a yearly or other periodic basis to determine if any standard needs to be altered.

Selection of a Specific Standard

The collection of data allows agency management to select the one or two specific standards that can best be attained on a continuing basis. The best standard allows agency management to balance the need for an efficient operation with the need for a stimulating, but not oppressive, work environment for direct-service employees. The most effective way to evaluate the agency's productivity is to develop individualized productivity standards for each discipline.

Yet another step that can be taken to ensure the selection of the most appropriate productivity standard is to discuss the need for such standards with the agency's direct-service providers. This process, while time consuming, ensures that each direct-service provider understands the need for productivity standards, has an opportunity to state an opinion on the productivity issue, and leads to greater voluntary compliance because providers have a sense of ownership in a standard that they assisted in creating.

Still another resource that can be used in the selection of productivity standards is a management engineering consultant. These individuals specialize in the measurement and attainment of efficiency, and they are likely to make specific recommendations that will enhance the agency's performance regardless of which productivity standards are selected. The process of analyzing past performance and determining which standard is most efficient and attainable may be less painful and more objective and effective when a management engineer assists.

Development of Enhancing Tools and Procedures

After selecting the specific productivity standards that the agency will use to measure its performance on a regular basis, agency management should again review the work flow within the agency and determine what efficiencies can be introduced to assist staff in attaining these standards. Any tool that enables routine activities to be handled more efficiently saves valuable staff time and allows staff to make more patient visits.

Some examples of efficiencies that may be developed are:

- Designing a message form that allows staff to readily communicate with each other without having to telephone
- Designating a member of the management staff to review each direct-service provider's visiting schedule each day to determine which staff could benefit from some additional help and which staff could provide that help
- Conducting a pilot project to determine whether dictation of clinical documentation or computerized on-site input is more cost-effective than writing each note in longhand

Implementation of the Standard

The implementation phase of the development of productivity standards is the appropriate time to introduce staff members to the chosen productivity standards and to the new tools and procedures that have been developed to assist the staff in meeting the productivity goals. Even those staff members who have assisted in the selection of the specific standard and in the development of new tools and procedures need to know exactly what is expected in the way of performance and exactly how they are expected to use any new tools.

The agency's managers must be certain that they have communicated effectively their desires regarding individual performance. Managers must also be prepared to daily promote adherence to the new standards and the use of the new procedures and tools.

At the outset, everyone must be prepared for less than favorable performance while the staff members become comfortable with the new forms, procedures, or devices that they will be using. A certain amount of time, perhaps two months, should be set aside for testing the new items. Each staff member should be absolutely clear about the deadline for the testing period and the beginning of the real implementation phase.

Evaluation

The final phase of the process of developing productivity standards is evaluation. This phase should occur after some meaningful data has been collected over a reasonable length of time. For example, three months of data collected after the close of the testing period is probably sufficient to make some reasonably accurate generalizations.

Two important tasks are involved in this final phase of the process:

- Identifying and explaining variances
- Verifying the accuracy of the selected productivity standard

The first task, identifying and explaining variances, requires the identification of all deviations from the standard by comparing actual data to the selected standard. Both favorable and unfavorable variances should be scrutinized and justified because either type of variance contributes significantly to the learning process.

The second task, verifying the accuracy of the productivity standard, is perhaps the most important step in the entire process, but it is the one most frequently overlooked. In this step, the managers of the agency need to review the agency's performance, variations, and justifications to assure themselves that the standard that has been developed is truly an accurate measurement of the agency's productivity.

Following the completion of this last task, the productivity standard may seem to take on a life of its own and become an entity that is difficult, if not impossible, to alter. As a result, the agency should review its productivity standards at regular and frequent intervals to determine whether the productivity standards the agency is currently using are still reasonable measures of agency efficiency.

Unique Answers to Unique Situations

The purpose of this chapter has been to introduce the reader to some critical operational issues, as identified by the executive staff of a large multihospital-based home health agency. The topics discussed, while diverse, are interrelated in that each one contributes to the success of a home health agency and each one affects the others. For example, decisions that are made about staffing affect the agency's productivity.

The one overriding principle to remember is that each agency must develop its own unique answers to each of the operational issues discussed in this chapter. Each agency has individual strengths and weaknesses that, taken together, create its own special identity. Using the solutions that another agency has developed to suit its own specific needs may not afford the "borrowing" agency enough individuality to function effectively. Each agency must examine its own circumstances and develop policies and procedures that will enable it to provide the best possible home care to the patients in its geographic area.

Notes

1. Meg Wise Christy and Cathy Frasca, "The Benefits of Hospital Sponsored Home Care Program," *Journal of Nursing Administration* (1983. 13:7-10).

2. Cathy Frasca, "Home Health Care Program Offers Comprehensive Services, *Hospitals.* (1981 Mar. 4:39-42).

3. JoAnn Parzick and Sister Mary Nolan, "POMR at Work in a Home Health Agency," *Family and Community Health* (1978 Apr. 1:101-113).

4. *Policy Manual* of South Hills Health System/Home Health Agency.

5. *Policy Manual.*

6. *Policy Manual.*

7. *Policy Manual.*

8. *Policy Manual.*

9. *Policy Manual.*

10. Wilma Meehan and JoAnn Parzick, "Psychiatric Home Care Nursing Team Helps Patients Overcome Depression," *Hospital Home Care* (1983 June. 2:77, 78).

11. Cathy Frasca and Melissa Weimer, "Establishing a Respiratory Therapy Program," *Home Healthcare Nurse* (1985 Feb. 3:8-12).

12. Melissa Weimer, "Home Respiratory Therapy for Patients with Chronic Obstructive Pulmonary disease," *Respiratory Care* (1983 Nov. 28:1484-89).

Chapter 6

Marketing

Roberta N. Clarke
Judith Walden

In an increasingly competitive environment, such as that in which home care now finds itself, marketing is a necessity. Marketing can be defined as "the analysis, planning, implementation, and control of carefully formulated programs designed to bring about voluntary exchanges of values with target markets for the purpose of achieving organizational objectives. It relies heavily on designing the organization's offering in terms of the target market's needs and desires, and on using effective pricing, communication, and distribution to inform, motivate, and service the markets."[1] Marketing is now generally accepted as a high-level management function on a par with the financial and human resources management functions.

This chapter begins with a discussion of market definition, with special emphasis on two vital players in the decision to use home care: the physician and the hospital discharge planner. After the home care agency has determined its market niche, it must look at its marketing strategy in terms of the four basics of marketing: product, price, promotion, place. However, sometimes an agency wants to take some immediate steps to improve the agency's image, visibility, and reputation even before it develops or implements a long-range marketing strategy. This chapter offers some practical suggestions for doing that and concludes with a description of two marketing programs, one for staff and one for the community.

Roberta N. Clarke, M.B.A., D.B.A., is an associate professor in the School of Management, Boston University, Boston, Massachusetts. Judith Walden, R.N., is president and executive director, Hospital HomeCare, Albuquerque, New Mexico. Contributing to this chapter is Lezlie Ann Schubert, R.N., community liaison nurse, Hospital HomeCare.

Market Definition

Defining the market for a hospital-sponsored home care organization requires deciding which segments of the market the organization is going to serve and, just as important, which segments it will not serve. Chapter 2 describes in detail the home care market segments.

Home care organizations make various decisions about which market segments they will serve. Some hospital-based or hospital-related programs serve only patients discharged from those hospitals. Others choose to provide home care services for anyone in the hospital's service area, whether that person has been a patient at the hospital or not. Some organizations provide only nonprofessional services, such as homemakers and home health aides; others, which are fast diminishing in number, provide only professional services, such as skilled nursing care. A few of the major home care corporations provide only high-tech home care products and the services needed for proper utilization of these products. Other home care companies provide no high-tech products and few, if any, pieces of durable medical equipment (DME), but instead choose to focus exclusively on services.

The way in which the market is defined affects the whole marketing strategy. Because no one agency can serve everyone well, an agency should focus its resources on serving fewer market segments and on serving these segments exceptionally well, rather than spreading limited resources too thinly and serving everyone poorly. For example, an agency choosing to serve the elderly, including the "old" elderly, with a full range of services may also choose not to provide child care.

One function of market definition is to provide a sense of the size of the market and some estimate of the share of that market that the home care agency is likely to capture. Information on market size, translated into absolute number of visits, is required for the budgeting process (see chapter 7). The targeted market share and number of visits projected also affects the budget for promotion. Conversely, the amount and nature of promotion affects the market share attained and the number of visits provided.

An important aspect of understanding the market is identifying the individuals involved in the decision to purchase home care services and assessing their roles in the decision-making process. Each decision usually involves an *initiator,* an *influencer,* a *decider,* a *buyer,* and a *user.* For example, a unit nurse in a hospital's orthopedics unit may initiate the purchase of home care services by suggesting to the patient's family that their elderly relative would be best served by receiving health care at home. The discharge planner may be a strong influencer in the decision to use home care and in the selection of a home care agency. The physician decides that the patient should receive home care and, strongly influenced by the discharge planner, may recommend a specific agency. Medicare is the buyer because it usually pays for the service, and the patient, of course, is the user of the service.

Different individuals play different roles in the decision-to-buy process, and sometimes one individual may play several roles. For example, the patient may be both user and purchaser if the patient wishes the services of a private-duty nurse. The discharge planner may be both initiator and influencer. However, except in the case of private-duty or demand services, the physician is usually the sole decider.

In some decisions to purchase home care, the patient's family actively participates by gathering information for themselves and deciding on which home care service to use independent of recommendations by the physician or discharge planner. More often, however, family members assume a somewhat passive role in the decision-making process and instead rely on the experts—the discharge planner, physician, or nurse—to guide them into what they expect is the right decision.

Figure 6-1, below, shows the roles played by those in the decision-making process in many first-time purchases of home care services. The person who benefits the most from the purchase of home care services, the patient, is usually not very aware of the availability of home care services and is one of the least influential persons in the decision-making process. On the other hand, the physician, who may be the most important person in the decision-making process because the physician must prescribe home care for reimbursement purposes, has a relatively low awareness of the services and receives limited, if any, financial benefits from prescribing home care.

In defining their market niche, home care agencies must not overlook the importance of physicians in the decision to use home care services. Agencies must also be aware of the influence of hospital discharge planners.

Figure 6-1. Levels of Awareness, Importance, and Benefits of Home Care to Decision Makers

	Level of Awareness of Home Care Services	Level of Importance in the Decision-Making Process	Level of Benefits Received through Purchase of Home Care Services
Unit nurse	Somewhat aware	Not very important	Low
Discharge planner	Highly aware	Very important	Medium
Attending physician	Somewhat or not very aware	Very important	Low
Patient's family	Not very aware	Somewhat important	Medium or high
Patient	Not very aware	Not very important	High

Physician's Orientation to Home Care

As a result of hospital cost containment efforts of the mid-1980s, physicians are becoming more aware of home care services. The effect of the prospective pricing system (PPS) and the subsequent earlier discharge of patients has sensitized physicians to the need for care after discharge. The same may be said for physicians under contract with health maintenance organizations (HMOs) and preferred provider organizations (PPOs): these physicians have financial and professional or peer group incentives to discharge patients from acute care settings as quickly as possible, thus increasing the need for the provision of both clinical and nonclinical services to the patient in the home.

However, in spite of this increased awareness of home care services, physicians still present a challenge from a marketing perspective. Physicians are hard to reach because they are so busy. Also, many medical service and product promotional efforts compete for their attention through all forms of media and direct mail as well as through visits from salespersons.

Hospital-sponsored home care services have the built-in advantage of having more ready access to physicians who are affiliated with the hospital. Yet even this connection is no guarantee that the physician will choose to use the hospital's home care services. Physicians with multiple admitting privileges may find that each hospital at which they have privileges is asking them to use that particular hospital's home care service. Also, physicians who have developed a satisfactory long-term relationship with a home care agency may not wish to disrupt that referral relationship. Thus, easier access to a hospital's physicians does not necessarily guarantee getting their home care referrals.

Also, hospital-sponsored home care agencies may have a disadvantage in a highly competitive market: physicians whose primary affiliations are with competing hospitals may be less prone to use the home care services of a hospital that is a competitor to the physician's hospital of primary affiliation. The hospital-sponsored home care service does not necessarily have better access to these physicians and may have to counter an enmity existing between competing hospitals that parallels the hostility between rival high school football teams.

The battle for physician referrals can be fought with a variety of tactics. One of the major national home care corporations has a written policy directing all local offices to be in frequent contact with the home care patient's physician to ensure that the physician is satisfied with the patient's care. Other agencies guarantee that they will minimize contacts with the physician by keeping the patient well-enough served so that the patient does not need to pester the physician with telephone calls. Some organizations send the physician brief weekly reports on the patient so that the physician is prepared to answer any questions if a family member calls. Other organizations use such tactics as sending thank-you notes for each referral. The likeliest way to capture physicians' referrals is to contract with the HMOs and PPOs that have enrolled the physicians' patients to be the primary organization providing home care services.

In trying to lure physician referrals, the home care agency must be aware that the Medicare-Medicaid Antifraud and Abuse Amendments of the Social Security Act prohibit the payment of remuneration, either in cash or in kind, for the referral of patients. *Accordingly, the structure and operation of any plan to provide recognition to physicians or hospital employees who make referrals to the agency should be reviewed by legal counsel.* The fact that a given practice is prevalent in the industry cannot be assumed to indicate its legality.

Discharge Planner's Role

The majority of a home care agency's referrals are likely to come from hospitals. Although some of these referrals clearly come from physicians who refer their hospitalized patients, most referrals come from the discharge planning efforts of the hospital and its discharge planner. The role of the discharge planner, historically a minor role from the hospital's perspective, has rapidly grown in importance as prospective pricing has dictated shorter lengths of stay and earlier discharges. Once considered a peripheral activity both clinically and managerially, effective discharge planning is now becoming intimately tied to a hospital's financial health.

The discharge planner has also gained importance in the eyes of post-hospital service providers, such as skilled nursing facilities, board-and-care homes, rehabilitation centers, and home care agencies. Because discharge planners may exert so much influence over the selection of specific providers within a class of providers, they have become the target for a multitude of promotional efforts.

A hospital-sponsored home care agency has a major advantage in promoting to its hospital's discharge planners because it has direct access to them as well as good-will based on institutional loyalty. This advantage is likely to result in a majority of the hospital's discharges to home care going to the hospital's agency. However some of the hospital's patients may still be referred elsewhere because of the ability of another agency to better meet the needs of the patient, geographic considerations, or time availability for the provision of services. Some home care organizations report that even when the hospital has an exclusive contract with an agency, the discharge planners may choose not to honor the contract terms because they resent being told where to refer their patients.

The relationship between a hospital-sponsored home care agency and discharge planners becomes even more difficult when these discharge planners work for competing hospitals. The same institutional rivalry that physicians may manifest may also be evident with discharge planners. Moreover, the home care agency becomes just one of many seeking to gain attention from discharge planners.

Home care agencies have sought to attract referrals from discharge planners through a variety of means:

- Providing a full range of services so that the discharge planner and the patient's family can engage in one-stop shopping instead of having to work with three different agencies to arrange for six different services.
- Providing verifiably high-quality services, such as trained homemakers, bonded employees, lower staff turnover, and reliable delivery of services.
- Providing services 24 hours a day, 7 days a week.
- Using aggressive selling techniques, including taking discharge planners to lunch or dinner or inviting discharge planners to by-invitation-only educational retreats. However, to avoid potential violations of the antifraud and abuse amendments, the agency should consult legal counsel.

Marketing Basics

To be successful, home care agencies, whether hospital-based or freestanding, must think about their operations in terms of the basics of marketing: product, price, promotion, place. Agencies must determine what *products and services* they will provide to the markets they have defined. They must determine the *price* of such products and services and *promote* the products and services they are providing to their potential customers. While they are making these decision, they must constantly keep in mind the advantages and disadvantages of the unique *place* in which they provide care: the home.

Products and Services

One of the major tasks in developing a marketing strategy for a home care agency is to decide what products and services will be provided. To do this, the agency must first look at how it has defined its market.

If the market is defined as home care for the elderly, then the provision and maintenance of sudden infant death syndrome (SIDS) monitors and the provision of new mother visits should not be included in the product and service line. If a major focus is on cancer patients in the early stages of the disease, then intravenous (IV) chemotherapy and related clinical and equipment maintenance services are necessary. If the focus shifts to the later stages of the disease, the product-service definition must shift to include the availability of 24-hour nursing care, even if a nurse is merely on-call rather than being constantly present. For this market, the services may also include bereavement counseling for patients and their families and special training for nurses in the provision of painkilling medications for the dying patient.

The range of services traditionally offered by home care agencies has been expanding in recent years. The original concept of visiting nurses has diversified into the provision of occupational, physical, respiratory, and stomal therapies; medical social services; specialized nursing (pediatric and orthopedic); and nonclinical service providers such as homemakers and home health aides.

This broadening of service lines has been accompanied by the introduction in the past decade of many product-related home care services. These services include continuous ambulatory peritoneal dialysis; IV therapy for the delivery of nutrition, antibiotics, or chemotherapy; wheelchair maintenance; SIDS monitor maintenance; and the provision and maintenance of other durable and nondurable medical equipment and supplies.

In defining its product and service line, the home care agency must make sure that two major premises are always in the forefront of any planning activities:

- What home care is really selling is *benefits.* Every person or organization involved in the home care experience benefits in some way.
- A home care agency is providing a *service.* All of the employees of the agency have an impact on how the agency, and consequently home care itself, is viewed.

Benefits Approach

Of major importance in defining the product and service lines is the recognition that a home care agency sells *benefits,* not merely products and services. Charles Revson, the late president of the Revlon cosmetics company, was known to say cosmetics are manufactured in the factory, but the store sells help and hope.[2] Every product or service delivers a benefit, and markets will often segment themselves according to benefits.

The benefits that home care is viewed as providing vary, depending on what group or groups make up a particular market:

- Insurance companies, employers, and alternative delivery systems want the benefit of low prices, which translate into paying out less of the premium pool for the care of insured clients.
- Hospitals see home care as a way to provide revenue that PPS, through the fixed payments for diagnosis-related groups (DRGs), has reduced. Home care allows hospitals to discharge appropriate patients earlier and may help hospitals reduce inpatient lengths of stay. The hospital may also perceive hospital-based home care as another service to which overhead can be allocated and as a source of potential profitability. In addition, hospital-sponsored home care may benefit the hospital because the hospital can stay in contact with the patient after the patient's discharge from the acute-care setting; such continued involvement may perhaps enhance the patient's use of the hospital for other clinical needs or for future hospital stays.

- For many patients, home care may be viewed as the only thing standing between them and a nursing home. The benefit of keeping patients from being institutionalized, usually for the rest of their lives for elderly patients, is enormous and not to be underestimated from the perspective of patients or their families.
- Family members of the patient may view home care as a way to alleviate guilt feelings, as a babysitting function, as a safety check, or as a means of keeping the family together.
- The benefits of home care for physicians have not always been clear. Physicians may see home care as a way to respond to pressures by hospital management to discharge patients earlier. A more charitable view is that physicians recognize and are attuned to the benefits that home care provides to their patients and their patient's families.

Because individuals buy products and services on the basis of the benefits they provide, the home care agency should clearly communicate these benefits. Most agencies tend to merely list in their promotional materials the products and services that they provide. Far more effective is the translation of these products and services into benefits. Such information is more likely to influence decision makers who are not aware of or familiar with home care services.

Service Approach

Although products represent an increasing share of the overall home care market, the majority of home care expenditures are still for non-product-related services. Services differ from products in part because they are intangible: services cannot be seen, touched, smelled, heard, or tasted. What is tangible about services are the individuals who deliver them. The way the service providers smile or frown, their tone of voice and manner of speaking, their carriage and appearance, and the respect or disrespect with which they treat patients and their families have a major impact on the way the service is viewed. If a home care visit is delivered competently in a clinical sense but unempathetically and coldly by the service provider, then the patient will probably view the visit negatively even though the service provider's clinical performance is correct.

Consequently, the marketing of any service requires attention to the way in which the specific individuals who provide the service present themselves and interact with patients and their families. This means that home care agencies must recruit, select, train, motivate, evaluate, and compensate staff on the basis, not only of clinical and technical skills, but also on their ability to present themselves to and interact with patients, families, physicians, and other potential markets.

Hospital-based home care agencies may not be unfamiliar with this concept because their hospitals may already have instituted a guest relations program for hospital staff. Guest relations programs recognize that an organization cannot assume that its staff will act empathetically without the proper incentives, training, and commitment of the leadership structure.

Guest relations programs typically also go to great lengths to point out that nonclinical providers are as important as clinicians in fulfilling the guest relations function of any organization. The person who first answers the telephone in the home care agency has the potential to affect the perceptions of more customers than does any individual clinician. Therefore, good marketing requires that *all* home care employees who routinely encounter patients, families, physicians, or other persons or groups who may be purchasers of home care be sensitized to guest relations.

Price

In most areas of health care, pricing is not very straightforward because of third-party reimbursement, regulations, retroactive denials, and the difficulty in pricing a service that is sometimes viewed as a right. Often, the price for home care services is set by parties from outside the agency. From a profit perspective, then, the agency can use only cost control and volume to achieve desired profitability for third-party reimbursed services.

Unlike most industries, in which price affects demand, health care relies heavily on third-party reimbursement; and consequently, the restrictive eligibility guidelines and the regulated limits on reimbursement may determine demand. Although the demand for home care is presumably greater than utilization figures indicate, restricted eligibility guidelines and limited reimbursement prevent patients from receiving as much home care as they, or their physicians, may like.

The one consumer market segment that is not affected by reimbursement concerns is the private-duty or demand segment. Long undertargeted, the private-duty or demand segment is expected to grow as more individuals with substantial personal resources enter their 60s and 70s and as diagnosis-related groups (DRGs) dictate earlier discharges. Because these persons are paying for home care out of their own pockets, they will be price sensitive, and so competitive pricing will be the norm for most private-duty home care services.

Patients or their families also pay out of pocket for certain DME and supplies, such as hospital beds, bedpans, monitors, and so on. Patients or families purchasing what they view to be low-risk products, such as hospital beds, commonly shop around; that is, they usually call a number of suppliers to find the best and presumably the lowest price. The home care agency that provides DME may find itself in price competition with large commercial outfits. If the competition's low prices cannot be matched, then the home care agency should try to offer some added value, such as greater convenience, guaranteed quick service, or free delivery, to justify the higher price.

Other price-sensitive buyers include organizational buyers, such as HMOs, PPOs, and employer groups. These buyers have, or should have, a strong commitment to home care, given their desire to foster early hospital discharges. They also have a profit incentive, which makes them price sensitive, particularly given the volume of services that they may be purchasing. However, even these large volume buyers may be willing to accept higher prices if they can work with one home care agency that provides a full range of services. Working with one agency is more efficient than working with many different agencies.

The concept of quality of home care services seems less of an issue for volume purchasers because few home care providers have actually differentiated themselves successfully on the basis of quality. In the absence of any other differentiating characteristics, volume buyers are likely to choose a home care provider because of price and convenience.

Promotion

One way to characterize promotion strategies is to distinguish between *push* and *pull* strategies. A push strategy relies largely on personal selling; and a pull strategy relies heavily on the use of impersonal media, such as advertising, direct mail, and billboards.

For example, one nonhospital-sponsored home care agency chose to rely on a push strategy that was managed by a full-time promotional person, who was originally trained as a health educator. This person developed a 15-minute video and oral presentation on the agency and its services. After getting the support of the medical director, the nursing director, the head of social services, and the in-service training director in each of the neighboring hospitals, she presented the video and oral program to medical and nursing staffs in each hospital at their regular meetings, to social service departments, and, when requested, at hospital in-service training sessions. Demand for the agency's services skyrocketed without their having spent any money on media advertising. However, significant sums were invested in paying for the promotional staff member and for related promotional expenses.

In contrast, some of the national and regional home care chains have engaged in extensive advertising, a pull strategy, both to recruit staff and to promote their services. Advertising, which requires a major investment and presumably could not be undertaken by agencies with insufficient budgets, should be viewed as a long-term effort and a long-term investment. Home care agencies that spend only enough to buy a few advertisements a year would probably be better off investing their money elsewhere.

A mixture of push and pull strategies is also used. In addition to advertising, national and regional home care chains are more likely to use personal selling to develop awareness and, subsequently, referrals. However, such a mix is costly.

One of the most common mistakes that a home care agency can make is to inadequately budget for promotion. The amount needed to effectively promote a home care agency depends in part on what the agency's competitors are doing. The amount also varies with the number of persons the home care agency is trying to reach and the frequency of exposure to the promotional messages that the agency wishes to attain. No matter how good a home care agency is, it may fail if its referral and promotional channels are inadequate.

Place

The key value of home care is its place of distribution—the home. The home is both a less costly place to the individual and group buyer and a more comfortable place for the patient. The place of distribution of home care is, by its nature, customer oriented.

However, the time availability of home care is not so customer oriented. Most home care agencies do not have even a 24-hour hotline or telephone service, let alone 24-hour delivery of service. Most home care is provided between 7 a.m. and 5 p.m. Unfortunately for the patient, not all medical and homemaking needs can be met during business hours, and so customers may be dissatisfied and possibly poorly served.

For example, terminal cancer patients may need nursing care night and day. If they choose to die in their homes, as many do, the hours during which nursing care is traditionally provided will not be sufficient. An elderly patient who lives alone and is recovering from a hip fracture may temporarily need 24-hour homemaking services. Ten hours of home care a day is not sufficient to keep such a patient out of a hospital or nursing home.

Even a hospital-based agency, which should have the edge in receiving referrals from its own hospital, will lose business if those referred patients need care during times when the hospital-sponsored agency is not operational. Alternative delivery systems prefer to work with one home care agency that can provide for all its needs, including 24-hour service, rather than having to work with two or three agencies, none of which fully meets patients' potential needs. Consequently, having home care services available 24 hours a day, 7 days a week, can be an enormous marketing edge and selling point for a home care agency.

Suggestions for Initial Marketing Efforts

The first steps in developing a marketing program are often the hardest, especially for small home care agencies in which the director assumes the role of chief marketer in addition to many other duties, including administration and even direct service. Newcomers to marketing are tempted to devote time, energy, and resources to attending seminars, reading articles, forming committees, and developing a long-range, comprehensive marketing plan.

Although these steps are essential in the marketing process, they usually involve long-range behavior. Most agencies want to begin immediately to take actions that will affect the agency's image, visibility, and reputation. Considering and implementing some of the following suggestions gives the agency the satisfaction of improving services and visibility and encouraging loyalty among consumers while a long-range marketing strategy is being developed.

Telephone Procedures

The agency should review its procedures regarding telephone referrals and calls for information on agency services. Is the first telephone contact informative and helpful? Are brochures about the organization and about general home care services mailed to all callers? Is a nurse available to answer questions and to take messages from physicians for staff members who are visiting patients? Do physicians have a hotline so that they can telephone the intake nurse directly? To check on the agency's telephone procedures, the agency director can have friends call the agency and evaluate the effectiveness of its intake procedure.

The selection of the agency receptionist or switchboard operator is extremely important. This person is often the first contact a patient or physician may have with the home care agency. The receptionist or switchboard operator should be professional, reliable, knowledgeable, and above all, friendly.

Nurse Marketers

Continuity-of-care or liaison nurses who convey a professional, organized, and helpful image can be effective marketers because of their personal credibility and access to physicians, hospital nurses, and discharge planners. To enhance their effectiveness, these nurses should identify appropriate referrals and be available for consultation when physicians are at the agency. Nurses can also provide ongoing education about the range of home care services through consultations with hospital clinicians, by passing out newsletters and handouts, and by hosting an annual "All about Home Care" program that includes refreshments.

Recognition

During National Home Care Week, Hospice Month, the agency's anniversary, or other specially designated times, the agency can recognize the efforts of discharge planners, physicians and their office staffs, head nurses, and department heads. A thank-you gesture is more effective at these times than at traditional gift-giving times.

Frequent referrers to the agency can be given such unexpected tokens as an inexpensive personalized gift, an invitation to an omelet breakfast, or a coffee mug inscribed "Top-Doc." Staff members from the home care agency can extend the gift-giving to discharge planners who have been helpful by refueling the candy jar or by giving a surprise balloon bouquet or flower arrangement. However, such promotional programs should be reviewed by legal counsel.

Organizational Identification

The agency can encourage the patient's identification of the home care agency by:

- Putting stickers with the agency's name and telephone number on the patient's telephone
- Putting the agency's name and phone number on a house-shaped magnet that can be kept on the patient's refrigerator
- Recording blood pressures on an agency card that patients can take to their physician
- Giving new patients of the home care agency a packet containing a booklet on home care services; a blood pressure card; medication schedules; brochures from voluntary health care organizations (for example, diabetes and heart associations); patient's bill of rights; names of nurses, therapists, and team leader or supervisor; instructions on how to contact the home care agency during an emergency; and other educational handouts for both patients and care givers

Categorization of Physicians

An agency staff member should categorize physicians according to referral patterns: frequent, moderate, occasional, and nonreferrer. The agency can then identify physicians who are supportive of home care but whose number of referrals do not put them in the category of "top-docs." Additional promotion directed to these physicians may help to upgrade them to "top-doc" category.

A yearly survey of physicians, especially those who are frequent and moderate referrers, can provide valuable insights. The "top-docs" can be interviewed individually. A separate survey sheet for physician's office personnel reinforces the importance of their role in the continuity of patient care.

Visits to Physicians

Home care clinicians can be especially effective in making information calls to physicians because they have the credibility of being direct-care providers. Encouraging staff members to make such visits by allowing them to factor the administrative time into their monthly productivity statistics and by providing brochures and instruction in making effective calls pays off in improved agency-physician relations and more referrals. Clinicians and other staff members involved in physician relations should be encouraged to write thank-you notes for selected referrals; send Christmas cards; and deliver "top-doc" mugs, pen lights, and other small, inexpensive gifts to physicians who consistently refer patients to the agency.

Public Announcements

The agency should send announcements of new personnel and services to the business section of the local newspaper. Feature editors and medical reporters of newspapers and television stations should be included on newsletter mailing lists. This regular reminder of the agency's presence may stimulate interest in a story. Also, developing a relationship with key media personnel who may have responsibility for health-related articles is important.

Public Presentations

The agency should offer to make presentations at clubs, senior centers, church groups, and professional associations on topics of current interest, such as the changing health care environment, high-tech home care, hospice and bereavement, and care of the care giver. This type of presentation is often more effective than direct promotional speeches about specific agency services because attendees gain information that they can use immediately. Promotional material about the agency and its services should also be made available to attendees of these presentations.

Such presentations meet the group's need for an informational program and the agency's need for increased community visibility and positioning as a referral source for services. When a need for home care services arises, attendees may remember the agency's presentations and seek out that agency for home care.

Employee Morale

Employee morale is often overlooked in marketing efforts. Employees are the agency's best asset in marketing the agency's services and so should receive the utmost support of administration. The agency can show this support by providing continuing education programs, employee newsletters, resource files for community services, and a forum for voicing their concerns.

Employees also enjoy an occasional thank-you gesture for their hard work. Administration may sponsor an ice cream social, a thank-you luncheon, and birthday cards. Complimentary letters from patients, families, and physicians should be posted, circulated, or reprinted in an employee newsletter.

Two Marketing Programs

The importance of marketing to both staff and the community cannot be overemphasized. The following sections provide information on a customer relations program for staff and a successful community education program. Employees of the home care agency need to be reminded of the importance of their role to the success of the agency. Taking advantage of every opportunity to educate the community about home care is in the best interests of the agency.

Customer Relations

One commonly held fallacy is that marketing should be done exclusively by the director, the community liaison nurse, marketing director, or the continuity-of-care nurses. Actually everyone in the agency, from the supply clerk to the clinicians and supervisors, has a role in marketing. Understanding that role can enhance each person's effectiveness in representing the home care agency.

Any activity undertaken by the home care agency that affects its customers in any way is a marketing activity. Such activities as how telephones are answered and billing procedures explained, what the nurses or therapists or aides say during the home visits or what they leave with the patients, how payments and collections are handled, how services or visits are scheduled, what atmosphere is created in the reception area, or how fast staff members respond to patients' or physicians' calls or to unusual requests all have an impact on the consumers of home care; and this list can be expanded upon by any staff member without any effort.

Focusing on these kinds of customer relations activities rather than on marketing activities per se has several advantages. Such activities help employees clarify their role in corresponding or interacting with others. The emphasis is less on selling services, which may be a difficult concept for some staff members, and more on identifying and meeting the needs of consumer groups.

One way to begin emphasizing customer relations is to schedule a workshop for staff members. Community or hospital resources who are experts in this area can be asked to serve as faculty.

At the beginning of the workshop, the agency's relationship with consumers should be graphically illustrated, as shown in figure 6-2, next page. This figure shows the variety of persons who influence referrals to the agency. Figure 6-2, or something similar, can also be used to explain the need for segmentation in marketing and to introduce the concept of needs-driven marketing.

Staff members can begin to understand needs-driven marketing by identifying agency strengths and matching agency services to appropriate target markets. The group can use figure 6-3, page 119, to discuss what resources

Figure 6-2. Persons Who Influence Referrals to a Home Care Agency

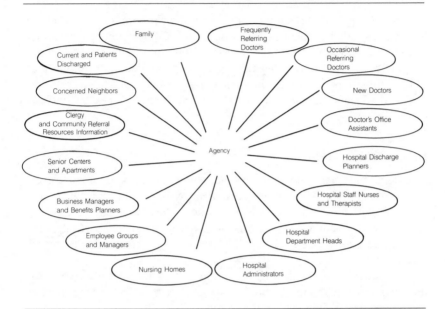

are available at the home care agency and how these resources can be used to meet the needs of various target markets. This exercise illustrates the need for flexibility in meeting the varied needs of consumers while also maintaining awareness of the agency's needs. Home care employees can share ideas on identifying and meeting needs.

This exercise also points out the need for tailoring the information about home care services to the various target groups. For example, "care in the comfort and privacy of your own home" may be a selling point to the general public, because most persons value comfort, privacy, and independence. For parents of ill children, however, the message can be altered to appeal to the mother's need for convenience and familiarity. Privacy needs may be less important for parents who have sick children; they may just want professional and good care. For parents of handicapped or medically fragile children who make daily trips to physicians and therapists, the convenience of home care may be an important selling point. The comfort and familiarity of home, which can blend life-style and motivational factors, may enhance compliance with the treatment program.

Community Education

A community education program can complement the marketing efforts directed toward physicians and professionals. Participating in health fairs, exhibiting at workshops, and speaking to clubs gives the agency representatives

Figure 6-3. Form to Use to Determine Agency Strengths and Services Appropriate to Various Markets

Target Markets	Services	Agency Resources (Our Needs)
Patient and family needs	• Care-giving skills • Information about the illness and its side effects • 24-hour availability if problems arise • Respect from staff • Visits scheduled at their convenience • Supplies delivered • Informing the doctor • Agency telephone number accessible • Knowing the primary nurse in charge of home care • Home care goals and treatment plans • Long-term community resources	
Concerned friends	• Courteous reply to calls for information • Pamphlets about home care • Suggestions for ways they can help	
Hospital administrators	• Excellent service given to patients • Discharge planners and other staff satisfied • Sound financial management • Marketing visible and consistent with hospital image	
Frequently referring physicians	• Excellent patient care • Prompt response to telephone messages • Communication that fits office practice (weekly update calls, calls to office nurse first, and so forth) • Opportunity to serve on medical advisory committee • Recognition for referrals (luncheons, mugs, thank yous, and so forth) • Input into annual evaluation survey • Opportunity to meet nurses and therapists	

the opportunity to talk with persons in the community about their concerns and needs and to gather ideas for new services and marketing strategies. Special events, such as an "All about Home Care" workshop or a fund-raising activity, can position the agency as a resource in the community.

Hospital HomeCare (HHC) in Albuquerque, New Mexico, hosts a "Coaching Care Givers" workshop three times a year. The free workshop offers family care givers, home health aides, and companions the opportunity to talk individually with nurses, therapists, counselors, and volunteers from the home care agency and from the hospital. Participants are encouraged to practice with equipment and supplies, which are set up in displays in the hospital's lobby. Selected techniques, such as transfers and body positioning, are demonstrated by nurses and therapists.

The workshop is marketed to several groups:

- Physicians receive a newsletter and flyer to post in their offices.
- Physicians' office personnel are visited personally to request that they mail flyers to patients and families who could benefit from such a program.
- An article is submitted for publication in newsletters of various businesses, churches, civic and service organizations, and social service and health care organizations.
- Flyers are posted in libraries, groceries, pharmacies, and other acceptable locations.
- Television and radio public service announcements are produced. Nurses and therapists explain home care services on radio talk shows while promoting the workshop.
- Care givers for current and past home care patients are encouraged to attend.
- Employee relations managers are asked to post the flyers in lounges and other visible areas so employees who have a need for this coaching can attend.
- Voluntary health care organizations and hospitals are invited to send information and representatives for a resources table; they then have an interest in the success of the workshop.
- Discharge planners, hospital department heads, and staff members are encouraged to post flyers around the hospital and to attend the workshop in the lobby. Their input is requested during the planning to ensure that they have an investment in the workshop's success.

Various handouts have been developed by HHC for distribution at the workshop. The handouts offer advice and suggestions for easing the stress of care giving. Some of the handouts that are available are "Taking Care of the Care Giver," "Understanding the Private Pain of Loss," "Managing Problem Behavior," and "Listening, Sharing, Helping."

At the end of the workshop, the physician's office staff and discharge planners are given packets of handouts to keep as resource materials for family members in care-giving roles. A "thanks to you, it was a success" note is sent to all parties who received the promotional information.

A community education program, such as the one developed by HHC, can heighten awareness of home care services and provide prospective patients and families who need the care but are not referred for one reason or another with the assurance that they can request services. Such programs help break through stereotypes by presenting home care in new ways. The agency can highlight high-tech care, maternal-child health care, postoperative care, and instruction in care-giving skills. These programs increase the visibility of the agency and encourage loyalty from physicians and their staff members, other health care agencies, hospital personnel, discharge planners, patients and their care givers, and agency employees.

The home care agency should be sure that all printed material prepared for distribution at such community education programs is professional and tasteful in appearance, easily read, and color coordinated. The wording should be specific to the material's purpose and directed to a particular target audience. Brochures can be developed around specific programs, such as pediatric home care and welcome home care for new mothers and infants or for specific audiences such as senior citizens and families of seniors who want information on the Medicare home care benefit. The agency's logo, name, address, and telephone number should be clearly visible on all printed material that is distributed by the agency. Name identification and promotion is extremely important in today's competitive health care environment.

Notes

1. Roberta N. Clarke and Philip Kotler, *Marketing for Health Care Organizations* (Englewood Cliffs, NJ: Prentice-Hall, Inc., 1986), chapter 1.
2. Andrew P. Tobias, *Fire and Ice: The Story of Charles Revson, the Man Who Built the Revlon Empire* (New York City: Quill, 1983).

Chapter 7

Budgeting and Financial Management

William J. Simione, Jr.

The home care market has a product component, such as durable medical equipment (DME) and pharmaceutical supplies, and a service component, such as direct patient care services provided in the home. This chapter is primarily concerned with financial considerations relative to the service component of the home care market.

The service component has two categories. The first category is called the *Medicare market,* which is composed of services that are traditionally reimbursed by the federal Medicare program. These services include skilled nursing care, physical therapy, speech therapy, occupational therapy, medical social services, and home health aides. These six services are defined in the Medicare regulations as *intermittent services.* Intermittent services can be reimbursed through the Medicaid program, commercial insurers, and private payers. Medicare currently reimburses for these services on the basis of cost or charge, whichever is lower. In some instances, these services can be reimbursed at lower than cost or charge when they exceed the cost limits established by the Medicare program.

The second category of the home care service component is the *private-duty or demand market.* Services in this category are normally reimbursed at a competitive charge that in most instances is not regulated. Some of the services included in this market are the private services of a registered nurse, licensed practical nurse, or home health aide; staffing for institutions; homemaker services; live-in helpers; companions; and chore services. Private-duty services are reimbursed through commercial insurance carriers, private

William J. Simione, Jr., C.P.A., is a partner in Simione and Simione, Hamden, Connecticut.

payers, and some Medicaid programs. Referrals for these services come mainly from physicians and institutional health care providers.

Private-duty or demand services are commonly referred to as *demand services* because, in most cases, patients dictate to the health care agency how much service they want. Medicare services are commonly called *need services* because the payer dictates the amount of services given on the basis of patient need and coverage requirements.

Financial Feasibility of Developing a Home Care Program

Before deciding whether to enter into the home care market, the hospital should research the following three areas:

- Alternative models and corporate structure (freestanding or provider based)
- Affiliations or joint ventures with another home care provider
- Reimbursement issues

Freestanding or Provider Based

In considering the home care market, either the Medicare or the private-duty or demand market, the hospital must decide whether the home care organization is to be freestanding or provider based. A freestanding agency is an entity set up outside the corporate structure of the hospital, whereas a provider-based agency is a department of the hospital.

The Health Care Financing Administration (HCFA) has specific rules concerning the freestanding or provider-based status of a home care agency. The prime element in HCFA's determination is the control factor: who in essence governs the home care agency.

Medicare Market

A hospital that wants to develop a home care agency that is certified under the Medicare program has certain reimbursement advantages if its home care agency is provider based. As previously stated, Medicare has established cost limits on the amount that it reimburses home care agencies for their services. Provider-based home care agencies have a higher limit than freestanding agencies because hospitals are granted an add-on to cover the higher administrative and general costs that are incurred. In addition, a hospital-based home care agency has portions of the hospital's costs allocated to the home care department through the hospital's cost report (see "Development of a Prospective Cost Report" later in this chapter). If the home care agency is freestanding, then some of these costs could not be allocated.

On the other hand, a provider-based agency's cost per visit may be higher in many instances than a freestanding agency's because of the methodologies used in determining costs. Price sensitivity is something that must be considered in marketing the services of this new entity.

Private-Duty Market

The private-duty or demand market is highly competitive, and therefore providing service at a low cost is desirable. Consequently, a private-duty agency should be freestanding and separate from the Medicare entity. If private-duty services are kept in the Medicare entity, Medicare costing methodology allocates an inappropriate share of general administrative costs to these private-duty services. As a result, the profit potential is reduced.

Purchase of Services

Another factor to be taken into consideration when deciding on a freestanding or provider-based structure for the private-duty or Medicare market segments is contractual agreements with the hospital for the purchase of services. Some of these purchased services include patient accounting, data processing, nursing administration, payroll and personnel, communications, administration, legal and accounting, and plant operations.

Medicare regulations state that if a Medicare-certified home care agency purchases services from a related entity, Medicare reimburses only the *cost* of those services. Prior to entering into these types of agreements, the hospital should carefully study the Medicare regulations concerning related organizations.

Affiliations or Joint Ventures

Depending on the objective and size of the hospital, the cost of starting a Medicare-certified home care agency can be a deterrent to a successful operation. To successfully operate such an agency, appropriate administrative staff have to be recruited or developed. The hospital may want to avoid these associated costs by considering an affiliation or joint venture with an existing home care agency for either the Medicare or private-duty market or for both.

Reimbursement Issues

A hospital must research all state and federal regulatory reimbursement requirements prior to establishing a Medicare-certified home care agency. Reimbursement issues differ from hospital to hospital and state to state. The following represents just a few reimbursement issues that should be explored:

- Cost limits
- Amortization of start-up costs
- Documentation requirements: statistical, financial, and clerical
- State regulatory requirements
- Requirements for home office cost reports, if needed
- Pending changing in costing methodolgy
- Related organizations

Two of the main financial areas that must be understood in operating a Medicare-certified home care agency are budgeting and cost reporting. The rest of this chapter discusses these two areas.

Revenue and Expense Budget

The following are the steps to take when developing a revenue and expense budget for a Medicare-certified home care agency. These steps must be performed in this chronological order so that a budget can be developed accurately.

1. Projection of service volume
2. Projection of full-time equivalents (FTEs)
3. Projection of expenses
4. Development of a prospective cost report
5. Development of charge structure
6. Projection of revenue

Projection of Service Volume

Whether the home care agency is a new or existing one, it still must evaluate trends and statistical data if it is to accurately project service volume. Various experts in the field of home care or direct service staff should also be consulted. Talking to persons who work directly with patients in the home is one way to find out about factors that may significantly affect volume projections.

New Home Care Agency

In the Medicare market, most referrals come from an acute care setting. Therefore, a hospital contemplating the development of a new home care agency must use statistical data from acute care institutions to project service volumes. The most useful data to use in calculating volume projections are discharges to home care by diagnosis and by payer source. If this information is not available, then certain assumptions have to be made from total discharges, and these assumptions have to take into consideration the type of services and other demographics peculiar to the agency's situation.

Figure 7-1, below, shows how service volumes can be computed. Discharges should be segregated between those over and under age 65. The utilization of services is usually higher among persons over 65 years of age.

After the total number of visits projected per year is calculated, then the type of service that will be performed should be established. Figure 7-1 shows a typical composite of the type of services offered. However, many factors, such as the changes in regulatory coverages, availability of the labor market, and the philosophy of the agency, can change this distribution.

Existing Home Care Agency

An existing home care agency can analyze historical patterns and trends and derive volume projections from data accumulated from its respective

Figure 7-1. Projection of Service Volume

	Over 65	Under 65
Total discharges per year	9,000	5,000
Percent to home care	10%	2%
Number of discharges to home care per year	900	100
Total number of patients discharged to home care	1,000	
Number of visits per patient	x 20	
Total visits per year	20,000	

	Percent*	Visits
Distribution of Services:		
Skilled nursing care	45.0	9,000
Physical therapy	10.0	2,000
Speech therapy	3.0	600
Occupational therapy	1.0	200
Medical social services	1.0	200
Home health aide	40.0	8,000
Total	100.0	20,000

* The percentages used in this example are for demonstration purposes only and should not be used unless the set of circumstances surrounding the proposed home care agency are similar.

statistical systems. Factors that could affect this analysis are changes in the regulatory climate, previous admissions to the agency, changing referral patterns, and changes in coverage criteria. These factors can dictate changes in the type and volume of service given by a particular discipline or service. For example, HCFA recently reinterpreted what Medicare will reimburse for home health aide services. Any projected volume of services provided by home health aides has to reflect this change. Similar coverage and reimbursement changes may also occur with Medicaid and commercial payers.

Figure 7-2, below, projects nursing service hours on the basis of the agency's historical data. In the example, only skilled nursing care is projected. However, this example can and should be used for every type of service.

Projection of Full-time Equivalents

Once service volume has been determined, the next step is to project how many direct-service field staff, or full-time equivalents (FTEs), are needed to deliver services. To do this, the length of time it takes to perform a visit must be determined. The hours per visit can be obtained from an ongoing accumulation of time data, or the agency can perform periodic time studies to obtain this information.

Figure 7-2. Projection of Nursing Program

	Visits		
	Actual 1985	Actual 1986	Projected 1987
Skilled nursing care:			
Medicare	10,000	12,000	14,000
Medicaid	2,000	2,000	2,000
Private insurance	1,000	2,000	2,500
Full fee	500	200	100
Part fee	500	700	500
No charge	1,000	1,100	900
	15,000	18,000	20,000
Hours per visit	1.3	1.5	1.7
Total service hours	19,500	27,000	34,000

The visit is composed of three parts:

- Preactivity and postactivity time (record keeping, office time)
- Travel time
- Activity time in the home

Visit time is determined by analyzing historical trends as well as other factors, such as the following:

- Case mix
- Duration of treatment
- Intensity of services
- Scope of services
- Service area
- Paperwork flow

Once the average visit time has been estimated, then the total number of visits for that Medicare service can be multiplied by the average visit time per service to get the number of visiting hours required for that program. To arrive at the total number of FTEs needed to perform that service volume, the number of visiting hours should then be divided by the number of available service hours per staff member. This formula is shown in figure 7-3, next page.

Projection of Expenses

After the number of FTEs required has been computed, then consideration needs to be given to building the support services required to administer the programs. The following are some of the expenses that must be anticipated:

- Salary and related expenses
  - FTEs: supervisors, administrative personnel, director of finance, business staff
  - Employee benefits: payroll taxes, health, retirement
- Contracted services: volume projections, price increases, limits on physical therapy
- Transportation cost: fluctuations with volume, last year's cost per trip, anticipated increases, projected cost per trip, administrative expenses
- Space occupancy: adequacy of space, computer room, increase in staff
- Other line items: office supplies, postage, insurance, dues and subscriptions, legal and accounting fees

Development of a Prospective Cost Report

Once the service volume and the number of FTEs and supportive expenses have been calculated, then a prospective cost report can be prepared. The

Figure 7-3. Projection of Full-Time Equivalents

Working Days:

Days in year		365
Less: Weekends	104	
Holidays	12	
Vacations	20	
Sick days (average)	6	142
Working days		223
Less: In service education	12	
Community activity	11	23
Number of days for service		200
Number of hours per day		7.5
Hours per staff		1,500

Full-time equivalents:

Projected Service Hours	÷	Hours Per Staff	=	Full-Time Equivalents
34,000	÷	1,500	=	22.7

reason for this step is that Medicare and some of the other payer sources reimburse on a cost basis. Without the information contained in this report, revenue from these payer sources cannot be projected.

The prospective cost report should be developed using the Medicare methodology that is outlined later in this chapter (see the section "Cost Reporting"). One outcome of this prospective cost report is the calculation of the anticipated cost per unit of service.

Development of a Charge Structure

From the projected cost per unit of service that was developed from the prospective cost report, an appropriate charge per unit of service can be formulated. Many commercial insurance companies pay for intermittent services based on the home care agency's charge per visit.

Some factors that should be taken into consideration when developing the charge per visit are:

- Competition in the marketplace
- Provision of third-party payer to pay the lower of cost or charge
- Cash flow
- Working capital
- State regulations

Projection of Revenue

The gross revenue needed to support the expenditure budget can be determined by payer source. Projected revenue is calculated by multiplying the anticipated amount that each payer will pay by the estimated visits projected for each Medicare service. When projecting revenue, the hospital must remember that Medicare reimbursement is calculated by multiplying the cost per visit developed in the prospective cost report by the number of anticipated Medicare visits as long as these costs do not exceed the Medicare cost limit.

Cost Reporting

Understanding the Medicare cost report from an administrative viewpoint is critical because the costs per unit can fluctuate depending on internal management decisions as well as external forces. For example, if new programs are added or deleted, the basis for determining costs varies and is reflected in the cost per unit. Also, increases and decreases in volume within a particular service affect the cost per visit or hour.

Medicare-certified home care agencies are required by regulation to file a Medicare cost report for their cost reporting year. This cost report determines the cost of services rendered to the Medicare program and is used for final settlement.

Three basic procedures have to be followed in preparing the home care agency's cost report. These procedures are:

- Allocation process
- Step-down process
- Cost-settlement process

Allocation Process

During the allocation process, an agency allocates the expenses on its trial balance sheet to three major categories of cost centers:

- *General service cost centers.* The general service cost centers consist of items that cannot be readily identified as part of a particular patient service or program. The cost centers included under this category are depreciation for building and fixed and movable equipment, plant operation and maintenance, transportation, and general administrative functions.

- *Reimbursable cost centers.* The cost centers included under this category consist of all services covered under the Medicare home care benefit. These services are skilled nursing care, physical therapy, speech pathology, occupational therapy, medical social services, home health aide, medical appliances, DME, and medical supplies.

- Nonreimbursable cost centers. This category includes all services and programs rendered by the home care agency that do not fit into the previous two cost centers. Although the following is not a complete list, it is a representative example of services that fit into this nonreimbursable cost center: homemaker service, respiratory therapy, private-duty nursing, clinic services, health promotion activities, day care program, home-delivered meals program, school nursing program, mental health program, and counseling service.

A home care agency must allocate all its expenses on the trial balance to these three categories of cost centers. Certain expenses can be completely allocated directly to a cost center. An example of this is a physical therapist's salary for a therapist who only works with patients needing skilled care. In this case, the salary cost is allocated directly to the physical therapy cost center.

In many instances, however, an expense has to be allocated to more than one cost center. An example is the salary of a physical therapist who performs not only skilled care services but also is responsible for supervising the agency's other therapies, such as speech and occupational therapy. A portion of this physical therapist's salary that is designated for supervision must be allocated to all three cost centers (physical therapy, speech therapy, and occupational therapy). This split is accomplished by using the physical therapist's time as a basis for allocating salary to the cost centers that this position benefits. For example, if a study of the physical therapist's time shows that he or she spends 50 percent of his or her time doing direct service in the physical therapy program, 30 percent supervising other patients, 10 percent in the speech therapy program, and 10 percent in the occupational therapy program, then the salary can be allocated accordingly.

When a certain expense or items of expense require distribution to more than one cost center, the only recommended statistical base that can be used is time study data. This situation has created many problems within the home care agency cost report because the allocation of many items requires the use of different statistical bases. An example of this situation is an intake, or admissions, position. At the time that the intake person is taking information on a referral over the phone, he or she does not know what services are going to be rendered to that patient, and therefore a proper distribution of the intake person's salary cannot be made to the appropriate cost centers on the basis of the time the intake person spends on a patient. Perhaps a more appropriate statistic to use in this case is the number of patients by service. However, any attempt to allocate salaried costs by the use of another statistic other than time requires prior approval from the home care agency's fiscal intermediary before the start of the cost-reporting year.

Step-Down Process

Somewhat different from the allocation process, the step-down method of cost finding involves allocating the costs of the general service cost center by sequence to the remaining general service cost centers and then to the reimbursable and nonreimbursable cost centers, using the HCFA-recommended statistical basis. Figure 7-4, below, shows the HCFA-recommended statistical bases for allocating general service costs.

Cost finding in a home care agency is not as complicated as is cost finding for the hospital, because home care agencies are limited to only the five general service cost centers. The five general service cost centers and their respective statistical base are listed in figure 7-4. If an agency wishes to change the recommended statistical basis during the cost-finding process, it must seek prior approval from its fiscal intermediary prior to the start of its cost-reporting year.

However, because home care agencies are limited to only these five general service cost centers, costs are sometimes inequitably allocated to cost centers that they do not benefit. An example of this situation is the use of net cost as an allocation base for administrative and general costs. Certain items within the administrative and general cost centers, such as the patient accounting function, will be allocated to cost centers that they do not benefit. Patient accounting should be allocated only to those services that require patient billing and collections and that have accounts receivable. Under this system, a cost center, such as health promotion, that does not require billing to individual patients absorbs part of the cost for patient accounting. Presently, HCFA is in the process of preparing a revision to the instructions associated with the cost report. This revision allows an agency to use discrete costing, if approved by its fiscal intermediary, and to develop unique

Figure 7-4. Statistical Basis for Allocations

General Service Cost Center	Statistical Base
Depreciation of building and fixed equipment	Square feet
Depreciation of movable equipment	Value or square feet
Plant operation and maintenance	Square feet
Transportation	Mileage
Administrative and general	Net cost

cost centers applicable to their agency. Such a revision gives some relief to the many inequitable allocations presently occurring in the home care agency cost report.

Cost-Settlement Process

After all of the costs are allocated to the appropriate reimbursable and non-reimbursable cost centers, a cost per visit of service is determined by dividing the number of visits rendered within that cost center into the total cost for that cost center. During the cost-settlement process, the total number of visits rendered to Medicare beneficiaries is then multiplied by the appropriate cost per visit to determine the actual cost of rendering services under the Medicare program. An example of this process is shown in figure 7-5, below.

Figure 7-5.   Example of Cost-Settlement Process for Skilled Nursing Care

Total Cost	÷	Total Visits	=	Cost Per Medicare Visit	×	No. of Visits	=	Medicare Reimbursement
$500,000	÷	10,000	=	$50	×	8,000	=	$400,000

Chapter 8

Legal Issues

Eileen A. O'Neil

Introduction

Because of the increased use of home care services and the sophistication of treatment currently provided in the home, the issues of consent to treatment and negligence take on special importance. With this broadened exposure to liability, patient care records play a crucial role in protecting the home care program if suit is filed for improper or inadequate care.

In addition, novel organizational arrangements for the delivery of services have raised other legal concerns. Home care providers must consider the impact of antitrust law as a result, in part, of the gradual erosion of protection previously given health care providers and to increased competition in the home care field. Contractual agreements between providers have become widely used for a variety of purposes, and these relationships in turn raise questions related to the Medicare-Medicaid Antifraud and Abuse Amendments of the Social Security Act.

This chapter summarizes the legal issues frequently encountered in hospital-based home care situations. However, the information provided in this chapter is merely a brief introduction to the law relevant to home care. For maximum legal protection, home care program personnel must also seek sound legal advice that is tailored to the relevant state law, current developments, and the agency's particular objectives.

Eileen A. O'Neil, J.D., is an attorney in Boston, Massachusetts, and holds a faculty appointment in health administration at the University of New Hampshire.

Consent to Treatment in the Home

The patient's right to determine the substance and direction of care is a critical legal topic in home care. The principles of the law of consent are essentially the same for all providers; however, the method by which hospitals, physicians, and home care agencies obtain consent from patients may vary. This section summarizes the legal tenets involved and then discusses several options that home care programs can use to fulfill their duty to ascertain whether the patient has been informed about treatment.

The patient's right to decide what to do with his or her body has a long-standing tradition in this country, although a substantial part of the litigation in this area has taken place in the past two decades. In 1914, Justice Cardozo succinctly summarized the patient's prerogative in the celebrated case of *Schloendorff v. Society of New York Hospital:* "Every human being of adult years and sound mind has a right to determine what shall be done with his own body; and a surgeon who performs an operation without his patient's consent commits an assault for which he is liable in damages."[1]

Over the years, the state courts and legislatures have fine-tuned this basic principle, and the result is a body of law that points out three elements of valid consent:[2]

- *Consent must be voluntary.* The patient must willfully and without coercion agree to undergo a certain procedure or treatment.
- *Consent must be competent.* The patient must be capable of giving consent. Each state differs on the issue of competency, and so the home care agency should obtain copies of relevant statutes. Generally, however, persons over the age of 18 have the right to give consent to treatment, but parental consent is required for the treatment of minors. Certain exemptions with regard to minors exist by specific state law. In most states, minors may consent to drug or alcohol treatment, and minors who are married or who have children are emancipated, that is, they are able to make their own decisions without parental involvement. Minors also have a constitutionally protected right to privacy, which enables them to consent to care for sexually related matters. On the other end of the scale, adults who have been adjudicated incompetent or incapacitated by a court no longer have the right to make their own health care decisions. This ability is vested in a guardian of that person by a court order. The laws relating to incompetency are also a matter of state determination, and so the home care agency should become familiar with applicable laws.
- *Consent must be informed.* Courts and legislatures have created this doctrine to ensure that, prior to giving consent, the patient has sufficient information to make an intelligent, or *informed,* decision. As with competence, the specifics of informed consent are a matter of individual state law. Generally, though, effective informed consent

requires that information on the following points be given to the patient:

- An explanation of the treatment or procedure must be given to the patient in lay person's language.
- The risks must be disclosed. If, for example, the patient is to receive chemotherapy in the home, the patient must receive information on the dangers of that treatment. Certain states require the provider to reveal all the risks that the reasonable patient would want to know (that is, the *material risk approach*[3]) in contrast with the risks that a reasonable provider would disclose (that is, the *professional standards approach*).[4] The significant difference between these two state standards is that, under the professional standards approach, the plaintiff would be required to use an expert witness to establish in court what the provider should have told the patient about a particular treatment.
- The patient has a right to know the medical alternatives to the suggested treatment. The risks and prognosis of each possible alternative should be discussed with the patient.
- The provider should discuss the option of foregoing all treatment and its consequences for the patient.

Although the right to determine the course of treatment generally belongs to the patient, whether or not the provider thinks the decision is wise, an emergency creates an exception to the provider's duty to obtain consent prior to treatment. *Emergency* is an objective term: the provider must make a *reasonable* determination that the patient's life or limb is in imminent danger and the patient is incapable at that time of giving competent consent. This *implied consent principle* is used daily in emergency departments when a patient arrives in need of care but is incapable of expressing a decision on treatment. Indeed, failure to render care in those circumstances would subject the emergency department staff to liability for negligence.[5] When the patient's life or limb is in immediate danger in a home care situation, the patient should receive care without regard to consent. However, the particular facts surrounding the incident must be carefully documented. When the patient's condition is not jeopardized by a delay in care, the patient or family member should be involved in any treatment decisions.

The possibility of lawsuits based on lack of consent arise when procedures that carry greater risks (that is, paralysis, loss of organ function, or death) are more prevalently used and when various reasonable alternatives exist. Many high-tech therapies fall into this category, as does the use of medications that may cause complications.

With increased exposure to liability comes the greater need for legal protection. Several risk management approaches are available to home care programs. The selection of the specific alternative to be used by the home care program should be based on administrative and medical staff perspectives.

The general rule to keep in mind is that in most states, the physician who prescribes the treatment has the primary responsibility in the area of consent. However, the home care program also has a role because, if the patient alleges lack of consent, both parties will be named as defendants in the suit. Thus, the agency's approach should be coordinated with physicians to be certain that the policy for securing consent prior to treatment is workable.

The agency may supply the physician with a blank consent form, just as hospitals do for surgical procedures. The physician then fills in the pertinent information, for example, an explanation of the treatment, risks, and alternatives. The advantage of using such a form is that the disclosed information is spelled out in writing. The disadvantage is that the agency is responsible for getting the form completed by the attending physician prior to presenting it to the patient for signature.

A way to get around this problem is for the agency to use a shorter form, in which the patient acknowledges by signature that he or she has been informed by the physician about the nature of the procedures and the risks and alternatives. The details of what was discussed by the physician are not included in this short form. If the patient has not been given the relevant facts, he or she would most probably tell the representative of the agency prior to signing the form. The physician could then be notified by the agency that the patient does not seem to understand the nature and effects of the treatment. The patient's record should indicate that the physician was notified.

Home care program staff can also ask the patient whether the physician has discussed the treatment and its risks and alternatives with the patient and dispense with the use of a form. The same benefits result from this policy because the uninformed patient would most probably respond that he or she was not informed. Documentation of this verbal exchange should be placed in the patient's health record. Also, the physician should be notified that the discussion with the patient occurred, and the fact that the physician was notified should appear in the patient's record.

The method used by the home care agency to ensure that the patient has given an informed consent to treatment should be acceptable to both medical staff members and home care staff. The basic idea is to protect both parties in their individual duties to the patients.

Closely connected with the patient's right to determine his or her own treatment are *living wills,* which are documents expressing the patient's wishes about whether extraordinary treatment is to be provided if the patient is unable to articulate at some future date. Some states have enacted statutes that define the requirements for a valid directive of this nature. Other states have allowed the state courts to determine who shall be entitled to make treatment decisions for the incompetent or unconscious patient. Because this area of law is rapidly evolving and because each state has quite different laws on the subject, the home care program should obtain a legal opinion on how to proceed when the terminally ill patient is being treated.

Negligence Issues in Home Care

Because liability for patient injuries applies to all types of health care settings, the home care program should be aware of situations that may result in negligence and of methods for reducing such exposure. This section provides an overview of negligence law, which includes malpractice (the negligence of a professional), and specifically focuses on acts or omissions in home care.

Standard of Care

Principles of *negligence,* which is the failure to prevent a foreseeable injury to a patient, have evolved through court decisions over centuries.[6] As the level of health care becomes more sophisticated, the duties of providers (professionals, paraprofessionals, and corporate entities) increases because the *standard of care,* a key component in proving negligence, increases to reflect the state of the art of practice.

In addition to proof of the existence of a standard of care, the plaintiff must prove the existence of two other elements prior to a finding of negligence by the court against the defendant. The injured patient must show that the defendant home care program, or its agents, failed to act reasonably (breach of the standard of care) and that this failure actually caused the patient's physical injury. With regard to this last requirement, the courts in most states will not impose negligence liability if the patient is not actually physically injured.[7]

Because negligence hinges on the standard of care owed to patients, a greater familiarity with this legal proof is an excellent step toward understanding liability and minimizing exposure to this area of law. Judges and juries typically lack the expertise to assess the obligations of health care providers, and therefore the standard of care of the *reasonable* provider is established in court through one or more of the following sources of evidence:

- Expert witnesses with the same or similar educational and occupational background of the defendant. Expert witnesses are called by any party to the lawsuit to testify about the provider's duty to the patient under the same or similar circumstances.
- State and federal government regulations, such as licensure and Medicare certification standards.
- National and state voluntary standards, for example, those of the Joint Commission on Accreditation of Hospitals.
- Internal policies and procedures adopted by the home care program regarding screening of staff and patient care policies, among other things.
- Direct promises made to patients by staff members of the hospital or home care agency.

The following examples show how each of these sources of evidence can be used to establish liability against home care providers:

- *Expert witnesses.* A nurse from a home care agency is providing care to a patient discharged from a hospital. The nurse fails to heed signs and symptoms of hemorrhaging. Later the patient is readmitted to the hospital with complications. The patient brings an action against the hospital and attending physician for early discharge following surgery and against the home care program and staff members involved. To support allegations that the injury was in whole or in part caused by the nurse, the plaintiff presents testimony from registered nurses who have home care background and experience but who are employed by other programs. These expert witnesses testify as to what a *reasonable* nurse would have done given the patient's symptoms. This testimony can help define for the judge and jury the defendant nurse's duty to the patient under the particular circumstances being adjudicated. Furthermore, other expert witnesses can be introduced to testify on the policies and procedures that the agency should have adopted to prevent injuries of the type at issue. The most logical expert for this type of testimony is a director of another home care program.
- *Government regulations.* Licensure standards in a particular state may require home care agencies to fully review a patient's plan of treatment with the attending physician every 60 days. An agency in that state fails to contact the physician for a 60-day review because the agency finds that the patient's progress under the care plan is excellent. Two weeks later, the patient is readmitted to the hospital with complications resulting from medications. The plaintiff in the case could argue that if the agency had complied with licensure laws, the adverse reaction could have been prevented. The injured patient would also have to show that the failure to review the plan of treatment caused the particular injury.
- *Voluntary standards.* Standard II for Home Care Services of the Joint Commission on Accreditation of Hospitals states that hospital-based programs must have a sufficient number of qualified personnel to deliver patient care services and to meet program objectives.[8] The plaintiff could argue that the defendant failed to meet this duty and that this lack of sufficient qualified staff caused the patient's injuries.
- *Internal policies and procedures.* In *Darling v. Charleston Community Memorial Hospital,* the hospital's failure to adhere to its own voluntarily adopted policy, which required consultation with specialists in certain circumstances, was also crucial in the plaintiff's successful suit for negligence.[9] This ruling could also apply in the home care setting. For instance, if an agency adopts a procedure that the physician should be contacted by the nursing staff in specific situations, liability can be imposed for deviation from the policy even when the

omission resulted from oversight. Again, the plaintiff must establish that the breach of agency duty caused the injury.
- *Promises made to patients.* One of the more vulnerable areas in hospital-based home care is the transition from the inpatient setting to the home. For example, discharge planners may, with the best of intentions, promise the patient that a home health nurse will visit the patient's residence on the day after discharge. However, because of a lack of communication, the home care program does not learn of the discharge for two days. Assuming that the patient suffers an injury as a result of lack of nursing care, the argument could be made that the hospital had a duty to follow through with the promise and that better communication is needed between discharge planning and the home care department to provide continuity of care. The more precise type of negligence in this situation is hospital abandonment of the patient.[10]

Two areas of particular concern for home care should be mentioned. First, with the increased use of high-tech therapies in the home, the skill and ability of the staff become more important as does in-service training to provide advanced nursing knowledge. Second, unlike a patient in the hospital who has consistent nursing attention, the home care patient and family must participate closely in monitoring the patient's condition. Patient education in this area may prevent problems that could ultimately result in a claim of negligence that resulted from lack of careful instruction of the patient.

Corporate Liability and Ostensible Agency

In addition to being liable for the actions of any employee or volunteer who causes an injury through breach of duty, the home care program may also be liable under the doctrine of *corporate liability.* Corporate liability arises when a corporate provider fails to have reasonable policies and procedures to protect patients or when the provider breaches its own adopted standard.

Another theory of liability for negligence is *ostensible agency.* In *Mduba v. Benedictine Hospital,* the hospital had contracted with a group of physicians to manage and staff the emergency department without hospital involvement.[11] When a patient was injured in the on-campus emergency area, the hospital was named as defendant by the plaintiff. In holding the facility liable for the negligent acts of the subcontractor physicians, the court reasoned that when the hospital holds itself out to the public as a full-service institution and provider of services, it is liable for the wrongful actions of its subcontractors.

Similarly, if the home care program holds itself out as a provider of durable medical equipment (DME) and sales and services are actually provided by another company, the home care program could be held liable if it appears to the public that services are under the aegis of the home care program. The careful selection of subcontractors and the use of a protective contract, which is discussed later in this chapter, is wise from a risk management perspective.

Patient Care Records

Patients' health records play a vital part in any discussion of legal aspects relating to home care. As with the patient's health records in the hospital, the health records of the home care agency include the patient's medical and health history and the dates and types of care provided in the home. These records are required for licensure and reimbursement purposes, and they are also an important protective tool for an agency faced with a lawsuit. This section discusses the principles of law governing access to health records and information by patients and third parties and the pretrial and in-court use of documentation.[12]

Multiple Providers and Patient Information

In home care, unlike most other segments of the health care system, several providers may participate in one patient's care. If that patient is injured, the not-unlikely result will be a suit naming all parties as defendants. Consequently, the exchange of pertinent information among the providers to maximize the quality of care when necessary and to promote continuity is recommended from a legal perspective. If, for example, a respiratory therapist from a DME supplier notes a change in the patient's condition, he or she should convey this information to the home care agency providing nursing care and to the attending physician.

The wisest policy is to have the patient authorize the release of information to other providers. However, even in the absence of a release, the facts should be disclosed, particularly if such disclosure prevents an injury to the patient.

One of the most critical aspects of hospital-based home care is the continuity between discharge of the patient by the hospital and the intake of the patient by the home care agency. The discharging hospital should provide any relevant information on the patient to the home care program to close potential gaps in care. Likewise, when a patient is readmitted to the hospital, the hospital should receive all pertinent facts. Under the JCAH standards, for example, the completed home care health records are to be made part of the patient's hospital health records.[13] If a home care program fails to do this, as a matter of routine or in occasional instances, the injured patient could argue that better continuity in providing medical information on the patient's health may have prevented the injury that resulted.

Because of the importance of current medical information on patients, case law has consistently favored disclosure to persons with an *interest*. In

Simonsen v. Swenson, a physician informed the manager of a hotel in which the patient lived that he may have a sexually transmitted disease.[14] The case may seem humorous because the ruling was made 66 years ago; however, the court's finding still has relevance: If the party to whom disclosure is made has a legal interest in the matter, then the disclosing party is not liable for libel or slander.

A more recent case, *Tarasoff vs. Regents of University of California,* held that, under certain circumstances, the provider has a duty to *not* withhold information.[15] In this case, a man being seen by a psychologist at the University of California hospital indicated that he was planning to murder a young woman, Tatiana Tarasoff. The man was later discharged. When he murdered the girl, the family filed suit against the facility for failure to warn the Tarasoff family of the impending danger. The court agreed with the plaintiff and held the defendant liable for its failure to inform the family.

Information Requested by the Patient

In home care, as in other areas of health care, the patient is legally the owner of the information in the health record, and the provider owns the actual documents. Many states have established, either by case law or statute, the method by which the patient may obtain his or her health records. In most such jurisdictions, the laws typically balance the patient's right of access and the provider's right to have adequate time to respond to the request by the patient or an authorized representative (for example, an attorney or family member to whom the patient gives this authority in writing). For example, Virginia law allows the hospital and physician 15 days to respond to a written request for records by the patient and in addition allows the hospital to charge the patient a reasonable amount for the work and duplication costs.[16]

Most states do not require patients to tell the provider the reason for wanting their health records. Sometimes patients are uncertain or dissatisfied about some aspect of treatment and so request their health record. The agency may find it in its best interests to tactfully inquire about the purpose of the request because rapport with the dissatisfied patient may clear the air. However, in most states the provider may not withhold information if the patient does not disclose the reason for the request.

Persons other than the patient or authorized agent do not have an independent right to obtain information. For example, insurance companies and attorneys do not have automatic access privileges. For this reason, and particularly when third-party payers are involved, the patient is asked to authorize the disclosure at the beginning of treatment. If a person identifying himself or herself as the patient's attorney requests any information, the agency should refuse to comply until permission to release the records is obtained from the patient. The exception to this general rule is a court order to produce the records (subpoena duces tecum). Failure to comply with a court order can result in a citation for contempt of court. Although the patient's authorization is not necessary in this instance, the home care agency should notify the patient when records have been subpoenaed.

A corollary question is often raised with regard to family members who want to know about the patient's diagnosis, treatment, or prognosis. The principal rule to keep in mind on this subject is that the information technically belongs to the patient, unless by law a relative or guardian has the right to know (for example, a parent with regard to a minor child). Several policy approaches are acceptable from the legal point of view. One approach is to discuss the patient with family members as a matter of course. Although this position is legally correct, it may unnecessarily strain the relationship with the family and patient. A second approach is to suggest to the inquiring family member that the physician be contacted for information. This position may simply be unrealistic, because the home care provider is most visibly involved in caring for the patient. A third approach may be the most expeditious and legally appropriate: at the beginning of the relationship, the home care agency should ask the patient whether health care matters should be revealed and discussed with family members. Thus, the decision on disclosure of information rests with the *owner* of the information, and the provider does not have to try to guess whether disclosure should be made. Not only is this position correct legally, it is an excellent way to promote good patient relations.

Use of Records in Discovery and at Trial

Because legal action can be filed several years after the date of injury or the discovery of that injury, the documentation in the health record speaks on behalf of providers who may not recall the precise details of the patient's care or who are unavailable to testify on behalf of the agency at the trial. Each hospital-based program director should be knowledgeable about the state's statute of limitations, which may differ from the record retention time under licensure laws. Thus, a licensure regulation may direct agencies to keep records for five years, but the statute of limitations allows a patient six years after discovering the injury to file suit. If an agency followed the licensure law as a guidepost, the records to establish that the patient consented to treatment or that reasonable care was given may not be available when a suit is filed. Records of minors should be kept until the minors reach the age of majority plus the number of years required under the statute of limitations.

A poorly documented record is almost as bad as having no record at all. Content of the records should conform with licensure laws, certification standards, and preferably, JCAH standards.[17]

A patient's attorney may obtain the patient's health records by a court subpoena for use in pretrial discovery and at the trial. A related issue is whether a patient's attorney may also have access to other provider records.

The general rule in virtually all states is that business records relevant to the issues in the case are accessible to litigating parties and may be introduced as evidence in the trial. However, in many states an exception has been made in favor of health care providers to encourage discussion of and remedial action on the overall quality of care without fear that the information will later be used against them in a court of law. This special privilege typically protects quality assurance discussions, documents, and minutes from meetings. This issue raises two separate questions:

- Whether the state allows the plaintiff to obtain during discovery quality assurance information by court order for purposes of preparing for trial.
- Whether the state permits the use of such records in the trial itself. Some states allow discovery but bar the use of these records in the trial.[18] Other states prevent access and use for both purposes.[19]

This issue of special privilege, like the statute of limitations, is a matter of state determination, and the agency should be familiar with the appropriate rule by statute or case law. Also relevant to this topic is whether the privilege, if it exists, extends to home care. Most laws grant the privilege to hospitals. This issue is particularly important for agencies that are based in a corporation other than the hospital entity.

Contracts in Home Care

The typical hospital-based home care agency enters into a variety of contractual relationships in the course of doing business. Agreements with patients, other providers (for example, physical therapists), and inpatient facilities are common. This section discusses basic contract principles and then looks at the various kinds of agreements.

Basics of Contract Law

At the basis of all contracts are certain principles that govern the formation of the relationship and the interpretation of the parties' terms. Overall, the nature of the relationship and the individual provisions are a matter of the intent of the parties. The broad exception to this rule is that a contract with an illegal purpose is not enforceable by a court of law. Similarly, when a contract in part violates public policy, that provision is void under law. In one case, a patient signed an agreement before she received dental care to refrain from filing a negligence action against Emory University.[20] She was injured during dental work and sued the university. The court in Georgia allowed the suit to continue, because the waiver-of-liability provision violated public policy in that state.

Contracts may be either written or implied, with some reservations, by the actions of the parties. To be enforceable, a written instrument is required for:

- Purchase of real estate.
- Purchase of goods over $500 in most states.
- Promise to assume the indebtedness of another, unless a duty to make payment exists by law. For example, parents are responsible for children's necessities.
- Agreement for a specific period beyond one year. Although these agreements must be in writing to be enforceable in most states, oral and implied contracts are equally binding for other arrangements. However, the overriding disadvantage of an oral agreement or implied contract is that the parties' promises and intent may be disputed.

The following provisions are frequently used in written contracts:

- *Preamble.* The preamble states the reason for entering into the agreement. Because this section does not necessarily reflect the duties of the contracting parties, any terms that the agency deems material should be contained in the body of the contract rather than in this section.
- *Specification of standards that the parties will honor.* For example, a contract with a physical therapist may refer to the ethical standards of that profession.
- *Substitution under the agreement.* Another way of phrasing this subject is whether the contract is assignable by one or more of the parties.
- *Duration of the agreement.* If the contact is to continue indefinitely, that fact should be stated in the contract.
- *Compensation for services or goods.* This provision should be specific and detailed, as many disagreements arise on this subject. Benefits, expenses, and so forth should be stipulated.
- *Purchases or actions on behalf of the other party.* This clause states whether either party to the agreement has the right to make purchases or act in any other way on behalf of the other party to the agreement.
- *Materiality-of-terms clause.* The parties should determine prior to executing the agreement which terms are important enough to justify termination of the agreement.
- *Nonwaiver clause.* This clause typically states that a party does not waive his or her right to enforce a provision of an agreement simply because he or she has allowed variances before. For example, if the contract requires monthly payment on a specific date and the recipient of payment allowed the bound party to make a late payment, the recipient does not lose the right to force compliance with the date specified in the contract.

- *State law.* The parties should select the state law that will govern the contract if the parties reside or work in different jurisdictions.
- *Modification-in-writing clause.* This clause usually states that any revisions, amendments, or additions to the content of the contract must be in writing to be enforceable.

Contracts with Patients

The most prevalent type of contract in home care is that governing the relationship with patients. The fundamental nature of the agreement is a promise by the agency to provide services for an indefinite period on the basis of patient need in exchange for the patient's promise to pay for the services either directly or through a third-party payer. Although the terms of this agreement need not be in writing to be enforceable, the home care agency should give a patient a written summary of scheduled times of service and types of services, applicable costs and charges, and any pertinent duties of the patient.

Generally, the provider is the party vested with the right to determine whether to accept a patient for services. However, once the relationship is formed, the provider has a duty to act reasonably, that is, in accordance with principles of negligence laws. In a hospital situation, discerning when the relationship between a hospital and an admitted patient begins is relatively easy. However, the situation is cloudier with regard to home care. Although the question has not been decided in court, a home care agency can assume that if the patient is told at discharge that home care will be provided and that promise is not carried out, then the court will find that the relationship was formed by the promises made and the patient's reliance on that promise, particularly if the patient sustains an injury from such reliance.

The contractual arrangement with the patient is usually terminated when the patient no longer requires service. In some circumstances, the provider may want to stop services when the patient still requires care. This action should be taken only with legal advice on the applicable state law, particularly with respect to the amount of notice of termination that must be given to the patient.

Contracts with Other Providers

In some situations, the home care agency may need to subcontract for services to patients. If the agency contracts with an individual therapist or a community-based agency, for example, the agreement should contain several important provisions, particularly in light of the possibility of agency liability for the actions of the subcontractor under the doctrine of ostensible agency as mentioned in the section on negligence issues. The following list of recommended provisions is by no means exhaustive of those included in well-drafted documents, and legal advice is suggested to ensure that the contract is complete and in compliance with any relevant state law:

- Contractor's duty to comply with all agency policies and procedures, state and federal laws and regulations, and general ethical standards pertaining to patient care.
- Contractor's submission of proof of liability insurance. The limits and coverage of this insurance must be acceptable to the home care program.
- Contractor's maintenance of records and documentation in accordance with agency standards and the delivery of such documentation to the home care program within a specific time after the provision of services.
- Duty of contractor to be available for services at certain times and on certain days.
- Method of compensation, including a provision on whether expenses for travel and meals are or are not to be paid by the home care agency.
- Right of agency to terminate the agreement on breach of specified contract provisions and an indication of whether termination occurs immediately or with notice of a specific period.
- A hold-harmless clause in favor of the hospital-sponsored home care program.

The agency may also want to refer to required contract terms for agreements with other providers as outlined in Standard I by the JCAH.[21] Also, because the Social Security Act allows percentage contracts for compensation only under rather strict circumstances, agencies should avoid such methods of compensation or obtain a legal opinion on whether the arrangement falls into one of the narrow exceptions to the ban.[22]

Contracts between the Hospital and Home Care Agency

Although no laws mandate the use of formal contracts between the hospital and home care program, a written document may be advisable in two situations:

- When home care personnel are used by the hospital to carry out hospital, and thus nonreimbursable functions
- When patients are referred by a hospital to its home care program

Home care personnel are being used to carry out hospital functions when the home care staff performs discharge planning functions for the hospital. Such activities are separate and apart from the intake-coordination activities required by the home care agency. In this instance, a contract between the hospital and the home care agency should delineate details of the discharge planning duties and the time required to perform such duties. Such a contract may avert adverse reimbursement challenges for the home care program if the Medicare fiscal intermediary argues that the time spent on intake activities was actually a discharge planning function of the hospital.

A contract between a hospital and its home care agency for referring patients to the home care agency can achieve two goals:

- The method of sending and receiving referrals can be delineated, thus reducing the potential gap between inpatient care and home care.
- The intent of the parties in establishing the referral pattern can be stated in the preamble.

Assuming that no anticompetitive purpose is mentioned, the contract may be helpful in explaining why patients were referred to the hospital's home care program if an antitrust challenge is made (see the discussion of antitrust in the next section of this chapter). Technically, however, if the home care program is part of the same corporation as the referring hospital, the document cannot be a contract in a legal sense. In this case, a written instrument is used not to bind parties together as much as to reflect the actions of the providers in sharing staff or making referrals.

A related question is whether Medicare law prevents a hospital or other provider from making referrals to a home care program. Part of the Medicare law provides that "any individual entitled to insurance benefits under this subchapter may obtain health services from any institution, agency, or person qualified to participate under this subchapter if such institution, agency, or person undertakes to provide him such services."[23] This section of the law has been frequently used to support the opinion that a hospital must notify patients of the existence in the area of providers other than its own home care agency. In at least one case, this issue has been litigated and the federal Court of Appeals, Fourth Circuit, denied the plaintiff, Home Health Services, Inc., any remedy against the University of South Carolina and a physician, who were allegedly steering patients away from the plaintiff.[24] In a brief opinion, the court stated that this particular section of the Medicare laws does not give a certified agency a substantive right of action against providers who do not send referrals. Again, this issue is quite distinct from antitrust scrutiny, which is discussed in the next section.

Provider Conduct and Antitrust Laws

A flurry of antitrust litigation in the health care field over the past decade has caused justifiable interest in avoiding difficulties in this area of law.[25] Providers have traditionally enjoyed a degree of protection from liability under antitrust legislation for several reasons. First, the learned professions, including medicine, were exempted historically.[26] Second, the health care market was presumed to function independently of the cardinal rule that competition is the key to a healthy business environment. Furthermore, the considerable presence of government regulation, at least since the 1960s, removed health care from the realm of normal market conditions.

More recently, however, legal decisions, increased competition, and a rethinking of the economic basis of the health care system have sent a clear message to health care providers that certain types of conduct may result in criminal prosecution or civil damage suits. For this reason, providers must exercise caution in their individual actions and in the relationships they form with other providers. Prudent hospital administrators must be familiar with the substance of the antitrust laws as well as with the mechanics of applying their provisions. Because of the degree of uncertainty in the area of antitrust and home care, hospital-based programs are advised to seek good legal advice prior to the formation of relationships or the development of a policy that may reduce competition in the field.

Restraint of Trade

In the health care sector, the most frequently litigated section of the antitrust laws is Section 1 of the Sherman Act, restraint of trade. This federal statute, enacted in 1890, makes illegal "every contract, combination . . . or conspiracy in restraint of trade."[27] Although the language of the law is broad, Congress did not intend to prohibit all business activities that may restrain trade. Rather, according to principles developed through court decisions, contracts, combinations, or conspiracies between two or more parties violate the provision when the relationship *unreasonably* restrains competitive conditions. This unreasonableness standard is also rather vague, and so to refine the scope of illegal conduct, the courts have taken two approaches in determining if an arrangement falls within the ambit of prohibited action: the *rule-of-reason test* and the *per se rules*. A major issue in health care during the past decade has been whether courts hearing an antitrust challenge will apply the broader rule of reason or, conversely, invoke the per se rules. The defendant provider stands a much better chance if the rule of reason is used by the court.

Under the more common rule-of-reason analysis in a restraint-of-trade case, the courts assess the facts and the actual effect on competition. Also relevant under this standard are the motives of the parties in formulating the agreement. The courts assess answers to the following questions:

- What are the circumstances of competition surrounding the arrangement, for example, the relevant business market?
- Who are the disadvantaged parties, for example, consumers, competitors, and so forth?
- What is the functional purpose of the arrangement, and what are the motives of the parties to the contract or agreement?

Under this type of analysis, the plaintiff filing the suit must prove that the conduct is anticompetitive in intent and effect.

In the per se test, the only relevant question for the court is whether the parties did engage in the behavior. In other words, if the arrangement falls into one or more specific categories, it is deemed to be automatically illegal even when the ultimate effect is beneficial to the competitive market and when the intent of the parties is in some fashion procompetitive. The violations under the per se rules are price fixing, division of markets, tying arrangements, and concerted refusals to deal and group boycotts.

Price Fixing

In typical business markets, courts have traditionally found a violation when competitors conspire to set the prices of goods or services either high or low, even where the impact on the field in question would be beneficial to consumers. Because the per se rules were generally not applied to health care, the Supreme Court decision in the case of *State of Arizona v. Maricopa County Medical Society* was a surprise.[28] In this case a group of practicing physicians, acting under the umbrella of a county medical society, were found liable for agreeing to a ceiling on medical service charges to patients. Rejecting the defendants' position that the arrangement ultimately served to foster competition in the medical world and to reduce costs to the public, the court found that the per se rule against price fixing between competitors had been violated. In the home care field, any direct or indirect setting of prices between agencies constitutes a parallel illegal act.

Division of Markets

A decision by competitors, or those who may become competitors, to divide markets is the second type of per se wrongful activity because the assumption is that competition is reduced as a result.[29] Thus, a hospital-based agency and a freestanding home care provider may be guilty of restraint of trade if they agree to minimize the competition between them by dividing the market according to types of patients or geographical boundaries.

A home care program may define its services area to exclude patients or markets: what it cannot do, according to the per se rule, is to agree with a competitor to do so. However, if providers are acting pursuant to a state or federal regulatory scheme, for example, a state planning body, the actions do not constitute a violation because protection against all potential restraint of trade violations arises through the state action defense.[30]

Tying Arrangements

Tying arrangements are a third type of per se illegal activity. Under this situation, a seller, through its market power, forces a buyer to purchase a less desirable product or service (the *tied* product or service) along with the desired product or service (the *tying* product or service). This action by itself is prohibited conduct.

In 1984, the U.S. Supreme Court handed down an opinion on an alleged tying arrangement between East Jefferson Hospital and a group of anesthesiologists.[31] The plaintiff in that case, Dr. Hyde, was not part of the exclusive agreement and was thus prevented from practicing as an anesthesiologist in the hospital. The Court of Appeals for the Fifth Circuit found that the contract was a per se illegal tying arrangement because the hospital forced patients to accept anesthesiology services along with hospital care. At the Supreme Court level, that decision was overturned on the basis that the conduct did not constitute a per se violation and that Dr. Hyde had not established the anticompetitive effect and motive of the defendants under a rule-of-reason analysis. Because the opinion has relevance in home care, with regard to increased use of exclusive referral agreements and agency selection of subcontractors, a closer look at the court's reasoning is warranted.

The court first viewed the arrangement from a per se perspective. The initial issue was whether anesthesia services and hospital care were two separate services that could be tied together in a sale. The court found that the two were indeed separate and that the hospital did not have sufficient market power (30 percent of the beds in the market area) to force patients to take both services. Because patients could elect to go to other area hospitals or could conceivably forego anesthesia once in the hospital for surgery, no per se violation was found.

The court then scrutinized the case under the rule-of-reason test. The court analyzed the actual effect on Dr. Hyde as an excluded party to the agreement and the intent of the hospital and anesthesiology group in forming the relationship. Finding that Dr. Hyde had other options in practicing his specialty in the area and that the hospital had a legitimate business motive in contracting with the anesthesiology group, the court entered a judgment for the defendant hospital. A segment from the court's opinion is instructive in explaining the court's finding: "There is no evidence that the price, the quality, or the supply and demand for either the 'tying product' or the 'tied product' involved in this case has been adversely affected by the exclusive contract between [the anesthesiology group] and the hospital. It may well be true that the contract made it necessary for Dr. Hyde and others to practice elsewhere, rather than at East Jefferson. But there has been no showing that the market as a whole has been affected at all by the contract."[32]

This case points to several practices for hospitals and home care agencies to pursue:

- Any exclusionary arrangement should be carefully scrutinized by an attorney with antitrust knowledge.
- The hospital and home care agency should document, either in the contract itself or in governing board meetings, the reasons for the action.

- When an exclusive referral pattern is present, a conservative approach is to inform the patients being referred that other options exist, if that is the case. The hospital is then free to discuss the advantages — high quality and continuity of care — of selecting the hospital-based program.

Concerted Refusals to Deal and Group Boycotts

Another type of per se violation under the restraint-of-trade section of the Sherman Act is concerted refusal to deal or group boycott. Although a strictly unilateral refusal to deal with a competitor or other party is not encompassed by this rule, a collective or group decision to exclude a party is illegal. Most of the litigation in this area involves physicians who are excluded from medical staff privileges at a hospital. The courts will not find per se illegality unless the plaintiff is able to establish that a collective decision to exclude was made, for example, when medical staff members and physicians on the board collude to refuse privileges.[33]

In the home care field, a possible violation can occur if a hospital-based agency and the hospital together agreed to not work with another agency. To prevent any per se violations, the home care agency should be passive and uninvolved in the decision regarding referrals.

Monopolization

Under Section 2 of the Sherman Act, Congress prohibited another type of conduct: the monopolization of a market or the attempt or conspiracy to monopolize.[34] Increased legal activity in the antitrust area with regard to health care has raised challenges based on monopoly. The question in these cases is whether the merger or acquisition vests too much market power in one provider.[35]

Section 2 of the Sherman Act does not prevent a hospital from starting a home care program even when other providers have already established themselves in the market. Indeed, the presence of more home care providers is favorable to procompetitive market conditions because patients then have a greater array of choices. The monopolization prohibition becomes relevant, however, in a merger between two home care agencies or between a hospital with a home care program and a competitor. A thorough legal analysis should determine if the corporate arrangement is monopolistic.

Price Discrimination

Under the Robinson-Patman Act, seller and buyers are prevented from engaging in discriminatory practices for the sale of commodities, but not services.[36] Because home care agencies purchase many commodities and increasingly engage in the sale of medical products, they should have at least some familiarity with the issues under this law.

The essence of the Robinson-Patman Act, passed by Congress in 1936, is that a seller may not discriminate in the price of goods sold to two buyers when the products sold are of similar quality and the sales take place in the same time frame and when the price differences may cause an anticompetitive effect. An exemption to this law is when the discrimination is cost justified[37] or is designed to meet a competitor's sale price.[38] Not only is the seller subject to challenge on this basis, but a buyer also violates the law if he or she tries to get a discriminatory price or knowingly receives a seller's discriminatory price.[39]

Another exemption is contained in the Nonprofit Institutions Act, which was enacted in 1938.[40] This act states that the price discrimination sanctions do not apply when not-for-profit charitable organizations purchase or sell goods for their own use. The ambit of this provision is revealed by a U.S. Supreme Court decision involving a challenge by a group of retail druggists against pharmaceutical manufacturers who allegedly engaged in price discrimination by selling drugs to a not-for-profit hospital in the Portland, Oregon, area.[41] The precise question in that case was whether the drugs bought at a reduced rate were actually for the hospital's own use. In its ruling, the court found that some resale of the drugs by the hospital was within the exemption, but other resales fell outside the scope of protection. Sales to inpatients, ambulatory care patients, hospital employees, and medical staff members for personal use were deemed hospital use, but sales to persons who were no longer patients of the facility or to physicians for use in their outside practices were not exempt.

When the home care agency sells products, legal advice should be obtained prior to offering different prices to different buyers, particularly when the sale is through a for-profit entity or when purchases are made by persons who are not patients of the corporation making the sale. Likewise, home care agencies that are purchasing goods for other than their own use should exercise caution when the seller offers a volume discount or any form of rebate.

Antifraud and Abuse under Medicare and Medicaid

Proximity in relationships between providers, coupled with heightened competition in the health care field, has resulted in increased concern about criminal sanctions under the Social Security Act. This section gives an overview of the federal statutes on fraud and abuse and provides examples relevant to home care. Two types of offense are the objects of the Medicare-Medicaid Antifraud and Abuse Amendments:

- Fraud or misrepresentation of a material fact designed to gain payment when services have not been rendered

- Remuneration, including kickbacks, to induce the referral of patients

Fraud or Misrepresentation

Making false statements or representation to obtain payment under Medicare or Medicaid is a criminal act. Conviction results in a felony punishable by a fine of no more than $25,000 or five years imprisonment or both.[42] The statute speaks to whoever "knowingly and willfully makes or causes to be made any false statement or representation of a material fact in any application for any benefit or payment."[43]

The elements of the crime are a misrepresentation of a material matter (that is, a fact that has the capacity to deceive) and the knowledge by the wrongdoer that the stated fact does not warrant reimbursement, as opposed to a legitimate mistake about whether a service is covered under Medicare or Medicaid.

The following cases illustrate two types of violations under the law. In *United States v. Cacioppo,* an osteopathic physician submitted claims to Medicare that contained statements he knew were false.[44] Evidence presented by the prosecution established that Cacioppo billed for patient visits that never took place and for treatments that were never given as stated. He was convicted of Medicare fraud in 1975.

In *United States v. Oakley G. Smith,* the president of a hospital included in the hospital's Medicare cost reports personal expenses for remodeling his home and personal supplies unrelated to hospital administration.[45] He was found guilty of making false statements of material fact to obtain payment under the federal program. Making the false statement, rather than receiving the reimbursement, is the subject of the federal proscription.

In addition to criminal prosecution, violators are subject to civil penalties. Under a separate section of the Social Security Act, the Secretary of Health and Human Services is empowered to assess the convicted provider a penalty of up to twice the amount of the wrongful claim but not to exceed $2,000 for each violation.[46] The act also authorizes suspension from participation in Medicare and Medicaid programs.

Remuneration

The second part of the law prohibits remuneration (including kickbacks, bribes, or rebates) by one provider to another for the purpose of inducing that person to purchase or lease any service or product.[47] Parties on both the offering and receiving end of the deal are subject to prosecution, and conviction results in a felony punishable by a fine of no more than $25,000 or five years' imprisonment or both.

Previously, the law only prohibited kickbacks (for example, cash, long-term credit arrangements, or gifts and supplies) given in return for referrals or purchases. In 1977 the language of the law was amended to broaden the scope of offenses. A new term, *remuneration,* was included, in addition to the terms *kickbacks, bribe,* and *rebate,* thereby increasing the types of conduct that are illegal.

The impact of this revision appears in a Third Circuit decision, handed down in April 1985.[48] In that case, A. Alvin Greber, M.D., was convicted of a felony for violating the Medicare-Medicaid Antifraud and Abuse Amendments. Greber, a practicing osteopathic physician, was also president of Cardio-Med, Inc., a corporation that he formed to perform diagnostic tests for physicians. Cardio-Med billed Medicare for these services and, on reimbursement, gave the referral physician "interpretation fees" for initial consultation services and explanation of test results to the physician's patient. At the trial, the prosecution presented evidence that physicians received these fees even though the Cardio-Med staff actually evaluated the data.

Under the old and narrower statutory language, the fact that a physician actually performed some service would have negated a finding of criminal conduct under the amendments, because the payment was not technically a kickback. However, Greber's conviction under the new provision makes it clear that a violation exists if the purpose of the monetary or in-kind remuneration is an enticement to induce referrals. In addressing the effect of the revised law, the court stated: "The text refers to 'any remuneration.' That includes not only sums for which no actual service was performed but also those amounts for which some professional time was expended. . . . That a particular payment was a remuneration (which implies that a service was rendered) rather than a kickback, does not foreclose the possibility that a violation nevertheless could exist."[49]

Two exemptions appear in the statute:[50]

- When a buyer is given a legitimate discount for services or products if the arrangement is disclosed and the result is cost-effective for the federal program.
- When the arrangement exists between an employer and its bona fide employee.

A similar example of possible illegal conduct is the subject of an Intermediary Letter from the Health Care Financing Administration.[51] Although the interpretation in the letter does not have the full force and effect of law, the relationship involves home care and is worthy of note on that ground. A respiratory therapist employed by a hospital was offered an arrangement with a DME company. When the therapist referred a hospital patient to the DME supplier for home care equipment, the therapist would have the opportunity to provide certain services for the patient in the home. The fees for those services would be paid by the supplier. The Intermediary Letter directs carriers to report all such relationships to the regional Office of Investigation so that the office can review the facts of these cases. The Intermediary Letter delineates the factors that may lead to the conclusion that this type of arrangement entails remuneration for referrals:

- Whether the therapist provides services for only those patients referred by him
- Whether the supplier typically uses therapists to perform similar functions for patients not referred by a therapist
- Whether unusual circumstances require the use of therapists in some cases
- Whether the practices of other DME suppliers in the area are similar

The position in the Intermediary Letter is that an "opportunity to generate a fee" in return for the referral of patients is a violation of the Antifraud and Abuse Amendments to the Social Security Act.

Because of restrictions under Medicare law, a home care agency should exercise extreme caution in entering relationships based on the use of percentage contracts to compensate a provider for services.[52] In a percentage agreement in which no services are performed, the illegal kickback is clear. In *United States v. Duz-More Diagnostic Laboratory, Inc.,* the government successfully prosecuted the corporate laboratory for offering the referring provider a kickback of 15 percent of the reimbursable amounts under Medicare and Medi-Cal.[53] The Federal Bureau of Investigation, posing as the owner of a nursing home chain, approached the laboratory and received an offer for a fee cut in return for patient referrals. The case makes the point that in this situation, the offer of a kickback, rather than an actual receipt of money, constitutes a violation.

As a general rule, agreements that entail an exchange of money with a possible referral source should provide only for reasonable compensation for services provided. Also, legal advice from an attorney familiar with the Antifraud and Abuse Amendments and any relevant state law should be obtained prior to forming any agreement.

Contesting a Decision by a Fiscal Intermediary

Because many home care services are provided to Medicare beneficiaries, hospital-based agencies should be familiar with routes of appeal of intermediary decisions. Two categories of appeal exist under Medicare law:

- Appeal based on the amount of reimbursement for covered services under the program
- Dispute of the intermediary's decision regarding beneficiary entitlement under Medicare

Amount of Provider Cost Reimbursement

To obtain cost reimbursement for services provided to Medicare-eligible beneficiaries, providers must file cost reports with the designated fiscal intermediary on a timely basis.[54] Within 12 months of the receipt of the provider's final cost report, the intermediary is required to send the provider a written *notice of determination* on the amount to be reimbursed under the Medicare program. When a discrepancy appears in the provider's cost report, an explanation must accompany the determination notice. This explanation gives the fiscal intermediary's basis for the difference (for example, applicable Medicare law, regulation, or policy and procedure).[55]

This notice of determination must also alert the provider of its right to appeal, either at the intermediary level or to the Provider Reimbursement Review Board.[56] If the provider decides not to appeal, the fiscal intermediary's determination of the amount of reimbursable costs is final and binding.[57]

If an appeal is desired, the provider must file a written request for a hearing within 180 days from the date of the notice of determination. This written request for a hearing must include the following elements:[58]

- Precise identification of the parts of the cost determination that the provider is contesting
- Explanation of the grounds on which the contest is based (for example, Medicare law, regulation, or policy and procedure)
- Documentation to support the provider's position on the matter

When the amount in controversy is greater than $1,000 but less than $10,000, the hearing is held by the intermediary, and the request for the appeal is filed at that office.[59] If the amount in dispute is $10,000 or more, the provider files an appeal with the Provider Reimbursement Review Board.[60] At this level, the provider has a right to be represented by counsel, introduce evidence, and examine and cross-examine witnesses.[61] Evidence is admissible even though it would not be admissible in a court of law.[62] The board determination on the issue is final and binding unless modified by the Secretary of Health and Human Services. If the provider is dissatisfied by the ruling, it may obtain a judicial review. This review action must be filed in U.S. District Court within 60 days from the final determination by the board or Secretary.[63]

Beneficiary Eligibility

Another type of appeal is based on beneficiary eligibility. This appeal may be available for the provider when the fiscal intermediary deems that Medicare does not cover the services provided. The procedure for appeal depends on whether the disputed coverage falls under Part A or Part B Medicare services.

When the eligibility issue revolves around Part A claims, the appeal right is essentially shared with the beneficiary patient. If the beneficiary exercises his or her right to a hearing, the provider is made a party to the proceedings.[64]

The provider's right to initiate the appeal requires the presence of two factors:

- The beneficiary must decide to forego an appeal.
- The ultimate liability for the denied services must rest with the provider.

If the services are covered under the Medicare waiver of liability provisions, the provider is barred from appeal because Medicare payment is made under these circumstances.

If the provider has the right to appeal, the provider must file a request for reconsideration within six months of the fiscal intermediary's initial determination.[65] This request must delineate the areas of disagreement and pertinent law, regulation, or policy supporting the provider's stand. Documentation must also be provided, including, for example, a written record of services rendered, statements of relevant parties, and medical opinion.

After reviewing of the record, the intermediary issues a *reconsideration determination.* If the provider believes this ruling to be incorrect, the provider may request a hearing to be held before an administrative law judge in the Bureau of Hearings and Appeals of the Social Security Administration if the amount in contest is $100 or more. The written request for a hearing must be filed within 60 days from the date of receipt of the reconsideration notice from the intermediary.[66] Court review of a contested issue under Part A is available to parties after an appeals council has made its decision and if the amount of controversy is $1,000 or more.[67]

For claims under Part B, either the beneficiary or the assignee, for example, the home care agency, physician, or other provider, is entitled to a fair hearing by the intermediary if the amount in contest is $100 or more.[68] Under this part of Medicare law, the beneficiary may also challenge the reasonableness of the charges because this amount affects the amount of coinsurance to be paid by the beneficiary.[69] A corresponding appeal under Part A is termed a reconsideration determination, but the process under Part B is called a *review.*

Although the filing date may be extended for good cause, the beneficiary or provider must request a review within six months from the date of the initial notice of determination.[70] As with other appeal rights under Medicare, the beneficiary or assignee has the right to produce evidence to support the claim and to present witnesses.[71]

If the conflict is still not resolved after a review, the matter may be appealed within six months to an impartial hearing officer provided by the fiscal intermediary, as long as the amount involved is $100 or more.[72] The decision at this level is final and binding unless the matter is reopened by the hearing officer.[73]

General Recommendations on Appeals

Although the place, conditions, and process of appeals vary, certain measures should be followed for any appeal of a fiscal intermediary decision:

- The provider should carefully review the intermediary's determinations soon after receiving a notice of determination to ferret out all potential controversy.
- The request for an appeal should be specific in setting forth each area of dispute, and supporting documentation should accompany the written request.
- All relevant and supporting evidence should be produced on appeal, including any witnesses who can provide relevant information on the issues.
- Because time is vital, the provider should either send the request for appeal by certified mail, with return receipt requested, or obtain a written verification of the delivery date of the request if it is hand delivered.

Notes

1. 211 N.Y. 125 at 129, 105 N.E. 92 at 93.

2. For an in-depth analysis of consent laws in effect at the time of its publication, see Arnold J. Rosoff, *Informed Consent: A Guide for Health Care Providers* (Rockville, MD: Aspen Systems, 1981).

3. Canterbury v. Spence, 464 F.2d 772 (D.C. Cir. 1972).

4. Bly v. Rhoads, 22 S.E.2d 783 (Va. 1976).

5. O'Neil v. Montefiore Hospital, 11 App. Div.2d 132, 202 N.Y.S.2d 436 (1960).

6. For a lengthier discussion of negligence liability, see Arthur Southwick, *The Law of Hospital and Health Care Administration* (Ann Arbor, MI: Health Administration Press, 1978).

7. See, for example, DiGiovanni v. Latimer, 454 N.E.2d 483, (Mass. Sup. Jud. Ct., 1983). However, exceptions to this rule exist, particularly when the conduct results in emotional distress. See Taylor v. Baptist Medical Center, 400 So.2d 369 (1983).

8. Joint Commission on Accreditation of Hospitals (JCAH). *Accreditation Manual for Hospitals* (Chicago: JCAH, 1985).

9. 33 Ill. 2d 326, 211 N.E.2d 253 (1965).

10. See Meiselman v. Crown Heights Hosp., 285 N.Y. 389, 34 N.E.2d 367 (1941), which involves a patient's discharge from the facility for financial reasons and an unfulfilled promise that home care would be provided.

11. 384 N.Y.S.2d 527, 52 A.D.2d 450 (1976).

12. For greater elaboration on these medical health topics, see note 6.

13. Joint Commission on Accreditation of Hospitals, p. 40.

14. Simonsen v. Swenson, 104 Neb. 224, 177 N.W. 831 (1920).

15. 118 Cal. Rptr. 129, 529 P.2d 553 (1974).

16. Va Code § 8.01-413 (1979).

17. JCAH, pp. 38, 63.

18. For example, Or. Rev. Stat. § 41.675(2) (1981).

19. See Tex. Stat. Ann. art. 4447d, § 3 (1976).

20. Porubiansky v. Emory Univ., 275 S.E.2d 163 (Ga. App. 1980).

21. JCAH, p. 39.

22. U.S.C. § 1395xx.

23. 42 U.S.C § 1395a.

24. Home Health Services, Inc. v. Currie, et al., 706 F.2d 497 (1983).

25. For an atlas of the development of antitrust liability, see Martin J. Thompson, *Antitrust and the Health Care Provider* (Germantown, MD: Aspen Systems Press, 1979).

26. Erosion of this defense began with Goldfarb v. Virginia State Bar, 421 U.S. 773 (1975).

27. 15 U.S.C. § 1.

28. 102 S. Ct. 2466 (1982).

29. United States v. Topco Assoc., Inc., 405 U.S. 596 (1972).

30. Park v. Brown, 317 U.S. 341 (1943).

31. Jefferson Parish Dist. No. 2 v. Hyde, 104 S. Ct. 1551 (1984).

32. Jefferson Parish Dist. No. 2 v. Hyde.

33. Rovinson v. Magovern, 456 F.Supp.1000 (W.D. Pa, 1978).

34. 15 U.S.C. § 2

35. American Medicorp, Inc. v. Humana, Inc., 445 F.Supp 589 (1977).

36. 15 U.S.C. § 13

37. 15 U.S.C. § 13(a).

38. 15 U.S.C. § 13(b).

39. 15 U.S.C. § 13(f).

40. 15 U.S.C. § 13(c).

41. Abbott Laboratories v. Portland Retail Druggists Assn, Inc., 425 U.S. 1 (1976).

42. 42 U.S.C. § 1395nn(a). Parallel Medicaid provisions appear at 42 U.S.C. § 1396(h).

43. 42. U.S.C § 1395nn(b).

44. United States v. Cacioppo, 517 F.2d 22 (1975).

45. United States v. Oakley G. Smith, 523 F.2d 771 (1975).

46. 42 U.S.C. § 1320a.

47. 42 U.S.C. § 1395nn(b).

48. United States v. A. Alvin Greber, 760 F.2d 68 (1985).

49. United States v. A. Alvin Greber.

50. 42 U.S.C. § 1395nn(b)(3).

51. Part B. I.L., 84-9, Sept. 1984, in Commerce Clearing House, Medicare and Medicaid Guide, ¶34,127.

52. 42 U.S.C. § 1395xx.

53. 650 F.2d 223 (C.A. Cal. 1981).

54. 42 C.F.R. § 405.453(f)

55. 42 C.F.R. § 405.1803(b)

56. 42 C.F.R. § 405.1803

57. 42 C.F.R. § 405.1807

58. 42 C.F.R. § 405.1811

59. 42 C.F.R. § 405.1809

60. 42 U.S.C. § 1395oo and 42 C.F.R. § 405.1835

61. 42 C.F.R. § 405.1851

62. 42 U.S.C. § 1395oo(c)

63. 42 U.S.C. § 1395f(1)

64. 42 C.F.R. § 405.710

65. 42 C.F.R. § 405.711

66. 42 C.F.R. § 405.717

67. 42 C.F.R. § 405.730

68. 42 C.F.R. § 405.801

69. 42 C.F.R. § 405.807

70. 42 C.F.R. § 405.807

71. 42 C.F.R. § 405.809

72. 42 C.F.R. § 405.8

73. 42 C.F.R. § 405.841

Chapter 9

Quality Assurance: A Management Tool

Barbara A. McCann
Anne L. Rooney

One of the greatest challenges home care providers face is to survive as a viable organization and provide high-quality patient care. This challenge involves monitoring internal practices and results of provided care and facing the particular demands of the local community.

In a market with many providers, the choice made by physicians, employers, insurers, and other purchasers may often be made on the basis of price rather than quality. Although this action disturbs many home care providers, purchasers often have no choice in the absence of a demonstrated means to assess the quality and the efficiency of home care services.

An effective quality assurance (QA) system in a home care program can meet both internal program demands and external market demands. Internally, the QA activities can provide crucial information related to allocation of resources, conformance with federal and state regulations, risk management, and most important, the effectiveness of the care provided and the competence of the home care staff. Externally, the outcome information from QA studies can be used as an effective marketing tool because it can provide demonstrated evidence of the results of care delivered for a particular price.

Many home care professionals have experienced difficulty in creating a QA system that is an effective management tool and not just another worthless paper exercise. Most often, problems are associated with developing

Barbara A. McCann is director, Accreditation Program for Hospice Care and Home Care Development, Joint Commission on Accreditation of Hospitals, Chicago, Illinois. Anne L. Rooney, R.N., M.S., is associate director, Accreditation Program for Hospice Care, Joint Commission on Accreditation of Hospitals.

and implementing a monitoring and evaluation system as opposed to a system that only reacts to identified problems. This chapter discusses monitoring and evaluation activities and their implementation in a home care program. An explanation of the steps in the monitoring and evaluation process is included as well as an example of a QA study in a home care program.

Monitoring and Evaluation

An effective QA program encompasses all services provided by a home care program. For example, the program should cover the effectiveness of nursing services and home health aide care as well as durable medical equipment (DME), which may be provided directly or through a contract. The activities are designed to objectively monitor and evaluate patient care on a regular basis. Through the monitoring activities, the home care staff can resolve identified problems in care and staff performance before they become serious and can also identify opportunities to improve patient care.

Before continuing, two words that are associated with QA activities need to be defined. *Quality* is defined by the Joint Commission on Accreditation of Hospitals as the degree of adherence to generally recognized standards of good practice for home care and the achievement of anticipated outcomes for a particular service or procedure. *Appropriateness* is the extent to which a particular procedure, treatment, test, or service is effective, is clearly indicated, is not excessive, is adequate in quantity, and is provided in the setting best suited to the patient's needs.

Characteristics of Monitoring and Evaluation

The quality and appropriateness of care is ensured through a planned and systematic monitoring and evaluation process. However, the interpretation of these descriptors when they are applied to a working QA system is often troublesome.

Essentially, QA is viewed as a monitoring process. This monitoring process has three purposes:

- It provides for routine collection of information important to the program.
- It describes the effectiveness of what is being done.
- It provides a structured way of identifying problems.

This monitoring process is combined with an evaluation of the care and services provided. The evaluation component of the QA activities provides:

- A forum for judgments about the data collected

- Patterns and trends in care and utilization
- A basis for taking action
- A means for evaluating the effectiveness of actions taken

The planned part of the monitoring and evaluation process simply identifies what kind of information is collected and how frequently it is collected.

Monitoring and Evaluation Process

The final component of QA activity is a systematic process. The process for QA is systematic when:

- The indicators of quality or appropriate care reflect all the services provided by the program.
- Information is collected and reviewed at regular, designated intervals.
- Information is reviewed using criteria that reflect current knowledge of clinical experience in home care.

The key factors in all of these descriptors is to ensure that the QA activities that are implemented are continuous so that improvements in care and performance of the home care staff can be sustained. Also, the results of these activities must be integrated, that is, the information is shared with home care staff and is coordinated, to the degree possible, with other institutions or agencies providing care to patients in the home care program. Clearly a process that demonstrates all of these characteristics will provide valuable information internally to management and the governing body and externally to purchasers of care.

Such a monitoring and evaluation process has nine steps.

Step 1. Assignment of Responsibility

The governing body is responsible for requiring and supporting a QA program. The management staff is responsible for ensuring the implementation and maintenance of a QA program for services provided either directly or under contract. A written plan is recommended to delineate:

- How the authority is delegated from the governing body and to whom
- Who is responsible for the implementing of the activities
- How the activities are to be carried out
- What the activities encompass
- How information from the results of the activities is provided to appropriate management staff and the governing body

When the home care program is a service of another organization, the organization's overall QA program should include provisions for the monitoring and evaluation of services provided by the home care program. However, the actual implementation of the activities can be conducted either by the individual home care program or by the organization's overall QA program. Typically, the home care service program is delegated responsibility for monitoring and implementing its own QA activities and reporting the results on a regular basis to the overall QA department of the organization. This method ensures that the indicators of quality care and the criteria used in the evaluation are specific to home care.

Step 2. Delineation of the Scope of Care or Service

Home care staff should identify:

- Services to be provided, for example, nursing and speech therapy
- Primary clinical activities to be performed, for example, intravenous (IV) antibiotic therapy and hyperalimentation
- Types of patients or families to be served, for example, major age groups or diagnoses such as AIDS, breast cancer, and chronic obstructive pulmonary disease.

Step 3. Identification of Important Aspects of Care or Service

The next task is to identify the clinical services considered most important in providing patient care. Those services or clinical activities that involve a high volume of patients, that entail a high degree of risk for patients, or that tend to produce problems for staff or patients and families should be deemed most important for purposes of monitoring and evaluation.

Step 4. Identification of Indicators

An *indicator* is a defined, measurable dimension of the quality or appropriateness of care or service. Indicators specify the patient care activities, events, occurrences, or outcomes that are to be monitored and evaluated to determine whether those aspects of patient care conform to current standards of quality and appropriateness. In the absence of current industrywide standards of practice, the home care program may set its own standards of acceptable practice.

Step 5. Establishment of Criteria

Criteria are used to evaluate the indicators and may be thought of as gauges against which the quality or appropriateness of an aspect of care, as defined by an indicator, can be measured. For a given indicator, criteria define what the home care agency considers to be acceptable practice.

Criteria should be objective and predetermined and should reflect current knowledge and clinical experience. However, they are not absolute standards of care. Rather they are tools for identifying practices that should be subjected to closer scrutiny by supervisory and other home care staff.

Criteria for each indicator can be identified or developed through a review of the literature or an examination of standards of care of professional practice, for example, community health nursing standards. No specific number of criteria need be selected for monitoring an indicator. However, the selected criteria should relate specifically to the indicator and should distinguish between acceptable and unacceptable care. In addition, criteria can include aspects of care that ensure compliance with federal regulations, such as patient or family teaching. Involving home care staff in the monitoring and evaluation process, particularly in the selection and approval of criteria, is part of a successful approach to monitoring and evaluation activities.

Step 6. Collection and Analysis of Data

To collect and analyze data, the individual or group responsible for monitoring and evaluation activities must:

- Determine data-collection methods
- Identify appropriate data sources
- Decide who will collect data, for example, an individual or group within the home care program or an outside agency or institution involved in the provision of home care services
- Determine sample size
- Set a time frame
- Determine who will analyze the data

Data to be collected should reflect all services actually provided by the home care staff.

Rather than create all new data sources and data-collection methods for purposes of monitoring and evaluation, the individual or group should attempt to use existing sources and methods when appropriate. Potential existing sources of useful data include:

- Patient records
- Medication sheets
- Incident reports
- 24-hour logbooks
- Team conference records
- Direct observation of staff or patients
- Utilization review findings
- Contractual arrangements when services are provided by an outside source

Ideally, data collection involves as little staff as possible. Many home care programs have found volunteers with a background in medical record review or a particular ability in the review of home care records to take over this function. These volunteers are trained in the use of the criteria and agree to support the confidentiality policy of the organization. The resultant reviews are objective and complete, and valuable staff time is spent in responding to the results of the review and planning courses of action.

Data collection can also be used to assist in the supervision of home care staff members and the evaluation of their competence on an ongoing basis. Figure 9-1, below, shows that the agency used three criteria to review a total of 35 records of four nurses. The results were tabulated by nurse and by criteria. Management staff looking at the information in figure 9-1 can clearly see that problems are present with regard to criteria 1 and 3. These criteria may need to be reexamined or forms changed. However, the management can also note that registered nurse no. 3 is consistently having problems. This information can be the basis for follow-up to determine if the results reflect problems in nursing care or in nursing documentation.

Step 7. Actions to Resolve Problems

After collecting and analyzing data, home care staff sometimes find that the care provided meets criteria and thus is acceptable. In those cases, the only action required is documentation of the provision of quality care. If a sufficient time elapses and no opportunities for improvement have been found, the indicators and criteria used should be reevaluated to determine their validity in measuring the quality and appropriateness of patient care.

Sometimes the results of data analysis point to an area of concern, a specific problem, or an opportunity to improve care or performance. When this occurs, a plan is formulated to resolve or reduce the identified problem

Figure 9-1. Example of a Tabulation of Criteria and Nurses Being Evaluated

Quality Assurance Study			Fourth Quarter 1986	
Criteria	**#1**	**#2**	**#3**	**Total**
RN				
#1	2/10	0/5	6/11	8/26
#2	1/5	0/10	2/10	3/25
#3	5/9	3/10	3/9	11/28
#4	2/11	1/10	0/5	3/26
	10/35	4/35	11/35	

or to take the opportunity to improve care. Then corrective action is initiated.

To be effective, corrective action must be appropriate to the cause of the identified problem. Further investigation may be required to determine the exact cause of the problem. A plan of corrective action should identify:

- Who or what is expected to change
- Who is responsible for implementing action
- What action is appropriate in view of the cause, scope, and severity of the problem
- When change is expected to occur

Step 8. Assessment of Actions and Documentation

A follow-up assessment, usually the same monitoring and evaluation activity that identified the problem, is conducted to determine whether the corrective action plan has resulted in resolution or improvement of the problem. Monitoring and evaluation activities are also continued to ensure that problem resolution or improvement is sustained, although the time frame of data collection or evaluation may change.

The results of continued monitoring and evaluation activities are documented to provide a record of the efficacy of the monitoring and evaluation process. Improvement, or resolution of the identified problem, does not necessarily result in the elimination of that particular monitoring and evaluation activity. The purpose of the QA programs and the monitoring and evaluation process is not just to resolve identified problems but also to maintain or improve the quality and appropriateness of care or services.

Step 9. Information Sharing

Information from monitoring and evaluation activities should be shared with home care team members. The integration of information can be accomplished by:

- Appropriately routing reports of monitoring and evaluation activities
- Routing minutes of meetings that address QA activities, including recommendations, actions, and conclusions
- Sharing information with other agencies or institutions providing services to home care patients

The type and frequency of reports depend on the organizational structure of the home care program and the home care program's policy.

Example of Monitoring and Evaluation

The seven characteristics of monitoring and evaluation and the nine steps in the monitoring and evaluation process can be illustrated by describing the monitoring and evaluation activities in a home care program. This section shows how the nursing service of a home care program implemented the monitoring and evaluation process.

Overall responsibility for the home care program's QA program was assumed by an interdisciplinary QA committee, as defined by the program's written QA plan. The committee was composed of representatives from each of the program's services, including contracted services. The patient care coordinator represented the nursing service. The home care director served as the committee chairperson and defined the specific program responsibilities of each service representative (step 1): to delineate the scope of their services, to identify important aspects of care, and to identify indicators and criteria, subject to discussion, modification, and agreement by their team members.

The patient care coordinator assumed responsibility for data collection and analysis. The nursing staff discussed findings and, when appropriate, made decisions on corrective actions during staff meetings. The patient care coordinator also assumed responsibility for ensuring that the necessary corrective actions were taken in regard to nursing services, for following up on those actions, for documenting monitoring and evaluation activities and their results, and for seeing that the monitoring and evaluation information from the nursing service was reported to the agency's QA committee.

The nursing staff agreed that the scope of services should include the following important elements of nursing services (step 2):

- The nursing assessment that identifies physical and psychosocial needs
- Patient and family education
- Psychosocial support of patients and their families
- Development of an appropriate patient and family care plan, with patient and family goals determined jointly with patients and their families.

Some important aspects of care, suggested by the patient care coordinator and agreed on by the nursing staff, include (step 3):

- Diabetic teaching and management (high volume, problem prone, high risk)
- Parenteral nutrition, antibiotic, and fluid replacement services (problem prone, high risk)
- Patient and family education regarding medication administration and side effects (high volume, problem prone, high risk)
- Management of Foley catheter care (high volume, problem prone)

The rest of this discussion focuses on only the first identified aspect of care, diabetic teaching and management, which is a common clinical activity performed in the home setting.

The nursing staff agreed on an indicator that would provide some of the information necessary for determining the quality of this important aspect of diabetic teaching and management (step 4): "Diabetic teaching and management is ongoing, is effective, and reflects nursing protocol." To monitor and evaluate this indicator, the nursing staff agreed on the following criteria (step 5):

- The nursing assessment for each diabetic patient includes a complete physical assessment, with emphasis on the following:
  - Visual acuity
  - Skin condition
  - Condition of feet, hands, and nails
  - Evidence of glucosuria or ketonuria
  - Evidence of neuropathies
  - Mental status and orientation
  - Evidence of infection
  - Symptomatology of hypoglycemia, that is, hunger, confusion, tremors
  - Symptomatology of hyperglycemia, that is, polyuria, polydypsia, lethargy, visual disturbances
  - Weight and vital signs
- A psychosocial and environmental assessment is completed for each diabetic patient and family and includes the following:
  - Patient and family understanding and acceptance of disease process and necessary life-style changes
  - Coping mechanisms and available support systems
  - Safety assessment, including a plan for the storage and disposal of insulin syringes, if applicable
- Problems identified in the initial and ongoing assessments are reflected in the patient plan of care 100 percent of the time.
- Nursing documentation reflects an education plan and ongoing assessment that includes the following:
  - Medication administration and compliance
  - Dietary compliance
  - Monitoring activities, for example, urine and blood testing at prescribed intervals
  - Understanding of disease process, including symptoms and treatment of hypoglycemia and hyperglycemia
  - Prevention of complications, that is, neurological changes, infections, skin ulcerations

The patient care coordinator reviewed, on a concurrent basis, all new diabetic patient records every other month. The coordinator used the preestablished criteria and maintained a record of cases not meeting criteria (step 6).

The findings of these monitoring activities were discussed at a staff meeting. After several months of monitoring, management could see that several nurses were not documenting a complete physical assessment and that in 75 percent of the patients reviewed, visual acuity and evidence of neuropathies were missing from the initial and ongoing assessments. The results revealed that several patients had difficulty with correct insulin administration. This difficulty is most likely the result of visual disturbances. After discussing these results, the nursing staff decided to implement the following plan of action (step 7):

- The nursing assessment form was redesigned to include a specific reference to visual acuity and neurological assessment.
- An in-service program was conducted by a diabetic nurse specialist. This program included an update on visual aids available for diabetic patients for use in insulin administration.

After implementing the revised nursing assessment form, the nursing staff continued to monitor and evaluate diabetic teaching and management, using the same criteria and data-collection and analysis methods. Two months later, the nursing staff was able to document significant improvement in meeting the established criteria (step 8).

All findings and other information were reported to the home care program's QA committee (step 9). To ensure sustained resolution of the problem and to continue the documentation of high-quality care, the nursing staff continued to monitor diabetic teaching and management every four months. When further problems or opportunities to improve patient and family care were identified, the time frame of monitoring and evaluation activities was changed as needed.

Figure 9-2, next page, summarizes the monitoring and evaluation activities for diabetic teaching and management that was followed by the nursing staff of a home care program.

Summary

Monitoring and evaluation, an integral part of the QA activities of a home care program, encourages both management and clinical staff to move beyond isolated problem identification and resolution to the evaluation of care on an ongoing basis and identification of opportunities to improve care.

To determine whether monitoring and evaluation activities are adequate, the home care agency staff should ask the following questions:

- Has responsibility for monitoring and evaluation activities been assigned?

Figure 9-2. Summary of a Home Care Program's Monitoring and Evaluation Activities for Diabetic Teaching and Management

Major Aspect of Care

Diabetic teaching and management

Indicator

Diabetic teaching and management is ongoing, is effective, and reflects nursing protocol.

Criteria

A. The nursing assessment for each diabetic patient includes a complete physical assessment, with emphasis on the following: visual acuity; skin condition; condition of feet, hands, and nails; evidence of glycosuria or ketonuria; evidence of neuropathies; mental status and orientation; evidence of infection; symptomatology of both hypoglycemia and hyperglycemia.

B. A psychosocial and environmental assessment is completed for each diabetic patient and family and includes the following: patient and family understanding and acceptance of disease process and necessary life-style changes; coping mechanisms and available support systems; safety assessment, including a plan for the storage and disposal of insulin syringes, if applicable.

C. Problems identified in the initial and ongoing assessments are reflected in the patient plan of care 100 percent of the time.

D. Nursing documentation reflects an education plan and ongoing assessment, which includes the following: medication administration and compliance; dietary compliance; monitoring activities; understanding of disease process, including symptoms and treatment of hypoglycemia and hyperglycemia; and prevention of complications.

Sample

Concurrent review of all diabetic patient records every other month.

Methodology

Diabetic patient records are reviewed by the patient care coordinator. Cases not meeting established criteria are aggregated and analyzed by the patient care coordinator and reviewed by the home care nurses.

Data Sources

Patient records.

- Has the scope of care or services been identified?
- Have the important aspects of care or services been identified?
- Have indicators of quality and appropriateness been identified?
- Have objective criteria been established to evaluate the indicators?
- Have relevant data been collected and analyzed according to a predetermined time frame?
- Have actions been taken to resolve identified problems?

- Has it been determined whether care has improved, has monitoring and evaluation continued, and does documentation of actions taken and the resulting outcome exist?
- Has the information from monitoring and evaluation activities been shared among staff members, with the governing body, and as appropriate, with outside agencies or institutions providing care?

Monitoring activities based on predetermined indicators and criteria as well as evaluation based on actions to correct problems or improve care can serve as a valuable management tool in ensuring a home care program's commitment to high-quality care. An effective QA program can provide the home care manager with crucial information and direction in such areas as staff performance, allocation of resources, and risk management. The importance of monitoring these areas is underscored because, by its nature, home care is decentralized and staff usually function independent of on-site clinical supervision. Therefore, in a time of increasing threats to the viability of home care programs and challenges that focus on proof of quality, QA will continue to play a major role in the effective management of the home care program.

Chapter 10

Risk Management

Patricia A. Peters

As an industry, home care has not yet been affected by the growing litigious environment of the 1980s, but the potential is there. The focus of this chapter is to identify areas in which providing organizations may be potentially at risk for patient or staff injury and liability. All risks cannot be eliminated, but appropriate attention and action can reduce or minimize the risk of patient or staff injury and enhance the delivery of high-quality, cost-effective services and products.

According to the American Society for Hospital Risk Management, risk management is "an insurance and quality control related discipline comprising activities designed to minimize adverse effects of loss upon a health care organization's human, physical, and financial assets through identification and assessment of loss potential, loss prevention and reduction, loss funding and risk financing, and claims control (professional/general liability and worker's compensation)."[1] Risk management is a process requiring skill and expertise from management, legal, financial, and insurance experts. This chapter concentrates on the management of loss prevention and reduction and claims control. These two components are referred to as risk management throughout this chapter. The legal, financial, and insurance components of risk management are complex and beyond the scope of this chapter.

Risk management interrelates with quality assurance and utilization review activities. Coordination of all three activities provides the home care program with the necessary components to minimize risks and liabilities.

Risk management activities cannot be executed in a vacuum. All levels of staff need to be cognizant of risk management goals and activities. Ideally,

Patricia A. Peters, R.N., B.S.N., is the director of home health services for Premier Hospital Alliance, Westchester, Illinois.

a multidisciplinary committee, led by a chairperson with direct or indirect authority, develops, implements, and monitors the risk management program. Realistically, because of the size of the staff in most home care agencies, this committee's responsibilities may include more than risk management. The committee may also function as the overseer for quality assurance and utilization review.

The structure of any home care risk management program depends on the services and products provided and licensure or insurance requirements. However, "an effective risk management program begins with an agency corporate policy that states the commitment to safe and efficient delivery of services and allocation of resources to ensure that the risk management effort succeeds."[2] Every state has laws regarding peer review related to discoverability and admissibility. A risk management program for a home care organization needs to protect staff and provide information consistent with the law of the state. For example, some states require that certain incidents be reported directly to the state or local public health department.

A discussion of risk management is best attempted by breaking down the subject into issues related to personnel, patients, and products. Each of these issues overlap, of course, and no one issue works in isolation.

Personnel Issues

The home care industry, which is a labor-intensive industry, requires personnel with many different types of skills and expertise. Care givers need to be comfortable and competent in providing care in a nonstructured, noninstitutional environment. Being able to improvise and demonstrate flexibility is vital because the environment in which home care personnel work is quite different from other health care settings. Each home presents staff members with an environment that needs to be evaluated for physical safety and for the support that the home provides to both the patient and care giver.

Some health care workers who function quite competently in a hospital setting are uncomfortable providing care in the home. The home environment creates a role reversal for the care giver. Home care staff are now guests in the patient's home; the patient or family allows the service or product to be brought to them. This situation is different from the inpatient setting, in which the patient goes to the health care facility for services, equipment, or products.

Qualifications

In hiring staff, specific criteria need to be followed to minimize potential liability. Job descriptions for every position should list job responsibilities and reporting mechanisms as well as required credentials, education, and experience. All personnel should be informed about any probationary periods and the criteria used for performance evaluations. Professionals should be asked to bring a current license to the job interview. Strict reference-checking procedures, both for professional and nonprofessional staff, should be enforced. Driving records should be verified for personnel who are expected to drive company vehicles. Having a clear picture of who is being hired minimizes the risk of potential poor or inadequate performance.

Just because a person has a license or experience does not necessarily mean that the person is qualified to provide any or all of the kinds of care that home care patients require. The expectation that a nurse with experience on an inpatient medical unit is competent to teach and manage a patient receiving home chemotherapy via an implant or a pump has many potential risks associated with it. The home care agency should establish an ongoing system whereby staff members demonstrate both theoretical and practical application of a skill, whether that skill is a new one or one not currently being used. Such a system does incur costs, but these costs are minimal compared with a patient's well-being or the costs of formal litigation.

Continuing Education

Staff members also need ongoing continuing education. New technology from inpatient settings is constantly being transferred into the home. Educational forums can provide staff members with a means of learning about and safely practicing new or infrequently used procedures.

For example, when the Hickman-Broviac catheters were introduced, nurses needed training on how to use and clean them. If the nurses did not receive proper instruction, they could not pass on correct information to their patients or, indeed, be able to evaluate if their patients had learned how to properly use the new catheters.

Scheduling and After-Hours Coverage

One personnel issue that can pose considerable risks to a home care provider is scheduling. The timely delivery of services or a piece of respiratory or medical equipment can play a vital role in the patient's health status and minimize potential patient injury. To minimize costs, many home care organizations use part-time or temporary personnel. If a provider guarantees that it will have staff in a home for specific hours, it needs to be able to schedule personnel to ensure the presence of that staff person. Temporary or part-time personnel often do not demonstrate the same loyalty as does a full-time staff person, who receives benefits, and so the agency must have backup personnel available to fill last-minute staff cancellations.

Along with staff scheduling, the home care agency's after-hours coverage should be clearly delineated. If the provider states that staff, whether professional care givers or personnel to deliver equipment, are available 24 hour a day, it must be able to guarantee that patients will receive a response within a reasonable time.

Transportation

Another factor that dovetails with scheduling is that of transportation. The home care agency must have adequate insurance coverage for company vehicles.

The most critical issue with regard to transportation relates to emergencies. Inclement weather can cause staff much difficulty. Regardless of road or weather conditions, patients need to be seen. To avoid the risk of compromising care, workable emergency procedures must be worked out.

Another issue is the transportation of patients or family members by staff members of the home care agency. Staff and clients need to be informed of the organization's policies on such transportation. Many home care nurses or therapists are asked to "drop off" patients or family members on the way to their next appointment. They must know how to respond to such requests.

Documentation

Documentation is another important issue in home care. Just as in inpatient settings, care that is not documented is considered not to have been given. "Detailed, well-maintained records are the first line of defense in litigation and the most accurate indicators of how well the home care agency is meeting its goals and implementing its policies."[3] Whether required by licensure or accreditations processes, reviews of patients' health records enable both management and staff to identify areas of compliance or noncompliance with agency procedures and standards for high-quality care. Multidisciplinary case conferences are one way to review utilization, the plan of care, and appropriateness of service.

The home care health record is subject to the same legal protections against disclosure as an inpatient record. All information relating to care and services, orders and communications from physicians, and case conferences need to be recorded objectively and filed in a timely fashion. Staff orientation sessions should include a description of the rights of patients to confidentiality, and patients should be informed of these rights. A breach of patient confidentiality by employees of the home care agency can increase the risk of lawsuits.

Insurance

The home care organization needs to have adequate professional insurance coverage for all staff members. However, adequate and complete coverage may be difficult to secure. To make the best decisions regarding insurance, the home care agency should understand the limitations of the policy, cancellation clauses, and scope of coverage. Because the insurance issue is so complex, the home care organization should consult with the hospital's risk manager or with someone else on the hospital staff who is fully acquainted with the insurance coverage.

Occurrences

Because the home care program depends so much on individuals and because human beings are not perfect, every home care program has experienced some unfortunate occurrences. An *occurrence* may be defined as anything that occurs outside of the scope of usual patient care.

Every home care program needs to have in place specific policies and procedures that delineate the reporting and handling of occurrences. Criteria for what an occurrence consists of needs to be established. Such criteria may be broad or specific, depending on the program's needs. Some programs choose to develop lists of specific occurrences that should be reported, for example, patient or staff injuries, reports of theft, vehicle accidents, or patients complaints about service.

Most insurer's require the home care agency to develop an occurrence or incident reporting system. Of course, monitoring everything that transpires in every patient's home is impossible. However, employees should be made to realize the importance of such reporting systems to the home care agency and to themselves. Employees should understand that the system is not punitive; instead it is designed for everyone's protection.

Regardless of what system is used, all staff members need to be aware of their responsibility as it relates to reporting occurrences. Staff responsibilities may include documenting the incident and notifying the appropriate persons by telephone and in writing. Occurrence reports, if used, should be forwarded to the risk management committee for tracking and evaluating actions and outcomes. Any repetitive occurrence needs to be addressed in both policy and educational formats.

In the program at Parkside Home Health Services, Park Ridge, Illinois, staff members complete occurrence reports for "anything unusual that occurs." The occurrences are reported to the manager of the area, appropriate actions are taken, and a copy of the report is forwarded to the chairperson of the Quality Assurance/Risk Management Committee. Two types of criteria have been established for the timeliness of reporting occurrences. Patient or staff injuries need to be phoned to the manager at the time of the occurrence, with a report to be completed later. Operational occurrences that do not directly affect patient care are only reported in writing. Occurrences are recorded by category and reviewed at the committee's monthly meeting along with all quality assurance activities. The committee makes recommendations if further actions, policies, or educational activities are needed. The committee's recommendations are presented to and approved by the administrative team that has the responsibility for operations.

If the reported occurrence is basically an internal operational issue, the committee requests that the staff who filed the occurrence report complete a problem-resolution form. This form is basically a quality assurance tool to encourage staff participation in resolving operational problems. The initiator, along with other pertinent staff members, form a team, work out a solution, assign responsibilities, set dates for implementing the solution, and actively participate in resolving the problem. Management is expected to participate, support, and monitor the process and outcome. The success of this program rests on the participation of all staff in a results-oriented process.

Exposure to Disease

Another personnel consideration that poses potential risk and liability is exposure to communicable diseases and improper disposal of toxic wastes. The risk of exposing other patients or the community to a communicable disease is a real problem. Policies and procedures need to be established and conveyed to staff and clients. Hospital-based home care programs often use the same disposal procedures for chemotherapeutic agents that are used by inpatient units.

High-Risk Circumstances

An important issue for home care personnel is the delivery of products or services in situations that pose a high risk to the care giver. Staff members should be supplied with complete information on the areas in which they will be working. Being a care giver in a high-risk neighborhood can present many potential problems, such as theft and rape. Another high-risk situation occurs when staff is confronted with an overprotective family pet or a hostile or aggressive family member.

Staff must be provided with adequate training, emergency backup systems, and escort service. Precautionary measures should be encouraged. Management needs to make sure that staff members understand that they can request that another staff member or an escort accompany them on any home visit if they are uncomfortable or afraid. Escort systems can be established with local community groups, off-duty hospital security staff, or local police.

Any injury, including more common injuries like back or foot injuries, need to be documented. Staff members should be supplied with medical examination and follow-up for all injuries, and the program should include a provision for worker's compensation.

Contract Personnel

In some home care agencies, products or services are provided by contract personnel over whom the home care organization has no direct control. All contracts or arrangements should include a clear delineation of the specific expectations and responsibilities of all involved parties. A statement of the scope of professional liability insurance should be included as well as a concise description of implementation, monitoring, and follow-up mechanisms as they relate to the delivery of products and services. The absence of any of these factors can put the home care program at risk. If a contract-service provider should have a problem or accident while rendering care, everyone should be quite clear about who assumes responsibility. Expected standards of care and practice need to be documented. The contract service or company should be supplied with policies and procedures of the home care agency that delineate its standards of practice.

Patient Issues

Historically, litigation occurs when patients are unhappy with the treatment they receive. Home care providers usually form a very special and unique bond with their patients. This bonding can be attributed to the setting in which care is provided as well as to the fact that the patient and family are actively involved in the care. Confidence in the provider is the strongest asset any program can possess against potential litigation.

In today's health care environment, patients are being discharged from the hospital earlier than in previous years. This tendency is true for all ages and kinds of diagnosis: jaundiced newborns are treated at home with portable bilirubin lights; young adults with Crohn's disease are able to be self-sufficient because of total parenteral nutrition programs; and older adults, who often have multiple health problems, receive a myriad of services and products.

When a home care company receives a request for service or products, it needs to screen the referral. Failure to communicate accurate information about the home care agency can put the provider at risk of accepting a patient for whom it cannot provide adequate or appropriate services. The home care provider needs to have available a clear statement of the scope and limits of its program and provide this statement to its referral sources and and to its patients. Written materials on the program's focus and in some cases even the plan of care should be given to the patient. Also, before accepting a patient, the home care agency should be sure it understands the patient's expectations.

To avoid the risk of miscommunication, the home care agency should have clear, concise admission and discharge policies and procedures. These policies and procedures need to state what services are available and who qualifies for them. All home care personnel, referral sources, and patients must be made aware of these policies and procedures. Accepting a patient with needs that cannot be fulfilled by the provider can put the patient's health and well-being in danger.

After a patient is accepted by the home care agency and a plan of care has been established, consistent verbal and written communication needs to flow between the patient, physician, and all care givers providing service. A breakdown in or lack of communication puts everyone in jeopardy. For example, if a patient's cardiac status changes, the visiting nurse contacts the physician and receives an order to change medication and decrease activity; a problem may arise if this information is not conveyed to the physical therapist who is working with the patient on a home exercise program. Staff members need a set procedure to follow in such situations. Careful documentation of all care plans, medications, and physician's orders help, but oftentimes one staff member may not have access to another care provider or to the health record before going into the home.

Abandonment

Occasionally, the original plan of care agreed upon between the patient and the care provider proves to be inadequate because of a change in status of the patient's health. In other words, the patient's needs change while service is being provided by the home care agency, and the provider finds that the additional services are either not acceptable to the patient or available from the provider. The liability issue in this situation is one of abandonment.

Home care providers need to possess a thorough understanding of what abandonment means: failure to continue to provide for the patient when care is still needed in a case for which the home care agency has assumed responsibility constitutes abandonment. In such situations, the primary concern is follow-up. Facilitating appropriate linkages to other available or necessary services, such as suggesting community care programs or alternative housing or, in some cases, obtaining a guardian, may be necessary to fulfill the home care agency's responsibility to its patients.

Emergencies

Staff members need to be cognizant of their responsibility to the patient when emergencies occur while they are present. Emergencies can present themselves in many forms. Staff members may arrive at a home to find that the patient has fallen, is unconscious, or has expired. The staff member's responsibility is to take appropriate action immediately and to remain with the patient until the patient is out of danger or until necessary services have been acquired. All personnel need to be aware of this responsibility, the procedures to be followed, the actions to be taken, and any follow-up that needs to occur. For example, if a fall occurs while a therapist is working with a patient and the patient appears to be injured, the therapist needs to notify the physician, summon needed assistance, and if the patient needs to be transported to an emergency department, stay with the patient until the patient is safely transported.

Sometimes a patient may experience some type of emergency when no home care personnel are in the home. Such a situation can involve anything from a fall to chest pain to confusion about medication regimens. From the day they are hired, every staff person must understand what actions should be taken in these situations. For example, the agency should have policies and procedures describing actions to be taken by licensed personnel when an emergency occurs and the proper documentation of the incident. Also, patients and families need to be taught what occurrences should concern them so that they can obtain quick and appropriate assistance. Many older adults who live alone fear falling and not being able to summon help. One option for these individuals is an emergency call system that they wear on their person. Regardless of what plan is established, home care staff members need to document the plan and any occurrences and notify the proper sources. The plan should be clearly understood by the patient, and that understanding needs to be demonstrated, verbally or in writing, and documented.

Patient Abuse

The home care agency must also consider the issue of patient abuse. Patient abuse can be physical or mental; it can take the form of theft or neglect. Patients may not report such problems until well after the fact because they are vulnerable and may be afraid of retribution.

To avoid such problems as much as is humanly possible, home care providers must screen all personnel carefully and supervise the care that is being rendered by going along with the care giver on a home visit and by visiting the patient when the regularly assigned care giver is not present. Appropriate actions need to be taken if any wrongdoing is suspected. Patients should be confident that they will not be the object of punitive action if they express concerns about their care.

Products

The delivery and use of pharmaceuticals and medical and respiratory equipment in the home has increased greatly. As a result, the potential risk or liability to the provider has also increased.

The pharmaceuticals used in the home include total parenteral nutrition, chemotherapy, antibiotics, and fluid and blood replacement products. Most potential problems resulting from the use of pharmaceuticals can be avoided if patients and their families receive proper instruction and are committed to providing such care in the home. Qualified staff who know how to properly administer products and who have good assessment skills should be the only persons caring for patients who use these products.

When products are being administered via a device, adequate backup techniques to use in an emergency should be taught to persons living in the home. For example, patients receiving continuous infusion chemotherapy via a pump, or their caretakers, need to thoroughly understand what actions should be taken if the pump malfunctions. Inadequate teaching could cause the patient undue physical harm.

The home care agency should also develop clear protocols for the administration of drugs that are considered experimental or new to home care use. The home care agency needs access to information on the use and stability of the drugs as well as the scope and limitations of the use of those drugs as set by the FDA and state and professional licensure.

Medical and respiratory equipment also require the provider's attention. With the increasing use of sophisticated life-sustaining equipment, such as respirators and apnea monitors, the potential for risk is high. Home care providers need to have policies stating what role and responsibilities they assume with regard to such equipment and what procedures must be followed for inspection, maintenance, and on-call assistance. Staff members and patients need to receive in-service instruction and be provided with an instruction manual for operating the equipment.

Emergency backup systems for the equipment need to be available in the home. Patients should not be totally dependent on external energy sources. Electric companies cannot be expected to extend special treatment to patients using medical equipment.

The home care provider needs to assume responsibility for emergency systems. For example, a second ventilator or apnea monitor with a battery pack or a portable battery-operated generator in the home reduces the risk and provides the patient with high-quality services. The cost involved is minimal compared to the potential loss of life.

Summary

Following is a list of potential risks and liabilities with suggested activities or systems to be implemented to reduce or prevent the risk. The items are listed in three major categories:

- Personnel
- Patient issues
- Products and services

Personnel Issues

Potential that staff are not qualified to perform certain activities	Verification of current licensure
	Check of employment references
	Assessment of skills by formal credentialing process
	Ongoing continuing education opportunities

	Provision of job descriptions that state specific duties and responsibilities
	Verification of the presence of adequate professional insurance coverage for the scope of the individual's practice
	Policy statement on staff members' rights and responsibilities
	Procedure for performance evaluations
Potential transportation problems	Verification of the adequacy of insurance coverage
	Verification of driving record
	Policy on patient transportation
	Documentation of emergency plan and communication of procedures in case of inclement weather
Potential staff injuries	Policy on reporting of occurrences
	Provision for workers' compensation
	Policy on employee physicals when hired and at regular intervals
	Staff educational programs, on, for example, lifting patients, handling toxic waste, infection control
Potential for inadequate or unsafe services being provided by contracted vendor	Legal contract with specific expectations of responsibilities stated, including monitoring, follow-up, and implementation of feedback mechanisms and utilization review program
Insufficient communication between care givers, patients, family, physician, and referral source	Standards for levels of communication
	Policy and procedure for communication with physician

	Regular mandatory patient care conference
	Documentation system that provides communication to patients, physicians, and referral sources
Potential exposure to infectious diseases	Policies and procedures for isolation techniques and assignment of staff caring for a patient with an infectious disease
Potential coverage or scheduling problems	On-call system in place
	Policy statement on availability and scope of products and services to be delivered during non-working hours
Inadequate or inappropriate documentation	Policy and procedures for documentation
	Quality assurance program and utilization review program that meet regulatory and accrediting body guidelines
	Understanding of requirements of fiscal intermediaries
	Standardization of forms
	Ongoing review of documentation system on forms
	In-service programs on documentation
Potential treatment errors	Policy and procedure for occurrence reports
	Ongoing monitoring of occurrences, actions taken, and evaluation of outcomes
	Standards of care
	Educational programs
	Policy and procedures for clinical treatments and procedure
	Adequate insurance coverage
Patient emergencies when staff members are present	Policy and procedures for actions to be taken, documentation to be completed, and communication that should occur

Potential abandonment issues	Thorough understanding of what could constitute abandonment: • Refusal to provide care after seeing that the patient needs treatment but before the treatment is begun • Refusal to attend a case for which the agency has already assumed responsibility • Failure to provide follow-up attention • Failure to arrange for a substitute during times of absence or unavailability
Potential exposure to combative patients and high-risk neighborhoods	Policy and procedures for safety precautions and actions
Inadequate care giver in the home (or no home support system)	Policy and procedures for admission Patient rights and responsibilities Knowledge and access to community resources
Patient emergencies when staff members are not present	Policy and procedure for teaching patients and care givers what actions are to be taken in case of an emergency, including documentation that patient has been taught and has demonstrated the procedure
No clear understanding by patient of provider's expectations or of patient's expected participation of care to be received	Statement of patient's rights and responsibilities Patient's informed consent for services and products, billing, and payment Documentation of interaction or patient agreement for treatment and participation Educational materials to be used when care givers or staff members are not present Documentation of all educational sessions and demonstrations by patients of procedures they have been taught

Personal losses reported by patient or family members during or after staff members have been in the home

Policy and procedure for occurrence reporting system

Adequate insurance coverage

Employee security check

Potential patient dissatisfaction

Regular surveys of patients on services and satisfaction

Products and Services

Improper utilization or malfunctioning equipment

Standards or procedures for equipment or product inspection and utilization

Emergency backup system

In-service educational activities for staff and patients

Provision of user's instruction manual

Implementation of quality assurance and risk management programs

Potential requests for administering experimental drugs

Policy and procedures on scope of program

Understanding of scope of state licensure and limitations of practice with regard to, for example, nurses and pharmacist

Appropriate educational preparation of staff

Potential requests from patients to bring equipment from home when they are rehospitalized

Hospital standards and policies

Procedure for biomedical checks

Staff educational programs

Improper disposal of toxic waste

Policy and procedure for proper disposal of toxic waste

Notes

1. Definition of risk management appears in marketing membership brochure of the American Society for Hospital Risk Management, Chicago, Illinois.

2. James Tehan and Sharyn Colegrove, "Risk Management and Home Health Care: The Time Is Now, *Quality Review Bulletin* (1986 May. 12(5):179).

3. Panel on hospital-sponsored home care held in 1986 by the Institute on Quality of Care and Patterns of Practice, American Hospital Association, Washington, DC.

Chapter 11

Government Policies and Programs

Marion M. Torchia

Despite evident public demand and a correspondingly rapid development of new services, government at all levels has been hesitant to support home care. The reasons for official reluctance are not difficult to understand: public money is chronically scarce, and legislators have been hesitant to create a new and hard-to-limit entitlement at a time of escalating health care costs and budget deficits. However, the results of governmental passivity have not been entirely positive. In the face of a widening gap in health care delivery, only a patchwork of home care programs, administered without coordination by a variety of federal and state jurisdictions, are now in existence. Home care is inadequately reimbursed and therefore often simply unavailable, and what is available may not match patients' needs. This chapter attempts to describe current public programs on the federal and state levels and to point out discernible trends in the development of public policy with regard to home care.

Federal Home Care Programs

Five programs constitute the preponderance of federal and joint federal-state involvement in home care.[1] Medicare and Medicaid, the two major health care reimbursement programs, account for the largest portion of expenditures on home care — well over $2 billion annually.[2] A series of health and social service programs for the elderly under the rubric of the Older

Marion M. Torchia, Ph.D., is the associate director for federal agency affairs, American Hospital Association, Washington, DC.

Americans Act (Title III) also includes in-home services. The Social Security Act's social services block grant (Title XX) and the Public Health Service's home health grants and loans program complete the picture.

Medicare

Established in 1965 as a nationwide health insurance program for the elderly and disabled, Medicare's primary purpose was to cover the costs of hospitalization and physicians' services. A limited home health convalescent benefit was an added feature. This benefit was envisioned as essentially a medical service that would be ordered by a physician as part of a plan of treatment.

A set of *conditions of participation* spelled out the standards that a Medicare-certified home health agency must meet.[3] To qualify for home health payments, individuals had to have been hospitalized for a minimum of three days and had to be homebound and in need of either skilled nursing care or specialized therapy on an intermittent basis.[4] Once these threshold requirements were satisfied, the patient was entitled to a strictly limited range of services: part-time or intermittent skilled nursing care; physical, occupational, or speech therapy; medical social services under the direction of a physician; part-time or intermittent services of a home health aide; and medical supplies and appliances.

A maximum of 100 home health visits per year was reimbursable under Medicare's Part A (hospital insurance), and another 100 visits were available under Part B (supplementary medical insurance). These requirements were relaxed somewhat in 1980 when Congress, in an attempt to seek alternatives to the institutionalization of the elderly in nursing homes, eliminated the prior-hospitalization requirement and the 100-visit limit and removed restrictions on participation by proprietary agencies.[5] However, the basic medical nature of the Medicare home health benefit and its emphasis on short-term, highly skilled care has never been changed.

In fact, the reforms of 1980 produced a cost-containment backlash because of the rapid expansion in the use of the home care benefit and in the number of health agencies participating in the Medicare program. Because federal administrators could see outlays increasing by an average annual rate of about 25 percent, they launched a concerted effort, which is still under way, to control this unexpected growth.[6]

Although the medical nature of the Medicare home care benefit has remained static, far-reaching changes have occurred in the Medicare program and in the American health care system as a whole. The enactment in 1983 of a prospective pricing system (PPS) for Medicare inpatient hospital services was among the most dramatic of these innovations. By paying hospitals a flat rate for each admission rather than a rate based on per diem costs, this new system accelerated an already evident trend toward shorter hospital stays, with the result that elderly patients are now being discharged at an earlier stage of recuperation and are more often in need of posthospital follow-up care. Ironically, in the face of increased need, the Medicare home care benefit is being constricted by means of stringent interpretations of eligibility and coverage rules and progressively lowered cost reimbursement limits.

Despite its fiscal difficulties, Medicare continues to exert a far-reaching influence over the development of the home care industry. Participation in the program has grown steadily—as of November 7, 1986, the Health Care Financing Administration (HCFA) reported a total of 5,949 Medicare-certified agencies.[7] As home care agencies have structured their services to meet certification requirements, the limitations of Medicare coverage have tended to become the limitations of the home care industry as a whole. This trend may be reversed to some extent if Medicare continues to tighten its payment policies and home care agencies are forced to look elsewhere for funds. Unfortunately, the real needs of the elderly may remain unsatisfied.

A unique set of structural problems plague the Medicare home care benefit. Statutory restrictions and inadequately defined requirements are reflected in the entire body of regulations: first in the conditions of participation, then in the eligibility and coverage rules, and finally in the claims review and payment process.

Conditions of Participation

The conditions of participation are a basic set of standards that delineate the organization of participating Medicare home care agencies, the qualifications of personnel and the nature of their responsibilities, and the procedures for coordinating and monitoring services. The intent of these standards is to ensure that agencies comply with relevant federal, state, and local laws; that they have clear lines of authority and assume full responsibility for patient care; that their staffs are properly licensed and professionally certified; and that records are properly maintained. These conditions are enforced through on-site surveys by state governmental units that act as Medicare's agents.

The linchpin of the Medicare conditions of participation is the physician's plan of treatment, which must be prepared for each patient and periodically updated. This plan of treatment must describe in detail all the services that the physician orders. This plan is used by HCFA to ensure proper patient care management and to document the medical necessity of the services provided.

Medicare's emphasis on the physician's role as guarantor of the quality of home care services is consonant with the original medical purpose of the home care benefit. However, Medicare policymakers have been ambivalent about the involvement of physicians in the program. Since 1981, physicians with a substantial ownership or management interest in a home care agency have been precluded from certifying that the agency's patients need home care. The reason for this prohibition was a belief that physician-owners had an incentive to overprescribe.[8] This deliberate distancing of physicians from home care agencies has generated tensions that remain unresolved. Physicians understandably resent the paperwork entailed in completing treatment plans, and they may also view independent home care agencies as interfering with the management of their patients.

The conditions of participation have recently been criticized for failing to guarantee the quality of home care services. In July 1986, the American Bar Association and the American Association of Retired Persons testified before the Select Committee on Aging of the House of Representatives. Each organization submitted to the committee its suggestions for stringent standards, sanctions, and enforcement mechanisms for home care.[9] If the public concern documented in their testimony persists, HCFA may be moved to modernize the home care conditions of participation and the survey process, as it is doing for hospitals and nursing homes.

Eligibility and Coverage Principles

Three key terms — skilled nursing, homebound, and intermittent care — that govern eligibility for home care have never been precisely defined by law or regulation.[10] Sensing a need to allow leeway for clinical judgment in individual instances, legislators have been reluctant to provide strict definitions; and HCFA has avoided promulgating regulatory definitions, relying instead on ad hoc instructions to the fiscal intermediaries responsible for paying claims. Ironically, in an atmosphere of fiscal constraint, these vague legislative requirements have proved vulnerable to stringent administrative interpretations:

- *Skilled nursing.* In its guidelines, HCFA has indicated that, to meet this requirement, a patient must need the services of a licensed nurse, either because a technical procedure is required or because the patient's condition is so unstable that a less technical procedure would be unsafe unless performed by a licensed nurse.[11] This definition eliminates from coverage severely ill patients who need only general nursing care.
- *Homebound.* This requirement can jeopardize the coverage of patients who are able to take walks, attend church, or be escorted to medical appointments.[12] Enforcement raises difficult privacy issues as well as problems of the legal liability of home care agency personnel, who may be required to attest to a situation they cannot verify.
- *Intermittent care.* The rationale for this requirement is that anyone who needs daily skilled nursing care belongs in a nursing home.[13] Interpretation of this requirement by HCFA has beome more stringent over the years, as "guidelines" have been transformed into de facto limits. Most recently the agency has announced that it intends to use the intermittent requirement to deny eligibility to beneficiaries who complement Medicare-paid care with services billed to other insurers.

Claims Processing and Payment

Inevitably, these criteria for eligibility have been interpreted inconsistently by the nearly 50 fiscal intermediaries who process home care claims. Congress, which has been unwilling to eliminate the requirements and has been cautioned by home care representatives not to tighten them, has chosen an easier course. The 1984 Deficit Reduction Act authorized HCFA to reassign all freestanding home care agencies to 10 or fewer specialized intermediaries.[14] As of October 1, 1986, the freestanding agencies were assigned to their new intermediaries. Whether the desired consistency of interpretation will be achieved remains unclear. In due course, HCFA plans to transfer hospital-based agencies to the new home care intermediaries. The transition will necessitate the development of new relationships between the hospital's and the home health agency's intermediary to coordinate claims processing, cost reporting, and auditing.

Medical Information Form

Taking another approach in its effort to streamline the home care program and limit costs, HCFA has been working to standardize the medical review process. A new set of medical information forms (HCFA 485-88) must now be used by all home health agencies in their correspondence with their intermediaries.[15] These forms, which replace similar tools used by individual intermediaries, are intended to include all the information needed for coverage determinations, including the details of the physician's treatment plan, a list of the services actually provided, the reasons for the patient's homebound status and need for skilled nursing, the extent of assistance available from family members, and an indication of any insurance other than Medicare. A form that is signed by the physician must be submitted for each patient at the start of care and every 60 days thereafter. Industry representatives cooperated in the design of the form and will continue to consult with HCFA as it is used. Home care agencies continue to experience problems securing physicians' signatures and verifying patients' homebound status.

Waiver of Liability

In 1972 Congress established a statutory *waiver of liability* to protect providers and beneficiaries from undue financial liability resulting from providing services that were determined after the fact not to be covered by Medicare because they were either medically unnecessary or custodial in nature. If the provider and beneficiary could not have known that the services would not be covered, Medicare would pay.

The waiver has been administered by means of a *favorable presumption;* that is, the provider was presumed entitled to payment if its past rate of denied claims was below a certain threshold, which was 2.5 percent in the case of home care agencies. In 1985, however, HCFA attempted to eliminate this presumption of good faith by regulation but was overruled by Congress. The Consolidated Budget Reconciliation Act (COBRA) of 1985 extended the waiver for at least a year, and the 1986 budget reconciliation act broadened its application to include payments denied on technicalities.[16]

Reimbursement Limits

Medicare home care agencies are reimbursed according to the cost-based system in use for hospitals before prospective pricing was introduced in 1983. The proportion of the home care agency's costs that are attributable to Medicare patients is subject to a set of Section 223 upper limits, which are set annually by HCFA at a level intended to represent the necessary costs for the efficient delivery of home care services.[17] Spurred by deficit-reduction directives from the President's Office of Management and Budget, HCFA has enforced increasingly stringent limits while making long-range plans to replace the system with prospective pricing or some other controlled payment method.

Effective July 1, 1985, these Section 223 limits were set for three years at successively lower rates: the first year, at 120 percent of the mean per visit cost; beginning July 1986, at 115 percent; and the year after, 112 percent.[18] Hospital-based agencies continue to receive an adjustment to take into account their higher administrative costs. These cost limits will undoubtedly impose a hardship on all agencies. Hospital-based agencies will be affected particularly severely because their costs are higher than average. In proposing the new schedule, HCFA noted that 80 percent of hospital-based agencies and 70 percent of freestanding agencies are expected to exceed the limit for at least one service.[19] An especially onerous change, whereby the limits would be applied to each particular home care service rather than to the aggregate of home health costs, was overturned by Congress in the 1986 reconciliation legislation.[20] Industry representatives successfully argued that aggregation is necessary because individual high-cost services must often be cross-subsidized if a comprehensive and financially viable program is to be offered.

Periodic Interim Payment

Under the cost reimbursement system, actual amounts due to providers are determined at year's end, and so Congress developed a system of *periodic interim payments (PIPs).*[21] Under PIP, biweekly payments are made based on estimates of costs and Medicare utilization. Theoretically, PIP should not be necessary under PPS. However, when PPS was enacted in 1983, PIP was retained to ensure an uninterrupted cash flow to hospitals. Now HCFA wants to base its payments on submitted bills and thereby save the cost of identifying and correcting overpayments and underpayments.

Home care agencies find PIP an important protection at a time when payment backlogs have become frequent, especially as a new medical review process is being implemented (Forms 485-88). To accommodate the needs of home care agencies, HCFA first relaxed certain requirements of timely claims submission so that agencies experiencing unusual delays because of the new form would not lose their eligibility for PIP and most recently exempted home care from its recently published rules eliminating PIP for hospitals that are paid under PPS.[22] Congress ratified the exemption of home health.[23] However, HCFA's long-term plan is clearly to replace PIP entirely; in its place, the agency intends to encourage the use of electronic billing to expedite claims and has committed itself to certain prompt payment guidelines.

Prospective Pricing under Medicare

Although HCFA has made it clear that cost reimbursement of home care has a limited life expectancy, it has as yet taken no definite steps to replace it. The agency may be hesitating for several reasons: the costs of home care depend more on an individual patient's condition than on diagnosis; as is often the case in a new industry, costs are extremely variable and may not yet have settled down; and no consensus about the appropriate unit of service to be paid for exists. A DRG-type system would require extensive research on the case mix of home care patients, and yet in 1985, HCFA abandoned plans to sponsor a demonstration project to test per visit, per month, and per patient episode payment methods.[24] Other prospective approaches, such as capitation and competitive bidding, may be the subjects of future experiments.[25]

Payment for Equipment and Supplies

The control of the cost of supplies and equipment associated with home care is important to HCFA. Routine supplies are treated as overhead items and are reflected in a home care agency's per visit costs. Home health agencies have the option of including nonroutine items, such as DME, in their Part A costs or charging for them separately under Part B. As the Section 223 limits have become more stringent, agencies have sought to avail themselves of the Part B option. However, HCFA has taken several steps to tighten its Part B payment rules. In December 1984 and July 1985, for example, instructions governing payment for rented DME were issued.[26] The view of HCFA is that Medicare should not be obligated to pay many times the purchase price of the equipment.

Under a little-used authority to set prices based on their *inherent reasonableness,* HCFA is establishing a new system of nationwide price limits for supplies and equipment used for enteral and parenteral feeding and is proposing price limits for oxygen use.[27] In addition, to carry out a requirement of the Deficit Reduction Act, HCFA is now requiring a coinsurance charge under Part A, ostensibly to place home care agencies and suppliers on an equally competitive footing because suppliers are already required to collect coinsurance.[28] The cost-cutting methods applied to Part B pricing may be transferred to the entire home care benefit.

Hospice Benefit

Authorized by Congress in 1982 and implemented by HCFA in regulations issued December 1983, the hospice benefit represents a significant innovation within the Medicare program.[29] Designed to provide palliative care to the terminally ill, the new benefit shifts Medicare's emphasis from specific technical procedures to total care of the patient's medical and social needs as well as the needs of the patient's family.

To qualify, a patient must be certified to be terminally ill and must waive the ordinary Medicare benefits related to a terminal illness. In return, the patient becomes eligible for a range of benefits not usually covered: palliative prescription drugs, medical social services, continuous home nursing, and respite care in an inpatient setting.

Because of its unique purpose and requirements, the hospice program is administered separately. Prospective hospices must be certified by HCFA as such and must undergo a specialized certification procedure according to special conditions of participation.[30] Nevertheless, the hospice program is basically an enriched home care program. Inpatient care is limited by statute to 20 percent of a hospice's total patient days.

As of July 1, 1986, HCFA had certified a total of 279 hospices; of these, 124 were based in home care agencies, 66 were based in hospitals, 79 were freestanding institutions, and 10 were located in nursing homes. The numbers are smaller than may be expected, given the existence of an estimated 1,200 hospice programs nationwide.[31] At hearings before the Senate Finance Committee in September 1984, witnesses suggested that inadequate reimbursement and restrictive patient management requirements may have discouraged would-be participants.[32] In response, Congress exempted certain rural hospices from the requirement that nursing services be provided directly by hospice staff and not contracted for; and in March 1986, HCFA proposed regulations implementing this exemption.[33] Finally, Congress responded to public consensus that the hospice concept is valuable by eliminating the sunset provision of this Medicare benefit and thereby extending the program's life indefinitely.[34]

Medicaid

Because Medicaid serves indigent persons of all ages, it provides a mix of home care services that are different from those covered by Medicare. States are required to provide nursing services, supplies, and home health aide services to eligible homebound patients, and many states also offer homemaker and social services.[35] Since the late 1970s, nursing home costs have threatened to engulf state health care budgets, and a major goal of the Medicaid home care program has been to provide support services to those elderly who would otherwise probably be institutionalized at public expense. Consequently, Medicaid-funded home care is broader and less tied to a medical model than is Medicare.

The 1981 Omnibus Reconciliation Act authorized a *home-and-community-based waiver program,* whereby states could waive traditional Medicaid requirements and provide in-home services to selected persons on an experimental basis if the states could demonstrate that the program would be cost-effective.[36] The program initially was enthusiastically received, and as of October 7, 1986, 47 states operated more than 150 projects.[37] However, as the first of these projects completed their three-year terms, the Office of Management and Budget demanded more precise evidence of cost savings before renewal applications were approved, and a number of projects have been terminated. Furthermore, the states themselves have hesitated to make too-extensive commitments to the program, lest their own expenditures increase uncontrollably. As a result, the waiver projects have remained small and localized.

Older Americans Act

In 1965 Congress created an Administration on Aging in the Department of Health, Education, and Welfare to carry out the provisions of the Older Americans Act, Title III.[38] A series of grants to the states are administered through a network of 57 State and Territorial Units on Aging and 660 Area Agencies on Aging. The purpose of these units is to coordinate community-based services that foster the economic and personal independence of the elderly. In 1982 approximately one-third of the program's $600 million budget was spent on in-home services, including homemaker and chore services and home-delivered meals.

Title XX Social Services Program

Title XX of the Social Security Act, which was reconstituted in 1981 as part of a social services block grant or general nonearmarked grant to the states, provides funds for household management, day care, home-delivered meals, and other support services for the elderly. The program is an important supplement to Medicare and Medicaid, but the federal government's adoption of the block-grant approach has, in fact, resulted in reduced federal funding and retraction of federal control. States are no longer required to provide matching funds or target services to the most needy. Furthermore, because Title XX is usually not administered by the same state agency that administers Medicaid, coordination of the two programs is generally nonexistent.

Public Health Service Home Care Grants and Loans

Authorized by the Orphan Drug Act of 1983, this Public Health Service grant and loan program provides seed money to foster the development of home care services for the elderly, the disabled, and the medically indigent, especially in areas where such services are in short supply and where transportation problems impede access to care.[39] About $3 million was awarded during fiscal year 1985: $2 million for the establishment and expansion of home health services, and $1 million for the training of home health aides. A total of $1.4 million was available in 1986.[40]

Legislative Achievements and Prospects

Throughout most of the 1980s, Congress exhibited a conservative, antiregulatory mind set, reflecting a Republican administration's commitment to reduce the scope of federal involvement in social programs and to replace regulatory standards and planning mechanisms with free-market competition. These ideological constraints, combined with intense pressure to reduce an escalating federal deficit, prevented serious consideration of a comprehensive new home care initiative.

Nevertheless, the major congressional committees with jurisdiction over health and social programs continue to hold hearings at regular intervals, and several Senate leaders have shown consistent interest in the subject: Orrin Hatch of the Senate Labor and Human Resources Committee has held numerous hearings; David Durenberger of the Senate Finance Committee's Health Subcommittee held an inquiry in June 1984; and in 1985 John Heinz, chairman of the Senate's Special Committee on Aging, examined the impact of restrictions on home care coverage and claims denials on the quality of care that Medicare beneficiaries receive.[41] On the House side, Congressman Edward Roybal's Select Committee on Aging has also scrutinized the administration of the home care benefit, looking in particular at the high incidence of denied claims and the alleged failure of the government to guarantee the quality of care.[42] These hearings, while not immediately fruitful, have created a factual basis for future action.

The 99th Congress, which met during 1985 and 1986, was conducted under the extraordinary pressure of the Gramm-Rudman deficit-reduction mandate, and the home care legislation presented to it was necessarily limited to one or two modest additions to benefits; several proposals for immediate relief from threatened cutbacks; and tentative, small-scale, structural adjustments of federal programs.[43] Even modest proposals tended to be pushed aside if they were construed as potential "cost items:" for example, proposals for Medicare coverage of home-administered IV antibiotics and for nutrition counseling services did not receive serious attention in committee.[44]

Nevertheless, the Consolidated Omnibus Budget Reconciliation Act (COBRA) of 1985, the massive legislation that authorized most of the health care spending in 1985, included several favorable home care provisions: temporary retention of the waiver of liability available to home health agencies, limitations on HCFA's price-setting authority for home care equipment and supplies, and the permanent authorization of the hospice benefit as well as a small increase in the hospice payment rates.[45] A proposal to pay for home treatment of ventilator-dependent patients, though not enacted, led to the chartering of a federal Task Force on Technology-Dependent Children, which over the next two years will examine alternatives to the institutionalization of these children.[46]

By mid-1986, consumer pressure seemed to be having an effect on an election-minded Congress, and the Omnibus Budget Reconciliation Act of 1986 contained a set of significant and valuable home care provisions, which, taken together, may signal a halt to cutbacks.[47] More important, these latest provisions were presented as meeting a perceived need, under the hospital prospective pricing system, for reliable posthospital follow-up care. Hospitals will now be required, as a condition of participation in Medicare, to have formal discharge planning programs. The Secretary of Health and Human Services is ordered to include in the annual report to Congress on the impact of the hospital prospective pricing system an evaluation of the adequacy of the procedures for ensuring the quality of Medicare posthospital services and an assessment of barriers to beneficiaries' access to those services. In addition, the Secretary must consult with an advisory panel of experts in home care and long-term care to develop a patient assessment instrument that will measure the need for posthospital care.

In this latest legislation, Congress, by extending the waiver of liability to claims denied on the basis of the intermittent-care and homebound requirements and by ordering the Secretary to promulgate clear definitions of these terms, has finally issued a clear call for reform of the home care medical review system. The law orders an experiment with *prior authorization,* which is a before-the-fact determination that home care is necessary, as a possible alternative to retrospective review and waiver of liability. In conjunction with this project, it orders an annual report on the frequency and distribution of payment denials. The law also extends the appeal rights of beneficiaries and permits providers to represent beneficiaries in such appeals of claims decisions by Medicare.[48]

Proposed extensions of coverage also received a somewhat more favorable reception in 1986 than the year before. Independent of the home health benefit and its particular restrictions, occupational therapy services delivered at home are to be reimbursed under Part B once Part A coverage is exhausted.[49] Under Medicaid, states are permitted to cover home respiratory services for ventilator-dependent individuals.[50] A proposal to subsidize home care for Alzheimer's disease victims yielded a major commitment, in the form of a $40 million authorization of a series of demonstration projects, to explore alternatives.[51]

Relief from a most onerous aspect of the Medicare cost reimbursement limits has also been granted. Beginning in October 1986, the limits must be applied in the aggregate, rather than by specific discipline; furthermore, the administrative costs of hospital-based agencies must continue to be recognized. The General Accounting Office must study the impact of the limits and the method of computing them and report its findings to Congress by 1988.[52] Also, home health agencies received permission to remain indefinitely on HCFA's periodic interim payment (PIP) system.[53] This last provision is a welcome protection against cash flow problems.

In summary, home care providers are encouraged by the renewed interest in home care on the part of Congress and the public and the beginnings of structural reform of federal home care programs. Although the problems of cost containment and deficit reduction have by no means been solved, the themes of quality and access to service are again being forcefully articulated. Providers are seeking closer alliances with beneficiaries to press for the continuation of this positive trend.

Trends on the State Level

State governments respond to federal initiatives in regulating and supporting home care by acting as agents of Medicare certification, cosponsors of Medicaid and the Social Security social services block grants, and managers of the state agencies on aging authorized by the Older Americans Act. They also implement the federal health planning law, under which some states require home health agencies to undergo certificate-of-need (CON) approval. In pursuing these activities, the states are by no means passive conduits of federal power; on the contrary, they try to shape the federal programs to their own policy objectives. Occasionally, they have moved in to fill a vacuum left by the withdrawal of a federal initiative or a cutback in federal funds. In addition to working to put federal programs into action, the states also regulate home care on their own authority, primarily through licensure laws and the regulation of health insurance.

State Review of Home Care Services

Federal-state cooperation in health planning had its origin in the Hill-Burton hospital construction legislation of 1946, which was intended to encourage the building of new facilities and to see that they were rationally distributed throughout the country. The Hill-Burton program and its successors, the Regional Medical Program (1965) and the Comprehensive Health Planning Program (1966), were based on a formal, state-managed health facilities planning process, which over the years developed more sophisticated information-gathering mechanisms and methods of soliciting public input and expanded its scope to include noninstitutional services. In 1972, state planning was given new "teeth" through the enactment of the Section 1122 program, which, in participating states, made Medicare reimbursement for capital expenditures dependent on a facility's compliance with the state's planning requirements. Finally, the Health Planning and Resources Development Act of 1974 (Pub. L. 93-641) put in place a full-fledged, three-tiered, federal-state-local planning program with federal funding and minimum federal standards of accountability.[54]

The energies of health planners have naturally been directed primarily toward the most capital-intensive facilities and costliest services, and home care has been somewhat of an afterthought. Nevertheless, motives other than cost containment, such as consumer demand for access to services and the desire of providers to protect their interests, have forced attention to this area. As of 1983, 38 of 52 jurisdictions had CON requirements for home care agencies; of these, 9 limited the requirement to institutional-based agencies, one (New Hampshire) made it necessary only for proprietary agencies, and one (New York) required it for public and voluntary agencies only.[55]

The purpose of the CON requirement is ostensibly a quality-related preference for a particular institutional form. However, CON has also openly been used to slow the entrants of new agencies into a marketplace that is perceived as already glutted: in Mississippi, a moratorium on new CON approvals was temporarily imposed in 1983 for this reason. The legality of this use of planning authority has been challenged on the basis of the antitrust laws. In one case, a state's criterion for approving new agencies — the full utilization of existing agencies — was struck down by a court that found it designedly anticompetitive.[56]

State Licensure Laws

State licensure of health care facilities has traditionally been concerned primarily with basic health and safety standards, minimum requirements for services, and qualifications for staff. States have been slow to license home care agencies. As late as 1978, only 16 states had such laws on the books; the number had grown to 25 by 1980.[57] In 1980, the Medicare program removed its requirement that proprietary agencies be licensed, thereby removing one motive for the institution of licensure programs.[58] In 1983, licensure programs numbered 30 nationwide.[59]

Licensure and Certification: A Two-Tiered Approach

A new state law in New York offers basic licensure or a more rigorous CON-Medicare-Medicaid certification as alternative pathways to approval for home care agencies.[60] The legislation was presented as a means of making high-quality home care available throughout the state. Certified agencies would be required to have services available 24 hours a day, 7 days a week; to provide nursing care directly by agency employees rather than under contract; and to provide a quota of charity care. For the first time, proprietary agencies operating in that state will be eligible for licensure. Those agencies that choose to do so may compete for an estimated 40 to 80 CON certificates.

At public hearings in October 1985, proprietary agencies attacked the certification requirements as discriminatory and the state's projections of need as unrealistically low. They view the charity-care requirement as particularly onerous in view of their responsibilities to their investors. This controversy may just be localized, or it may be an indication of a nationwide trend toward more direct regulation of home care services.

Future Prospects for Home Care Policy

Although the prevailing public anxiety about budget deficits in the late 1980s does not favor expanded funding of home care, an underlying public demand for governmental action remains. Demographic and social factors, combined with the basic restructuring that is occurring in the delivery of health care, have already made home care a necessity. The signs are that Congress and the state legislatures have begun to realize this and that creative attention is being given to designing a coherent home care policy.

Notes

1. For an overview of these programs, *see* Chai R. Feldblum, "Home Care for the Elderly: Programs, Problems, and Potentials," *Harvard Journal on Legislation* (1985. 22:193, 195-254).

2. In 1983 outlays under both hospital insurance (Part A) and supplementary medical insurance (Part B) totaled $1,388 million, according to "Twenty years of Medicare and Medicaid," *Health Care Financing Review,* table 26 (1985 annual supplement, Dec. 1985, page 43). Vendor payments for home health services under Medicaid in 1984 were $756 million, according to *Social Security Bulletin, Annual Statistical Supplement, 1984-85,* table 154 (Medicaid).

3. 42 C.F.R. 405.1201-1230, Subpart L.

4. 42 C.F.R. 405.235-236.

5. Omnibus Reconciliation Act of 1980 (Pub. L. No. 96-499), effective July 1, 1981.

6. "Twenty Years of Medicare and Medicaid."

7. Data as of Nov. 7, 1986, from file entitled "Providers and Suppliers of Services" that is maintained by the Health Care Financing Administration's Office of Survey and Certification.

8. Mandated by the Omnibus Reconciliation Act of 1980 (Pub. L. No. 96-499 § 930); regulations at 42 C.F.R. 405.1633. Recently published interim final regulations contain important clarifications of this conflict-of-interest prohibition. An exemption is provided for home care agencies that are the sole community provider. *Fed. Reg.* 23541-46 (June 30, 1986).

9. *The "Black Box" of Home Care Quality.* A report presented the chairman of the Select Committee on Aging, House of Representatives, 99th Congress, Second Session and prepared by the American Bar Association, Aug. 1986 (Committee Pub. No. 99-573) and "Home Health Benefits under Medicare: A Working Paper," prepared by Shela Leader for the Public Policy Institute of the American Association of Retired Persons, Washington, DC, July 21, 1986.

10. Social Security Act 1814(a)(2)(D); 1835(a)(2); 1861(m).

11. *Medicare Home Health Agency Manual* (HCFA Pub. No. 11), ch. ii, § 204.

12. *Medicare Home Health Agency Manual,* § 204.1.

13. *Medicare Home Health Agency Manual,* § 204.1.

14. Pub. L. No. 98-369, § 2326.

15. *Medicare Home Health Agency Manual,* §§ 234.6-234.8.

16. Consolidated Omnibus Budget Reconciliation Act (COBRA) of 1985, Pub. L. No. 99-272, § 9205; Senate Finance and House Ways and Means committee reports, July 1986; Omnibus Budget Reconciliation Act of 1986, Pub. L. 99-509, § 9305.

17. Pub. L. 92-603, § 223 (1972); Social Security Act, § 1861(v); regulations at 42 C.F.R. 460.

18. Fed. Reg. 27734-51 (July 5, 1985).

19. Fed. Reg. 20178-90 (May 14, 1985).

20. Onmibus Budget Reconciliation Act of 1986, Pub. L. 99-509, § 9315.

21. Social Security Act, § 1815(a).

22. *Intermediary Manual,* Transmittal No. 1254; Fed. Reg. 29385-94 (Aug. 15, 1986).

23. Omnibus Reciliation Act of 1986, § 9311.

24. In Dec. 1983, HCFA awarded a contract to Abt Associates, Inc. (Cambridge, MA) to test the various payment methods in more than 100 home care agencies (HCFA Contract No. 500-84-0021). The project never progressed beyond the design phase. Abt Associates, Inc. (Cambridge, MA), "National Home Health Agency Prospective Payment Demonstration: Summary of Payment Methods," unpublished paper, Feb. 1985.

25. In June 1984, HCFA awarded a contract to the Center for Health Policy Studies (Columbia, MD) for competitive bidding models and a research plan to test them (HCFA Contract No. 500-84-0033).

26. For rent or purchase guidelines, *see Medicare Carriers Manual,* Transmittal No. 1067, Dec. 1984, and Transmittal No. 1109, July 1985.

27. On HCFA's enteral and parenteral, *see Medicare Intermediary Manual,* Transmittal No. 1131, July 1984; for oxygen coverage rules, *see* Fed. Reg. 13742-50 (Apr. 5, 1985). For regulations on inherent reasonableness, *see* Fed. Reg. 5726-28 (proposed rule) Feb. 18, 1986) and 28710-17 (final rule with comments) (Aug. 11, 1986).

28. Pub. L. No. 98-369, § 2321.

29. Pub. L. No. 97-248, § 122; Fed. Reg. 56008-5636 (Dec. 16, 1983).

30. 42 C.F.R. 418.50-418.100.

31. This estimate is based on a 1983 survey by the Joint Commission on Accreditation of Hospitals, cited in "Background Materials on Medicare Hospice Benefit," p. 7. Prepared for the Committee on Finance, U.S. Senate, Sept. 9, 1983.

32. Senate Finance Committee, Subcommittee on Health. Hearings on the implementation of the Medicare hospice benefit, Sept. 17, 1984.

33. Pub. L. No. 98-369, § 2343; Fed. Reg. 7292-95 (Mar. 3, 1986).

34. Pub. L. No. 99-272, § 9123.

35. 42 U.S.C. §§ 1396-1396p (1982); 42 C.F.R. 440.70 (1983).

36. Pub. L. No. 97-35, § 2176.

37. Unpublished HCFA data, Oct. 1986. At the outset of the program, HCFA funded a survey of their initial responses. National Governors' Association, *An Analysis of Responses to the Medicaid Home- and Community-Based Long-Term Care Waiver Program (Section 2176 of P.L.97-35),* HCFA grants 18-P-97923/3-3/03 and 18-P-98078/5-01, June 1983.

38. 42 U.S.C. 3001-3037a (1982).

39. Pub. L. No. 97-414; Fed. Reg. 6253-55 (Feb. 14, 1985).

40. Fed. Reg. 24231-32 (July 2, 1986).

41. Hearings on the Community Home Health Services Act of 1981 (S. 234), before the Senate Committee on Labor and Human Resources, Mar. 4 and Nov. 10, 1981; Hearing on Community-Based Home Care Programs, before the Senate Committee on Labor and Human Resources, July 13, 1983 (S. Hrg. 98-525); Oversight Hearings on Home Care for Chronically Ill Children before the Senate Committee on Labor and Human Resources, Aug. 9, 1983 (S. Hrg. 98-455) and June 18, 1985 (S. Hrg. 99-132). Hearing on the Medicare Home Health Benefit, before the Subcommittee on Health of the Senate Committee on Finance, June 22, 1984 (S. Hrg. 98-957).

    Senator Heinz's Special Committee on Aging held a series of three hearings on the impact of prospective pricing on the quality of care (Sept. 28, Oct. 24, and Nov. 12, 1985). The Oct. 24 session focused on "Medicare DRGs: Challenges for Post-Hospital Care." In Aug. 1986, Heinz met with his constituents at a public hearing in Philadelphia on the problem of home health claims denials.

42. "Health Care Cost Containment: Are America's Aged Protected?" Hearing before the House Select Committee on Aging, 99th Congress, 1st Session, July 9, 1985 (Comm. Pub. No. 99-552). Rep. Claude Pepper (D-FL), chair-

man of the Select Committee's Subcommittee on Health and Long-Term Care, has published a report entitled *The Attempted Dismantling of the Home Care Benefit* (Comm. Pub. No. 99-552), Apr. 1986. *See also* note 9.

43. The formal title of the Gramm-Rudman-Hollings legislation is the Balanced Budget and Emergency Deficit Control Act of 1985 (Pub. L. 99-177), enacted Dec. 12, 1985.

44. H. R. 1215; H. R. 215.

45. COBRA of 1985, §§ 9205, 9304, and 9123. Sec. 9505 incorporated a hospice benefit into Medicaid at the option of the states.

46. S. 1249; COBRA, § 9520.

47. Omnibus Budget Reconciliation Act of 1986 (Pub. L. 99-509), § 9305.

48. Omnibus Budget Reconciliation Act of 1986, §§ 9313, 9341.

49. Omnibus Budget Reconciliation Act of 1986, § 9337

50. Omnibus Budget Reconciliation Act of 1986, § 9408

51. Omnibus Budget Reconciliation Act of 1986, § 9342.

52. Omnibus Budget Reconciliation Act of 1986, § 9315.

53. Omnibus Budget Reconciliation Act of 1986, § 9311.

54. For an overview of the federal health planning program, see James B. Simpson and Ted Bogue, *Guide to Health Planning Law: A Topical Digest of Health Planning and Certificate of Need Case Law* [U.S. Department of Health and Human Services, Office of Health Planning (HRP-0906594), Oct. 1985], section 2, pp. xi-xxxviii.

55. "Certificate of Need Issue Heats Up: State Hospice Laws Moving In: Survey of the 50 States' CON and Licensure Laws," in *Home Health Line,* (pp. ii-xiv, May 30-June 6, 1983). This document is a special nationwide compilation on the status of home health licensure and certificate of need.

56. For a discussion of the antitrust issues as related to CON, see James B. Simpson, "State Certificate-of-Need Programs: The Current Status," *American Journal of Public Health* (75:10, 1225-29 Oct. 1985). On page 1229, note 21, Simpson cites Dept. of Health and Rehabilitative Services v. Johnson and Johnson Home Health Care, Inc., 447 So.2d 361 (Fla. Dist. Ct. App. 1984.

57. Abt Associates, Inc., *Home Health Services: An Industry in Transition.* (Submitted to HCFA under contract No. 500-84-0021, May 3, 1984) p. 23.

58. Omnibus Reconciliation Act of 1980.

59. See note 55.

60. New York State: Chapter 959 (signed Aug. 6, 1984). Emily Layzer, "Will New York Proposals Have National Impact?—New York Home Health Proprietaries Gear Up for Certification, Tough Proposed Rules Discourage 'Brokering,' Mandate Charity Care, Add DME Responsibility," *Home Health Line* (10:245-48, Sept. 9, 1985). Layzer, "New York Proprietaries Term Proposed CON Rules 'Patent Discrimination,'" *Home Health Line* (10:309-12, Nov. 4, 1985).

Chapter 12

Development of a Durable Medical Equipment Business

Larry Brothers

The durable medical equipment (DME) area of home care is concerned with the product needs of the home care patient. It is also concerned with the services that are required when these products are used by the patient. This service component in essence determines the quality of the business. Although the supplier is generally reimbursed only for the sale or rental of medical equipment and supplies, the service component, that part of the program that is nonreimbursable, is the one aspect of the business that determines its success or failure. Professional staffing, delivery services, and complimentary equipment and supplies are examples of services that DME companies provide to their customers.

The DME business depends on a relatively small group of referral agencies and individuals. Hospital discharge planners, social workers, and physical and respiratory therapists must be confident that the products and services supplied by the DME dealer are of high quality. Most patients requiring home care product services are identified on discharge from hospitals. A much smaller percentage of referrals is provided from other sources, such as home care agencies, physicians' offices, and clinic operations.

Growth of the Industry

The DME industry has historically consisted of many small businesses serving local communities. Neighborhood pharmacists generally provided and

Larry Brothers is vice-president, Kensington Health Enterprises, St. Joseph Health System, Flint, Michigan.

met the medical equipment needs of their clientele. In fact, a significant percentage of the DME businesses of the 1980s is descended from neighborhood pharmacy operations.

As the number of services provided to patients in the home increased, so did the development of specialized home care companies. The expansion of local pharmacies into specialized home care companies became commonplace. Home oxygen therapy was the first specialized home care product line that saw major growth in the late 1970s. The growth of home oxygen and other respiratory services mirrored the growth of the field of respiratory therapy. The growing awareness of the causes of pulmonary disease, the dramatic changes in treatment modalities, and the considerable research performed in pulmonary medicine also contributed to the growth of home oxygen therapy. Unlike many of the hospital-performed respiratory treatment techniques, which became overutilized, home oxygen therapy is well documented as a means of improving the quality of life and reducing mortality in patients with chronic obstructive pulmonary disease.

The growth of the DME industry attracted the attention of large corporations, who entered the market through acquisition and merger programs. Many small businesses, unable to acquire sufficient capital to meet the increased demand for home care services, became early acquisition targets for the national chains. The interest of national corporations in the DME market indicates that they recognize it as a viable part of the health care industry.

In the early 1980s, hospitals emerged as a new force in the DME industry. Pressured by declining occupancy, increased competition, and major changes in the reimbursement structure, hospitals saw that alternative health delivery programs could help stabilize their market. *Market share,* a term little used by hospitals in the 1970s, now became a term for survival in the 1980s. Hospitals could no longer wave good-bye to patients at the discharge area and hope they would return the next time hospitalization was needed. Hospitals must now concern themselves with the health care needs of consumers, not just with the hospitals' needs.

The new, more diversified role of hospitals in the 1980s has not been welcomed by all segments of the health care community. Entry by hospitals, usually through a subsidiary corporation, has generated a real concern on the part of the DME industry. Providers of DME recognize that the overwhelming majority of DME referrals are generated by hospitals for discharged patients. Many DME companies perceive hospitals as their greatest threat to survival because of their close relationship with the patient.

The number of hospitals independently developing DME entities is actually less than rumored by the DME professional organizations. However, the threat of hospital domination of the DME industry spawned a new DME corporate model, the joint venture company. Companies, both independent and national chains, began aggressively courting hospitals to develop formalized business ventures, usually through the establishment of a corporation or partnership. The DME company offers equipment, expertise, and capital investment in exchange for the hospital's referrals and an equivalent capital investment. Many observers view these relationships as merely a purchase of the referral base of that hospital.

Hospitals were deluged with proposals for DME joint ventures. All this activity caused hospitals that were not even actively considering the development of DME programs to research the possibilities of starting a DME project by themselves. Many of the joint venture proposals presented to hospitals detailed phenomenal profit margins that certainly piqued the interest of even the most prudent administrator.

However, most hospital administrators found that although DME is potentially a profitable business, it must be approached like any other business, with sound research, planning, and development. After looking into the DME business, many hospitals discovered that a DME business could, in fact, be started with minimal outside assistance. They found that giving control and ownership responsibility to other parties was not necessary. However, not all hospitals have the internal expertise to develop a DME business. For some hospitals, joint venture programs, referral arrangements, and partnerships may be the best alternatives.

In the mid-1980s, the DME industry is evolving into an industry composed of three competing forces: the independent DME business, the national chains, and the hospital-based programs. These forces will compete and shape the industry through 1990, and it will be the quality of services, products, and personnel that will determine which companies are successful.

Products and Services

The products and related services required by some home care patients are generally provided through one of four defined DME service divisions:

- Home respiratory division
- Medical equipment division
- Medical-surgical supply division
- Nutritional support division

Home Respiratory Division

The home respiratory division usually ranks as one of the most profitable revenue centers for most DME companies for several important reasons. The equipment in the home respiratory division is usually rented rather than purchased because the equipment used to provide oxygen and respiratory services requires considerable maintenance, calibration, and periodic monitoring. At present, insurance carriers do not reimburse DME companies for maintenance services on patient-owned equipment. Most patients would indeed be at risk if their equipment malfunctioned or did not perform to specification. Many DME providers refuse to sell some types of home respiratory equipment because of the potential liability that could result from equipment failure. If the equipment is purchased rather than rented, necessary preventative maintenance procedures could not be performed unless a service contract was also purchased. Obviously, many consumers using this service have medical conditions that do not allow sufficient margin for equipment malfunction or error.

Another reason for the profitability of the home respiratory division is that it provides services to a large segment of the chronically ill, persons who have chronic obstructive pulmonary disease (COPD). Therapies enable the client to live not only a more productive life but also a longer one. Hospitals that offer pulmonary rehabilitation services, pulmonary clinics, or other special incentives for the COPD patient are in a good position to develop a substantial home respiratory service.

One point that must be emphasized is that although the home respiratory division generally has a favorable reimbursement forecast, its service component is much more substantial than for other divisions of a DME business. Patients using home respiratory equipment must be visited on a regular basis so that at least minimal maintenance functions can be performed. High-quality DME programs employ registered respiratory therapists and certified respiratory therapy technicians with home care training to administer the required home respiratory services. A highly trained professional staff can provide patient education, rehabilitation services, physical assessments, and laboratory services. A hospital-related DME program may be better able to provide these services because it can use trained personnel on the hospital staff.

Because of the importance of trained personnel, hospitals often become involved in DME under the shared-service model. This model establishes a contractual arrangement between the DME company and the hospital for the use of the hospital's professional staff. This arrangement allows the expertise of the hospital staff to be employed in the home care setting. Respiratory therapists who have continuous exposure to educational programs and critical care environments are generally better prepared to deliver home care services. However, because respiratory home care has evolved as a subspecialty within the field of respiratory therapy, specialized training designed to prepare the respiratory therapist for home care duties must be provided before any service is delivered. The use of professional staff, especially in the shared-service model, does contribute to the higher operating cost of the home respiratory division. In addition to the increased salary cost, this division also has professional liability insurance and higher transportation expenses than do other DME divisions.

The home respiratory division can be divided into three categories: home oxygen therapy, home respiratory therapy, and apnea monitors.

Home Oxygen Therapy

Oxygen therapy accounts for the majority of services provided by the home respiratory division. Three primary methods are used for delivering oxygen to patients at home: oxygen concentrators, liquid systems, and cylinders. The appropriate system for each patient must be carefully evaluated. The ultimate choice is the patient's, with the advice of the physician and home care supplier.

Oxygen concentrators are considered the most cost-effective oxygen delivery system for the home care patient. An oxygen concentrator is an electrically powered device that extracts oxygen from room air by using molecular sieve material. Major technological improvements have occurred in the past few years. Improved reliability, lighter weight, decreased power consumption, and quieter operation are all factors that have improved oxygen concentrator performance. However, despite these improvements and manufacturer's claims, these units still require considerable maintenance and are subject to malfunction. Preventative maintenance and repair services should be provided by trained biomedical technicians.

The advantage of using oxygen concentrators is that the monthly cost to the patient is fixed, or generally not dependent on use. Also, oxygen concentrators are the easiest home oxygen system to use, and some of the newer models are somewhat transportable.

The disadvantages are that highly mobile patients may find the oxygen concentrator and its supportive portable oxygen cylinders too restrictive for an active life-style. Also, those patients who live in remote areas or areas subject to power outages must have sufficient cylinder backup. Most companies now provide a cylinder backup at no charge for patients using oxygen concentrators. Minor complaints from patients are the slight increases in the electric bill and the audible hum identified with oxygen concentrators, although most of the newer units have minimized these complaints substantially.

Concentrators are not cost-effective for those patients who use their oxygen intermittently or for an hour or so daily. Cylinder oxygen is a more cost-effective method of administering oxygen to these patients.

Because the size of an oxygen concentrator has been cut almost in half in the past four to five years, units can be delivered by an individual respiratory therapist alone, without the services of a truck driver or delivery technician. All follow-up visits are more easily scheduled on a regular basis and provided by the trained respiratory therapist.

Liquid oxygen systems provide the greatest advantage to the patient who is physically active, mobile, or in some cases still employable. These systems are lightweight and portable.

Liquid oxygen systems are technically no more than advanced designs of a thermos bottle. A vacuum-bottle system maintains the super-cool temperatures required to keep oxygen in a liquid state. Most systems designed for home care employ both a stationary unit, which is a large reservoir, and a small portable system that usually enables the patient to be ambulatory for up to eight hours. The small portable system is filled from the large stationary system in the patient's home. The stationary system is generally filled on a weekly basis from a service vehicle designed to fill a number of liquid oxygen reservoir systems.

The ambulatory capability with the liquid oxygen system represents the greatest advantage for those patients requiring home oxygen therapy. However, only a small percentage of those patients identified as needing home oxygen therapy can fully realize the advantages of the liquid oxygen system.

The disadvantages of the liquid oxygen system are its higher cost, the weekly reservoir refills, and more difficult operating procedures. Also inherent with any liquid system is that as much as 50 percent of the product may be lost through evaporation as the liquid oxygen warms and converts to gaseous oxygen. Flow rate, duration of use, and ambient temperature affect the amount of product lost in this evaporative process.

Of concern to the supplier is that liquid oxygen programs are somewhat more expensive to implement compared with the oxygen concentrator and cylinder components of home oxygen therapy. A specialized delivery vehicle is required for refilling liquid systems, and so the company must have a sufficient volume of patients to make the provision of this product worthwhile. Although liquid systems are somewhat more expensive than the oxygen concentrators, competition has closed the margin between the two systems.

Oxygen cylinders are the traditional method of oxygen delivery. Oxygen is compressed under high pressures into either steel or aluminum cylinders of various sizes. Depending on the size of the cylinder, the unit is referred to as a stationary or portable oxygen system. All cylinders require a regulator to adjust flow rate and a carrying case if the unit is portable. Large cylinders must be secured with chains or cylinder stands to prevent them from tipping over. Oxygen cylinders and other high-pressure gas cylinders present certain hazards and patients must be thoroughly educated in the proper handling of compressed gas cylinders.

The advantages of oxygen cylinders over other forms of home oxygen delivery systems are that the number of cylinders required is easily and clearly determined. Because reimbursement for most home oxygen therapy is based on gaseous cylinder equivalents, the costs can be determined in advance.

The disadvantages of using oxygen cylinders include the hazards associated with high-pressure cylinders and the need to consistently refill the cylinders when they are empty. Oxygen use should be clearly determined to prevent unscheduled cylinder deliveries by the supplier or interrupted oxygen service by the patient.

Those organizations evaluating whether to become involved in the oxygen delivery business should take note of the following:

- The organization should look at types of systems offered by current suppliers in a service area. If current systems are well established, a new provider may have difficulty in changing referral patterns.
- New suppliers should avoid liquid oxygen systems during the start-up phase of the company. The increased operational costs and scheduling requirements may present too many problems for a new organization. Generally, only 5 percent to 10 percent of those patients who qualify for home oxygen therapy are sufficiently ambulatory to justify their use of liquid oxygen systems. Referring this small percentage of patients to another supplier for this service may be more cost-effective. In some areas, liquid oxygen systems are so well entrenched that a new supplier may be required to implement this service initially if it wants to be competitive. Implementing a liquid oxygen program effectively requires special planning.
- As a result of the 1985 Medicare oxygen eligibility requirements, a significant percentage of home oxygen patients will not qualify for home oxygen therapy reimbursement in the future. In addition, a grandfather clause for all existing home oxygen patients expires sometime during 1986.

Home Respiratory Therapy

Many of the treatment therapies used for respiratory therapy in the hospital can also be offered in the home care setting. As in the hospital, these treatment therapies must be medically justified and should conform to the basic treatment criteria developed in the hospital setting. However, with the more judicious use of treatment therapies in the inpatient setting, the number of home care referrals has decreased somewhat over the past few years.

The treatment therapies generally found within the home care setting are intermittent positive pressure breathing (IPPB), small-volume nebulizer treatments, high-output nebulizers; and mechanical ventilation.

Intermittent positive pressure breathing (IPPB) is a treatment therapy that hyperinflates the lungs while delivering aerosolized medication. The use of this treatment therapy, which peaked in the 1970s, has declined through much of the 1980s. Many hospitals report that IPPB treatments have declined as much as 50 percent in the past two years. However, IPPB is still considered a viable clinical treatment therapy by many physicians. Therefore, in most instances, the home care supplier is required to offer this service. The use of IPPB requires the expertise of a respiratory therapist and periodic home care visits.

Small-volume nebulizer treatments are also used to deliver aerosolized medication to the patient's lungs. This treatment therapy, which is dependent on patient effort and cooperation, has generally replaced IPPB in both the inpatient and home care settings. Most professionals recommend these services be provided to the patients on a rental basis. However, for many patients, especially the younger patient who requires few supportive services, the purchase of the small volume nebulizer may be more cost-effective. Rental is still advised for those patients who require periodic monitoring by a registered nurse or respiratory therapist.

High-output nebulizers are devices that produce aerosols for humidification purposes. This type of device, which is generally driven by an air compressor, is used to humidify expired gases for tracheotomy patients. It may also be used for patients who have had upper airway disorders or surgical procedures. An ultrasonic nebulizer is also used to produce aerosols. High-frequency sound waves produce the finest of particles for use not only in humidification treatments but also in the administration of various medications. The use of ultrasonic nebulizers in the home care setting has declined with the decreased use of this therapy in the inpatient setting.

Home mechanical ventilation requires the highest level of technological and professional support provided to the home care patient. Professional commitment to the family and patient must begin weeks before discharge and continue throughout the course of the disease. Intensive training and preparation of the family is essential to the successful delivery of this service. Psychological preparation of the patient, family, and home care staff is also recommended for the successful implementation of the home care plan.

Mechanical ventilators used in the home care setting differ somewhat from those used in the hospital. Mechanical ventilators employed in the home are portable and have simple and tamper-resistent controls and battery-operation capability. The use of hospital ventilators in the home is usually not successful because the sophistication of this equipment generally confuses the patient and family and may discourage them from implementing the entire home care plan. In addition, battery operation, which is essential in case of electrical failure, is a feature generally not found on most ventilators used in the hospital.

Implementation of a mechanical ventilator program is not without its risk, however, and so entering this aspect of the DME business is not recommended until other aspects of the DME or home care business are well established. The level of technical expertise and professional commitment must be exceptional. Professional liability concerns are real and must be carefully weighed. The risks in this type of program have prevented many DME suppliers from providing this service. However, hospital-based DME programs should have the technical expertise necessary to implement this type of program.

Apnea Monitors

A home apnea monitor program is a specialized high-tech DME program. The unit, which monitors respiratory movements and heart rate, is usually placed on infants who are under 1 year of age and who are at risk for sudden infant death syndrome (SIDS). This high-tech program also requires special clinical expertise and commitment because of the potential liabilities of working with high-risk infants. Professional staff with pediatric experience should participate in this program. Both technical training in the use of the monitors and cardiopulmonary resuscitation must be taught to the infant's family before the infant is discharged from the hospital. Also, the psychological preparation of the family should be included as part of the training program. Although this program may be implemented by any DME supplier, those programs that are associated with hospitals having a neonatal service are more successful, both financially and in terms of high-quality patient care.

Because of their potential lifesaving capability, apnea monitors require periodic calibration and preventative maintenance by biomedical technicians. Technological advancements in recent years have improved the monitors themselves. They are much more reliable and portable and produce fewer false alarms. However, the importance of intensive educational training of the family to ensure that the equipment is properly operated cannot be overemphasized. Most service calls connected with the apnea monitor program result from poor preparation of the family or a lack of understanding of the procedures required for the proper operation of the unit.

Medical Equipment Division

The medical equipment division has the most diversified and most numerous products of the four DME divisions. The extent of the products offered is a function of market demand, clinical services, and the medical specialties practiced in the locale. Many low-volume items must be carried to effectively service referred clients, and a small number of less frequently used products may account for a disproportionate time commitment on the part of the supplier.

Medical equipment division products are generally less technical than those found in the other divisions and can be handled by nonprofessional personnel with technical training. Product categories offered by full-service medical equipment divisions are:

- Ambulatory aids
- Bathroom aids
- Hospital beds and accessories
- Wheelchairs and mobility equipment
- Decubitis care equipment

- Patient lift devices
- Pain control devices
- Blood glucose monitors
- Blood pressure monitors

Ambulatory Aids

Ambulatory aids refer to canes, crutches, and walkers. Most suppliers report that ambulatory aids represent a significant percentage of referrals in the medical equipment division. In many cases, the DME supplier is required to instruct or reinstruct the patient on the use of this equipment. Therefore, a physical therapist should be retained in a consultant capacity for in-service training. The physical therapist may also be called on infrequently to provide patient instruction in the home, although this service is generally provided by home care agencies after a physician referral.

Although somewhat differentiated by brand name, the generic categories of canes usually include the standard, offset handle, quad base, and pyramid. Quad-base canes account for the majority of referrals in most locations. Canes are generally purchased by the patient.

Suppliers should plan on maintaining the inventories of at least two or more manufacturers to meet the needs of the patients and community referral agencies because canes are generally purchased. Minor differences in design or construction often generate considerable debate among physical therapists, who are commonly loyal to one brand. A supply of replacement handles and cane tips should also be maintained to support these products.

A variety of walkers should also be stocked, primarily because of variations in patient size. Walker categories include the nonfolding, folding, wheeled, and a few specialty devices. Like the other ambulatory aids, walkers are generally purchased because of their relatively low cost and duration of use. However, when the duration of use is expected to be less than two months, rental is more cost-effective. Inventory requirements depend on referral patterns, although most suppliers find that one or two brands of walkers account for 90 percent or more of their business.

Crutches also are offered in a variety of configurations, from the standard wood crutch to various aluminum specialty crutches. Crutches are usually rented because use is expected to be for a short term. Specialty crutches are generally purchased. Replacement parts for crutches should be kept in stock.

Bathroom Aids

Commodes and bath aids also represent a significant number of referrals to a DME company, second only to the ambulatory aid category. Many dealers represent more than one manufacturer of bath aids to offer a wide selection of products to their patients and referral sources.

For sanitary reasons, the majority of these items are purchased rather than rented. Referral patterns usually dictate that a small number of items account for the vast majority of purchases.

Commodes are covered benefit items by most insurance carriers. Many of the other products in this category are not covered. Bathroom-assist bars, elevated toilet seats, and bath benches are not covered benefits by most carriers.

Hospital Beds and Accessories

Hospital beds do not represent the same volume of referrals as the other categories. Unlike ambulatory aids and commodes, which are usually purchased by the patient, hospital beds are rented. Because income from rentals provides a financial base for a DME business, hospital beds may be the most significant nonrespiratory item offered by the DME supplier.

Hospital beds are usually classified as manual, semielectric, or fully electric. Manual beds are adjusted with a crank. Electric beds are adjusted with patient-controlled motors. Semielectric and full electric beds differ only in the power capabilities of the height adjustment.

Reimbursement for hospital beds varies significantly between the manual and electric varieties. Physician documentation of patient need often determines the reimbursement level. Independent of documentation of need, suppliers in some locations provide only electric models as a marketing ploy or in response to the unjustified demands of referral sources. The reimbursement for hospital beds generally includes all required accessories. Bed rails and mattresses are generally included, if required in the rental rate. Over-bed tables are not a reimbursable benefit, although many suppliers may include them as a complimentary piece of equipment.

Trapeze units or patient-assist devices are frequently used in conjunction with the hospital bed. Trapeze units may be floor based but are more conveniently attached to the hospital bed. Also like the hospital beds themselves, the trapeze units are generally rented because of the relatively short time they will be needed.

A variety of traction apparatuses is also used in conjunction with the hospital bed. Traction requirements vary significantly with the needs of the patient. Although most traction equipment is of the basic variety, sophisticated orthopedic traction equipment may be employed in the home care setting. Many suppliers lack the expertise to administer more sophisticated traction applications. Hospital-trained orthopedic technicians may be helpful to DME companies when special applications are requested.

Wheelchairs and Mobility Equipment

Wheelchairs represent a diverse product category, with numerous options and modifications available. Most dealers maintain a basic wheelchair inventory for rental clients and also stock a number of specialty wheelchairs for custom applications or special patient needs. The basic rental wheelchair should be capable of being easily modified to offer a variety of arm and leg rests. An adaptable wheelchair line enables the dealer to serve a diverse population with a relatively small inventory.

Those DME programs that serve rehabilitation institutes, pediatric hospitals, or other specialty centers are required to stock more diverse and specialized wheelchair lines. Some patients from these centers may require customized features, and providing these kinds of services may necessitate the employment of staff trained in wheelchair modification. Custom wheelchair preparation is a DME specialty service and is not recommended for new companies or those without a sufficient patient base for this service. Obviously, most custom wheelchairs are purchased by the patient rather than rented. Sports wheelchairs and custom electric wheelchair applications represent additional specialty areas.

Decubitis Care Equipment

Decubitis care equipment is designed to prevent or treat tissue breakdown resulting from confinement to a bed or wheelchair. Various devices use air, gel, water, or foam to reduce pressure on affected body surfaces. The reduced pressure improves blood flow and prevents pressure sores from developing.

Prevention rather than treatment of pressure sores is preferred. Treatment of pressure sores is difficult, painful, and a long-term process that in some cases requires admission to a hospital or skilled nursing facility. Representatives from DME companies may be justified, however, in suggesting decubitis care equipment for patients confined to bed or wheelchairs.

Patient Lift Devices

Patient lift devices are used to transfer paralyzed or flaccid patients for short distances. Most units employ a variety of seats or slings that are adaptable to most patient needs. These units are particularly useful when a patient is cared for by a single individual. Care givers must be well trained in the operation of these devices because improperly used devices may cause severe injury to the patient. Also, some homes have insufficient hallway or floor space to accommodate the use of these units.

Seatlift chairs are effective for the partially ambulatory patient. A patient who can use a seatlift chair may not need to rent a hospital bed. A number of unscrupulous DME dealers have promoted the seatlift chair as Medicare-funded furniture. In response, the Health Care Financing Administration (HCFA) has now launched a study on the effectiveness of the seatlift chair. The results of this study are expected to effect reimbursement or coverage for this item.

Pain Control Devices

Pain can be controlled by using transcutaneous electronic nerve stimulation (TENS) devices. The units are usually rented for the first month to evaluate the effectiveness of the technique. Subsequently, they are purchased or returned. Patients also require supply items on a continuing basis. As TENS is becoming more accepted, many facilities are reporting a substantial growth in their pain control departments.

Blood Glucose Monitors

The use of blood glucose monitors is also a rapidly growing home monitoring program. Many diabetics have found this program helpful in monitoring and controlling their disease. A small drop of blood is placed on a paper monitor strip, which is inserted into the blood glucose monitor. The monitor then analyzes the reaction of the blood with the chemicals contained on the monitor strip and indicates the blood glucose level. Measurement of the blood glucose level allows patients to adjust their diet or insulin in response to their life-style.

Blood Pressure Monitors

The increased use of blood pressure monitors is also indicative of patients' assuming more responsibility for their care. Even though blood pressure equipment is not generally a covered benefit, sales appear to be brisk throughout the country. Growth in this area is expected to continue.

Medical-Surgical Supply Division

The medical-surgical supply division is primarily concerned with the sale of home care supplies. Home care supplies may be delivered in conjunction with other DME services, but most often these items are purchased in a showroom or store environment. Although this division is dependent on walk-in trade, the DME business is not generally dependent on a showroom environment. Suppliers find that patients exhibit brand loyalty, and advertising may be effective in developing this portion of the business.

This division is divided into five distinct departments:

- Incontinent and urology supplies
- Ostomy supplies
- Surgical dressings
- Orthopedic supplies
- Miscellaneous supplies

Incontinent and Urology Supplies

Incontinent supplies and adult diapers represent a rapidly growing market, especially as the public becomes more educated and enlightened concerning incontinent disorders. If this business is to succeed, showroom staff must be especially sensitive to the problems of the incontinent patient.

A variety of urinary catheters and irrigation trays are necessary to support an active urology service. In many areas, advanced urology techniques are being performed in the home care setting. Product support by the DME dealer of new techniques allows the urological patient greater freedom and a reduced number of hospital or clinic visits.

Ostomy Supplies

A significant commitment to a diverse line of specialized products is necessary to develop an ostomy department. The various sizes, styles, and types of appliances dictate a substantial inventory investment. Many suppliers find it necessary to offer two or more ostomy lines to satisfy client preference. Ostomy patients rarely change appliance brands. Personalized service ensures customer loyalty.

New technology has improved ostomy appliances to allow the patient to have a more active life-style. Several professional athletes serve as role models for ostomates, and their lives demonstrate that ostomy procedures need not be restrictive.

Surgical Dressings

A selection of surgical dressings, gauzes, and bandages are usually included in the showroom facility. Although few DME companies report significant walk-in trade, a full-service DME dealer must offer these products.

A careful selection of products to be offered reduces inventory cost and improves profitability. Communication with local hospitals and home care agencies more clearly identifies product needs for home care. Some home care agencies have reported specialty supply markets developing for wound care and burn and respiratory services.

Orthopedic Supplies

Orthopedic supplies are also seen in most DME showrooms. A DME dealer should maintain a basic inventory of slings, cervical collars, and braces.

Few DME dealers have a significant enough referral base to gain proficiency in custom prosthetic and orthotic devices, which are generally considered as a separate health care business. A DME company should develop relationships with reputable prosthetic and orthotic firms for the referral of specialty patients. As prosthetic and orthotic dealers often receive requests for DME services, they may in fact refer the patient back to the DME company for high-tech needs.

Miscellaneous Supplies

Surgical support hose are offered in many locations. However, like many other product services, this line is offered for the convenience of the patient and referral agency. Other products that are seen in a DME showroom include patient convenience products, rehabilitation and occupational therapy supplies, and a selection of heat therapy devices.

Nutritional Support Division

Nutritional support programs have received considerable attention for several reasons. First, many sources have reported substantial profits from offering these services. However, carriers have subsequently reacted to these reports in the form of reduced reimbursement levels and more stringent eligibility requirements. This division can be the most profitable division, but it also presents the greatest financial risk. Second, hospitals are eager to discharge appropriate patients earlier, and some of these patients may need nutritional support therapies if they are to leave the hospital. Sophisticated technology for nutritional support permits shorter inpatient lengths of stay and greater treatment opportunities in the home setting.

Organizations considering entry into the nutritional support area need to determine the projected use of home nutritional support services in their community. Insurance coverage, physician confidence, and the ability of families to accept this type of patient ultimately determine the volume of services in the home. Thus, differentiating the potential market for home care services from actual use of such services is important. The high cost of these services precludes the participation by most individuals in such a program without adequate insurance coverage.

The DME division that has received much media attention in recent months has been the nutritional support division, which consists of four product services:

- Enteral nutrition support therapy
- Parenteral nutritional therapy
- Intravenous (IV) antibiotic therapy
- Chemotherapy

Enteral Nutritional Support Therapy

Enteral nutritional support therapy refers to the administration of nutritional supplements to a patient with gastrointestinal problems. This therapy is fairly well tolerated by patients in the home and requires a minimal amount of support care after initial patient instruction. Patient education begins while the patient is still hospitalized. However, the DME company must have professional staff capable of answering questions from the patient and family.

The administration of the appropriate nutritional supplement is prescribed by the physician. The nutritional supplements themselves are regulated to meet the patient's current caloric, electrolyte, and other nutritional needs. In many cases, adverse reactions can usually be controlled by changing the formula of the nutritional solution. Most formulas today are premixed and easily prepared and administered by patients or their families in the home care setting. Formulas are also now available to aid patients with nutritional problems not related to gastrointestinal problems. Malnutrition, chronic obstructive pulmonary disease, and special electrolyte disorders are now treated by a variety of nutritional supplements.

Parenteral Nutritional Therapy

Parenteral nutritional therapy uses intravenous solutions for the administration of fats, sugar, nutrients, and electrolytes. The parenteral solutions themselves are prepared by a licensed pharmacy and administered through a special indwelling catheter to patients in a home care setting. These therapies are used for patients with severe problems of the gastrointestinal system. Parenteral therapy is closely monitored by laboratory testing, and solution formulas are adjusted in response to the test results.

An effective parenteral therapy program usually requires a close working relationship among the DME supplier, pharmacist, physician, and representative of the home care agency. Those suppliers that have an affiliated pharmacy operation are usually able to provide a more coordinated program than are other independent suppliers. Hospitals with both affiliated DME and home care agencies may have an even more coordinated service. Several national home parenteral services have also developed expertise in this specialized area. These companies may have improved operating efficiencies because of a larger patient volume.

Sufficient volume or need for this service must be related to reimbursement issues. Coverage must be guaranteed before initiation of therapy to ensure that both patient and supplier have confidence in the arrangement. Coverage for home parenteral therapy remains somewhat volatile and inconsistent among carriers. Medicare has attempted to provide a more consistent administration of its program by using two national intermediaries. However, considerable change in the guidelines for reimbursement are expected over the next few years.

Antibiotic Therapy

The use of home IV antibiotic therapy is also growing rapidly but is somewhat limited because Medicare does not reimburse for this service. However, other carriers have realized considerable cost savings when patients use home IV antibiotic therapy rather than staying in the hospital.

The IV antibiotics are administered over several hours through a small IV catheter controlled by an infusion pump. Newer mini infusion pumps are usually battery powered so that patients can remain ambulatory.

Chemotherapy

Related to the home IV antibiotic program is the chemotherapy program. Chemotherapy agents are infused through an intravenous catheter. The infusion rate is again controlled by a mini infusion pump. The role of the DME supplier in home chemotherapy is to provide the necessary equipment in the form of an infusion pump, supplies, and IV administration sets. Specialized pharmacies must prepare the chemotherapy agents and bill for these drugs.

Operational Issues

During the planning and development of a DME company, several operational issues must be considered before the business plan can be completed. The two major issues are the staffing model and facility selection. The product services provided by the company determine the type of facility required and the level and type of personnel required.

Staffing

Although the industry has not yet established standard job descriptions or titles, the job functions unique to the DME industry can be classified as follows:

- Customer service representatives
- Professional staff
- Technical staff
- Billing staff
- Management staff

The administrative and financial functions common to the DME business do not differ significantly from those in other health care businesses. However, management should have a thorough understanding of the job duties and responsibilities of the positions unique to the DME industry.

The *customer service representative* is critical to the operation of a DME business. This individual is responsible for all referral activity and for the coordination of patient services. The individual not only is required to perform a variety of office procedures but must also excel in communication skills. Sensitivity to the needs of the ill and elderly are required personal traits. Background or experience in a medical discipline or medical setting is recommended for this position.

A DME company employs a *professional staff* of respiratory therapists or respiratory therapy technicians. The level of expertise required in the professional staff should be commensurate with the clinical services offered by the DME company. Job requirements for the professional staff should meet or exceed those required by local hospitals. Home care training or experience is desirable. Many respiratory therapy programs now have special courses in respiratory home care. Depending on the level of activity, some home care companies employ physical therapists, occupational therapists, or orthopedic technicians. However, the respiratory therapist has often been trained to perform basic functions common to the other disciplines.

The *technical staff* of a DME company consists of the home care technician or warehouse employee. This service employee is instructed on specific technical tasks to support the professional staff. Usually this individual assists the professional staff in difficult deliveries, delivers oxygen cylinders, refills oxygen reservoirs, and performs a variety of warehouse duties. This individual is not qualified to perform any professional services.

Billing is done by a billing clerk, who is responsible for reporting the various patient services performed to the appropriate insurance carrier. This individual may also field questions from patients concerning their bills and communicate various reimbursement policies to them. Familiarity with professional office billing is essential.

The *DME manager* coordinates the referral process, professional operations, warehousing, and billing. and so must have expertise in each of these areas. Professionals with hospital supervisory experience often are excellent candidates for this position. Experience with home care personnel helps the manager to be aware of many of the issues and problems affecting the home care patient. Nursing, physical therapy, and pharmacy are all acceptable backgrounds for DME managers. Large DME programs may employ a manager for each of the DME divisions.

In summary, the DME business has not matured sufficiently to have developed formal and standard job descriptions. The job duties vary considerably from office to office and depend on individual expertise. Personnel with both the necessary clinical background and understanding of the business aspects of this field are limited. In today's market, the quality of services is so dependent on reputable, experienced personnel that many companies are aggressively recruiting these individuals.

Facility Selection

Selection of the ideal DME facility is determined by a number of factors. In some locations, retail space availability and the financial capability of the organization influence the selection process. As with any new business, phased-growth plans should be incorporated into the long-term business strategy. However, the organization should not incur unreasonable costs by acquiring space that will not be effectively used. Generally, three areas must be identified in facility planning: a showroom floor, office space, and warehouse space.

Allocation for showroom space is most dependent on the services offered by the medical equipment division. Sufficient floor space should be allocated for display areas and floor stock. Shelving requirements should be proportionate to the services and items provided. Areas for community service projects, health care screening, and family consultation should be considered. A fitting room is required if the DME program provides orthopedic supports, braces, or surgical stockings.

A prime retail location is not required for a successful DME business. Even companies with substantial showroom traffic often do not experience the sales volume to justify a prime retail location. Proximity to a hospital campus may be more critical to the success of a DME business. If a prime retail location is desired, then the administrative and warehousing functions should be located elsewhere.

Adequate office space should be provided for administrative, financial, billing, and professional activities. Space allocation for computer services must be considered for all DME programs.

Warehouse space must be segregated into rental and sales areas. Rental inventory and supplies require a relatively small storage area. A specific area for storage of hospital beds may allow for more efficient use of floor space in the warehouse. Rental inventory space requirements are easily defined, as in-house inventory changes minimally in response to volume.

Sales inventory space must support both the showroom and home care activities. Turnover of products and accessibility to manufacturers and suppliers are important determinants in the level of inventory maintained. Most observers believe that inventory levels grow to meet space availability. Observers also think that like many businesses, many DME suppliers maintain far too much inventory.

Reimbursement

Reimbursement for DME services represents a great challenge for companies. Past abuse of the system by suppliers and reports of windfall profits have prompted carriers to more closely regulate the industry. Medicare has been the most aggressive in its regulatory response to the DME industry. As Medicare represents 70 percent to 80 percent of the DME suppliers' gross revenue, these regulations have a significant impact. In addition, other carriers usually follow Medicare-instituted guidelines. The growth of all home care and the associated cost shifting also has contributed to the regulatory efforts of Medicare.

Briefly, the DME program is reimbursed under the Medicare Part B benefit. As with other Part B benefits, the client must elect coverage and pay a premium for Part B benefits. The Medicare Part B program also has a deductible amount that must be met yearly. Medicare reimburses 80 percent of approved charges. The patient has a 20 percent copayment responsibility. Many patients have Medicare supplemental benefits from private carriers that are designed to cover the copayment amount.

Recent Medicare changes with regard to the DME program have resulted in equipment being classified as either expensive or inexpensive. *Inexpensive equipment* is defined as equipment having a purchase price of less than $120. Under the Medicare rent or purchase guidelines, inexpensive equipment should generally be purchased rather than rented. If the claim is submitted as a rental, rental payments cannot exceed the purchase price of the equipment.

Expensive equipment, which is defined as equipment with a purchase price of more than $120, may be rented or purchased by the Medicare participant. If the expected duration of use indicates that the equipment should be purchased rather than rented, the Medicare intermediary will recommend the purchase of the equipment. When that recommendation is made, continued rental payments are applied to the purchase price of the equipment. Again, rental payments cannot exceed the purchase price of the equipment. However, rental payments made prior to the determination are not subtracted from the maximum reimbursement amount.

Oxygen therapy equipment and other high-tech items have been excluded from the rent or purchase guidelines. The high-maintenance requirements and services necessary to administer these product services generally prohibit the sale of this equipment. However, stringent eligibility requirements for home respiratory patients and patients requiring enteral or parenteral services were also implemented in 1985. Blood gases and other laboratory tests must document the clinical need for home oxygen therapy. Extensive physician documentation is required for enteral or parenteral services. Medicare does not provide coverage for IV antibiotics or chemotherapy.

Reimbursement for the DME industry was completely restructured during 1985, and intermediaries have been slow to respond to changes instituted by HCFA. This situation has caused considerable delay in claims processing and subsequent cash-flow problems for many DME businesses. Although the major impact of these reimbursement changes occurred in 1985, fine tuning of the reimbursement mechanisms will continue throughout 1987. Major revisions in parenteral and enteral programs are scheduled for release in 1987. Program initiatives affecting the oxygen therapy program, and specifically oxygen concentrators, were implemented during 1985. Liquid oxygen services were not considered during this initial revision. However, the use of liquid oxygen has been targeted for program review.

Financial Considerations

The amount of capital required to develop a DME business depends on the product services selected, staffing model, facility location, and volume.

Program options must be selected prior to the development of detailed financial pro formas.

However, the most important factor in determining required capital costs is volume. Detailed research into referral patterns and statistics must be performed. The use of guaranteed referral sources and accurate estimates of projected market penetration are also required.

As with any capital-intensive industry, the accuracy of volume projections presents a good news and bad news situation. Programs considerably more successful than projected are also more profitable but in turn require more investment capital. As with any other program, insufficient development capital is the major cause of business failure.

Capital requirements are easily and accurately determined once volume and product services are known. A DME program serving a 500-bed hospital with a phased program plan requires $200,000 to $300,000. A program serving a hospital with 100 to 150 beds may require $80,000 to $100,000. Again, small hospitals with active clinical services and home care departments may outperform much larger institutions. The importance of accurate discharge planning statistics cannot be overemphasized.

A Final Word

A DME program can be an important part of a hospital's diversification strategy. To be successful, the business must be managed as a DME business and not as a hospital department. Risk can be controlled by developing a well-researched business plan. The business plan should contain a phased program approach consistent with the financial capabilities and expertise of the organization. Quality must be demonstrated for product services offered. Companies affiliated with health care institutions must reflect positively on the community, or the community will react negatively to the hospitals' new health care strategy.

Chapter 13

Contracting with Health Maintenance Organizations

William D. Cabin

Health maintenance organizations (HMOs) were originally developed in the 1920s primarily by proprietary companies, such as Kaiser, as not-for-profit, full-service health care delivery systems for their employees. The function of these early HMOs was to prevent health problems and provide access to relevant care for employees working at construction sites or manufacturing locations and for their families. The HMO provided this health care at a set premium rate. Covered care was provided by a specified group of physicians and hospitals that were under contract to the HMO. Other early HMOs were not-for-profit experimental ventures that were sponsored by a clinic or community group.

The use of HMOs as a mechanism for health care cost containment did not occur until the 1960s, when the federal government became interested in HMOs. At the same time, the Department of Health, Education, and Welfare (now the Department of Health and Human Services) was funding research on prospective pricing systems for inpatient hospital services under Medicare. The federal government, and other payers as well, looked at HMOs and the developing Medicare system of diagnosis-related groups (DRGs) as a means of reducing health care costs.

When the federal government created the federally qualified HMO in 1973, only 72 HMOs were in existence nationwide. The HMO Act of 1973 gave federally qualified HMOs preferential access to employees, loans, and grants and exemption from restrictive state HMO laws. The legislation was followed by a series of demonstration projects that examined the application

---

William D. Cabin, J.D., M.A., is an independent health care consultant affiliated with Home Health Associates, Totowa, New Jersey.

of the HMO concept to Medicare beneficiaries. In 1982 Congress passed the Tax Equity and Fiscal Responsibility Act of 1982 (TEFRA), and in 1985 regulations were adopted creating the so-called Medicare HMO and competitive medical plan (CMP). The goal of the Medicare HMO and CMP is to enroll Medicare beneficiaries and channel them to appropriate and less costly forms of care, thus saving the Medicare program millions of dollars.

Because of the emphasis on cost containment, HMOs have experienced tremendous growth. Between 1973 and 1983, the number of HMOs increased from 72 to 283, and as of December 1985, an estimated 480 HMOs had more than 21 million enrollees. Although most HMOs still cater to the nonelderly population, HMOs have rapidly entered the Medicare HMO program. As of October 1986, only 20 months after the final Medicare HMO-CMP regulations were published, the Office of Prepaid Health Care of the Health Care Financing Administration (HCFA) estimated that nearly 200 HMOs had become Medicare HMOs; this figure represents about 42 percent of all HMOs. A total of about 900,000 Medicare beneficiaries were already enrolled in an HMO.

Administrators of home care agencies must be aware at the outset that the motivating force for most HMOs is containing costs and generating surplus revenue, or profit margin. The ability to meet this bottom-line goal requires the HMO to keep its actual per member, or enrollee, cost of care lower than the payments made by various payers (Medicare, Medicaid, employers, or insurers). This prospective fixed-rate payment structure of HMOs forces home care agencies and other providers to be price competitive in seeking an HMO contract. The HMO will look for proof that home care agencies or other providers can decrease the HMO's use of forms of care, such as hospitalization and treatment by specialists, that cost more. This emphasis has increased as HMOs are used for Medicare beneficiaries and as the HMO industry itself has become increasingly a for-profit industry. As of December 1985, the private consulting group Interstudy (Excelsior, Minnesota) estimated that approximately 52 percent of all HMOs were for-profits, and these HMOs handle approximately one-third of all HMO enrollees.

This chapter discusses the contract negotiation procedure between hospital-based or hospital-related home care agencies and HMOs. It describes the process of:

- Assessing the HMO to decide whether to submit a proposal
- Developing the proposal
- Negotiating the contract

Assessing the HMO

The first stage of the process is to assess the nature of the HMO to determine what, if any, home care products and services are salable to the HMO.

What is salable to one HMO may not be salable to another. Salability depends on factors such as the HMOs structure and governance, its client population, its investors, its emphasis on elderly versus nonelderly members, and the clinical profile and utilization patterns of its members and participating physicians. Before developing an actual proposal to an HMO, the home care agency should gather relevant information on these and other areas to convince the HMO of the agency's ability to reduce inpatient and specialty physician utilization by HMO members. This section examines areas relevant to such an assessment.

Structure and Governance

The home care agency needs to find out who owns the HMO, what staffing model is used by the HMO, whether the HMO is federally qualified, and what state regulations apply.

Ownership

The home care agency should determine who owns the HMO. If the HMO is owned, in part or completely, by physicians, a clinic, or a hospital that is antagonistic to the home care agency, the agency may not want to submit a proposal. On the other hand, a linkage between the agency and one or more hospitals that have an ownership interest in the HMO should help obtain acceptance of the agency's proposal. Such relations also may make it easier for the agency to use its regular rate schedule even if some other home care agencies have rates that are somewhat, but not appreciably, lower. Any connection with an investor should be mentioned in any proposal submission.

Extensive physician ownership may also affect the predisposition of physicians to use their offices, clinics, group practices, or other outpatient facilities instead of home care. Acquiring ownership and HMO utilization data aids the home care agency in detecting the actual or potential existence of such practices by physicians. If such a predisposition is detected, the home care agency may want to include a paid home-visit component in its proposal.

Model Type

The home care agency should determine the staffing model used by the HMO. The staffing model varies depending on the organization of the HMO's physicians. The *staff model HMO* employs salaried physicians at central locations. The *group model* usually has physician group practices or a clinic as its base. The *IPA (individual practice association) model* uses an organization of group practices and physicians in private practice.

Physicians involved in HMOs that do not use the staff model may have a greater incentive than staff-model physicians to use home care to contain hospital utilization because cost and utilization rates directly affect their revenues from the HMO. Many HMOs set aside 10 to 20 percent of the contractual fee due to a participating physician in a *withhold pool* pending a year-end review of the physicians' hospital utilization. If the physicians meet or better the established HMO per member targets for inpatient utilization, they receive their withheld funds; if they exceed their targets, their share of the pool remains with the HMO to cover the loss. Some HMOs are developing incentives that give physicians their withhold-pool funds plus a bonus if their inpatient utilization is less than their target.

The nature of the HMO model also affects the accessibility of home care agency staff and clients to the HMO. The more centralized the location of the HMO's physicians, the greater the access. Thus, HMOs based on staff and group practice models that have specific clinic sites may be more accessible to home care agencies. The distance of the HMO's key referral sites from the home care agency affects mileage and time costs for the provision by the home care agency of on-site home care coordinators.

Federal Qualification Status

The home care agency should determine if the HMO is *federally qualified.* A federally qualified HMO must meet certain requirements in such areas as enrollment, coverage, management, board composition, quality assurance, and fiscal viability.[1]

In addition, federally qualified HMOs can force employers having 25 or more employees in the HMO's service area to offer one staff-model or group-model HMO and one IPA-model HMO in addition to whatever other insurance coverage the employer offers. This requirement is called the *dual choice requirement.*

Federal qualification may help the agency assess the HMO's credibility and market potential. It is not, however, an indicator of the quality of services.

Home care agencies should be aware that federally qualified HMOs are required by law to provide home care as one of their basic health care services. The HMO may provide this home care itself through contracts with individual health care professionals or use a home care agency. The policy of HCFA, which as of late 1986 is still being reviewed, is that the home care agency used by the HMO must be Medicare certified.

State Requirements

The home care agency should ascertain if the state laws governing HMOs mandate home care benefits and the nature of that mandate. As of October 1985, 16 states require HMOs to have a home care benefit, according to the Blue Cross and Blue Shield associations.[2]

Services and Enrollment

The home care agency needs to find out what the HMO's service area is, what services are covered by the HMO, what kinds of clients are enrolled in the HMO, how eligibility for home care is determined, and what supplemental coverage, if any, is supplied by the HMO. Knowing whether the HMO's members are primarily over or under 65 years of age helps the home care agency determine the kind of services it may want to include in its proposal. For instance, if the HMO has a membership with many families, the home care agency may want to propose programs for maternity patients who are discharged early or programs for well children or children with special medical problems. The home care agency's proposal can also be affected significantly by whether such Medicare eligibility criteria as being homebound or requiring intermittent care are used by the HMO.

Service Area

The home care agency should determine if the HMO's service area coincides with the agency's service area. If it does not, the home care agency may want to consider forming a consortium of agencies and submitting a proposal to cover the entire service area.

The home care agency must also determine if the HMO expects the agency to serve only the agency's service area or beyond. Providing services beyond the agency's service area affects costs and therefore may affect the agency's desire to participate. If the HMO has locations statewide or nationally and the home care agency is linked to a statewide or national hospital or health care system, a statewide proposal should be considered.

Covered Services

The home care agency should obtain a copy of the HMO's coverage policies. An HMO may offer more than one policy, and the policies may vary as to covered services and the use and levels of copayments, deductibles, and other requirements. Home care agencies particularly want to see how home care services are defined, including any limits on the number of visits allowed, the length of visits, or total length of stay in the home care program. Also, the home care agency should ascertain how approval for home care is obtained, who makes these decisions in the HMO, whether a prior authorization system is used, how requests for additional care are handled, and what type of utilization review is included for home care.

Some HMOs cover only skilled nursing and several therapies (physical, speech, or occupational), but not home health aides. Some HMOs allow registered nurses and licensed practical nurses to provide care; others do not. The limits on therapy services may vary. Some HMOs may also cover therapies as a separate item, thus creating a benefit that competes with the home care agency. Also, other competing services may exist. For instance, some HMOs cover home care but also have a separate benefit covering house calls made by physicians or home visits by nurses based in a physician's office or group practice location. Most HMO coverage policies list such exclusions, and some of them may be relevant to the decision by a home care agency to submit a proposal.

The nature of coverage or exclusions also may influence whether the agency submits a proposal by itself for one type of home care service, such as skilled care, or becomes part of a package proposal with other providers that covers a range of home care services and products. In the latter situation, the home care agency may want to submit a proposal as a broker for a broad range of covered or noncovered services, for example, skilled care services, durable medical equipment (DME), pharmaceuticals, and intravenous (IV) therapies; or the agency may want to submit a joint proposal with other providers. Thus, knowing if custodial care, private-duty nursing, DME, oxygen equipment and oxygen, medical supplies, pharmaceuticals, and other services are covered by the HMO is important.

If the home care agency is tied to a related organization that supplies certain products or services, then it may want to structure its proposal to include these products and services. This decision may be particularly relevant to a home care agency that is part of or related to a diversified hospital, hospital system, or broader health care system. The home care agency should keep in mind that a contract to provide only covered services can also give the agency a preferential referral position for providing noncovered home care services to HMO enrollees on a private-duty basis.

Enrollment

The home care agency should determine the size of the HMO's enrollee population, including the names of specific employers contracting with the HMO. For instance, an agency may prefer to work with an HMO that has 20,000 enrollees and is sponsored by two major local hospitals rather than an HMO that is based in one small clinic and has 2,000 enrollees. This kind of information is particularly important if the home care agency wants to contract with more than one HMO.

The home care agency should also determine if the HMO is a *Medicare HMO* because this determination affects the size and nature of the actual and potential enrollment population.[3] If an HMO is not a Medicare HMO, its patient population is largely non-Medicare and under 65 years of age. Such a patient population is a new one for most Medicare-dependent home care agencies. As a result, the agency may have to offer new services or programs, such as early maternity discharge and well-child and other pediatric home care, in its proposal to the HMO.

Home care agencies should be aware that to become a Medicare HMO, an HMO must provide at least all Medicare-covered home care services. The same requirement holds for the HMO's provision of other health care services normally provided its Medicare enrollees under their regular Medicare coverage, for example, hospital and physician services, skilled nursing care, and DME. The Medicare-covered home care services may be provided by the HMO directly, by contract with individual independent contractors, or by contract with a home care agency. If a home care agency is used, it must be Medicare certified. The policy of HCFA is unclear on whether a Medicare-certified agency must be used if the HMO also chooses to provide supplemental home care services, that is, coverage beyond the Medicare home care benefit.

Eligibility Requirements

The home care agency should determine what eligibility requirements for home care are mandated by the HMO. For instance, must the patient be homebound or in need of skilled care? Must care be medically reasonable and necessary? Is prior hospitalization required? Is prior authorization required? Is physician certification or recertification needed? The eligibility requirements also affect the degree to which the home care agency must modify its existing admissions procedures.

Medicare Supplemental Coverage

The home care agency should ascertain if the HMO issues a Medicare supplemental insurance policy and, if so, the nature of the policy and the number of subscribers. Such policies may be issued by an HMO or related company whether or not the HMO is a Medicare HMO. The existence, use, and nature of such a policy affects the potential population. For example, a non-Medicare HMO still may gain significant access to the elderly population by sponsoring a Medicare supplemental coverage policy just as any other insurer could. Thus, although the elderly may not enroll as Medicare HMO enrollees, they may use the HMO's participating providers for supplemental coverage. In addition, if a Medicare HMO also has a Medicare supplemental coverage policy, it has even more comprehensive control over determining the nature and extent of the care given to elderly population.

Working Relationships

The home care agency needs to find out how the HMO works with other providers, what the HMO thinks about exclusivity arrangements, and how it handles information collection and billing.

Other Participating Providers

The home care agency should obtain a list of hospitals, physicians, and other providers that have contracted with the HMO. This list is a potential reference source for evaluating the HMO's performance, particularly if the home care agency is linked to a hospital that participates in the HMO. The list also allows the agency to assess the extent to which its own hospital and physician referral base may be expanded by an HMO contract or threatened if the contract goes to a competing home care agency.

A linkage between the HMO and a hospital already participating in the HMO may favorably affect the politics and economics of obtaining a contract. In fact, executive officers of hospital-sponsored or hospital-related home care agencies should request the hospital administrator to notify the agency when an HMO approaches the hospital for a participating provider contract. The home care agency then has an opportunity to acquire assessment information and to negotiate its potential contract as a package with the hospital's services. Because most HMOs usually seek hospital and physician contracts before seeking other provider contracts, this notice also gives the home care agency a head start in preparing its proposal and, possibly, in acquiring the home care contract.

Exclusivity

The home care agency should ascertain whether the HMO intends to sign an exclusive contract with only one home care provider, with or without a competitive bidding process, or sign a series of nonexclusive contracts. The agency should also find out if the HMO requires the agency to contractually agree to not sign contracts with other HMOs. Any such proposal requirements should be reviewed by legal counsel for possible antitrust implications.

In nonexclusive contract situations, the HMO lets the individual physician decide on a home care agency. Usually, a designated HMO employee gives the physician data on the home care agency's prices. As a result, the home care agency should find out if that employee approves the physician's referral or only provides relevant data. Some HMOs will not sign any contract with a home care agency; instead these HMOs leave the decision to the individual physician and patient.

Information Base and Billing

The home care agency should determine the nature of the HMO's collection, maintenance, and retrieval of information and its electronics data processing (EDP) capabilities. The nature and compatibility of EDP systems affects access to records and enrollee identification information and affects the time it takes to process claims.

A hospital-sponsored or hospital-related home care agency may find the hospital's EDP system more compatible with the HMO than the agency's system. The agency may thus be able to piggyback on the hospital's system. Such compatibility may also facilitate the agency's access to HMO enrollment and utilization data, thus aiding the assessment process.

The home care agency should also determine whether the agency may use its existing billing and plan-of-treatment forms or whether other forms must be used.

Developing the Proposal

Once the assessment process has been completed, the home care agency should be in a position to write an effective proposal. In developing the proposal, the home care agency must remember that the HMO may not know or be convinced of the value of home care in containing HMO expenditures. Thus, the agency's proposal should *sell* the ability of home care to control costs. Specific examples of how home care has safely reduced hospital inpatient use should be included. Not only should the proposal sell home care, but it must also contain one or more attractive service and pricing options that the home care agency can provide the HMO. This section discusses some suggested elements to include in a proposal.

Description of the Home Care Agency

A basic description of the home care agency should include, but not be limited to, the following:

- Number of years in business
- Certification, licensure, and accreditation status
- Not-for-profit or for-profit status
- Size of service area
- Range of services
- Related organizations
- Linkages to other health care providers

The discussion of the range of services and available programs should be as specific as possible and should include any time frames for duration of visits by Medicare service, for example, skilled nursing, home health aides, therapies (physical, speech, or occupational), and medical social services. The description should also mention whether the home care agency has coverage 24 hours a day, 7 days a week, and both scheduled and on-call coverage.

Home Care Policies

The home care agency should indicate that the following home care policies will be mutually established with the HMO:

- Definition of home care
- Eligibility requirements

- Admissions and discharge procedures
- Billing policies and procedures
- Utilization review reporting requirements

Patient Records

A brief description of the system used by the home care agency for patient health records should be included in the proposal. Also included should be the fact that the home care agency will instruct appropriate HMO staff on how to use the the home care agency's system.

Potential Savings

The home care agency should develop specific examples, at least by admission category, of potential savings to the HMO from the use of home care. The examples should stress that home care can:

- Reduce inpatient admissions and average length of stay
- Result in a reduction in the chances of HMO physicians losing their withhold-risk pool when such an arrangement exists
- Increase the available year-end size of the HMO's inpatient fund and the HMO's and the physician's market share

The *inpatient fund* is the fund of monies allocated in the HMO budget to cover inpatient hospitalization costs. As inpatient use decreases below the budgeted target, the amount of surplus in the fund increases. This surplus minimizes the need to use the withhold pool to cover inpatient fund loses, increases the physicians share of withhold pool funds, and creates an additional surplus fund that the HMO may split with the physicians. The use of the interrelated inpatient and withhold pool funds between the HMO and physicians in surplus and deficit situations varies among HMOs.

In essence, the home care agency should show specifically how it can help the HMO achieve or exceed its cost and utilization targets. In developing such projections, the home care agency should use credible data about hospital inpatient and home care utilization and costs. Failure to use credible data may result in unrealistic expectations and jeopardize the home care agency's ability to obtain, renew, or expand its contract with the HMO. The sequence in making projections should be:

- Establish assumed hospital admission rates (usually per 1,000 HMO enrollees) by admissions category (broad categories such as obstetrics, surgical, and pediatrics)
- Establish possible average reductions in length of stay (for example, a half day per case) by admissions category when home care is used

Hospital-based agencies are in an advantageous position to obtain the data on admission rates by admission category because of the availability of hospital data. Such data can give a good approximation of projected HMO enrollee utilization. The best source, of course, is the HMO's own internal data.

After collecting this data, the home care agency should develop a specific admissions rate example. The elements to be included in the admission rate example are:

- Projected inpatient admission rate for the HMO.
- Projected number of HMO member months for services. Member months are the total number of months in which all HMO members are enrolled in the HMO in a given year.
- List of admission categories
- Projected admissions per admission category
- Projected length of stay (LOS) by admission category

The accuracy of the data assumptions in the specific admissions rate example would be enhanced if the agency could obtain actual data from the HMO itself, an affiliated hospital, or one of the national trade associations (such as Group Health Association of America or American Medical Care and Review Association) or private research groups (such as Interstudy in Excelsior, Minnesota) that specialize in the HMO field.

With this data, the home care agency can calculate the projected percentage of the reduction in hospitalization costs to the HMO. The projected reduction in LOS multiplied by the average cost per hospital day results in a projected first-year gross reduction in hospitalization costs to the HMO.

The home care agency next translates the projected reduction in hospitalization costs to a projected net savings in the HMO's inpatient fund (that is, the amount allocated by the HMO for inpatient services) and the resultant savings or profits to the HMO and at-risk physicians. The net savings can be reasonably estimated by reducing the projected reduction in hospitalization costs by about 30 percent.

The home care agency may want to go even further and calculate the cost of the home care necessary to achieve the projected savings. This figure can be achieved by multiplying the estimated number of home care visits by the rate per visit. Then the home care agency divides this figure by the projected number of member months to get a projected cost to the HMO per member per month. Another figure the HMO may find useful is the projected number of home care visits per 1,000 enrollees.

These types of calculations are suggested because many HMOs have actual projections of the number of home care visits per 1,000 enrollees and the costs of home care visits per patient per month. Thus, the home care agency will be speaking to the HMO's own cost and utilization projection targets for home care and showing a positive impact on hospitalization targets. The agency should indicate in the proposal that these projections are conservative and are based on home care for noncatastrophic or non-critical care diagnoses or conditions.

The home care agency may also want to discuss potential savings on catastrophic or critical care diagnoses or conditions (for example, patients requiring extended care). Data is available to show the cost savings of home care in such cases.[4] The point to stress, particularly to Medicare HMOs, is that although most HMOs have a *stop-loss arrangement* with an insurer to cover such situations, the cost of care may force the insurance company to raise its premium to the HMO, a situation that may be avoided or minimized by the use of home care. *Stop-loss insurance* is insurance an HMO secures to cover the cost of care to any enrollee above a certain amount per year: a typical figure is $25,000 to $30,000. Thus, the HMO's loss is stopped once the cost of care to any enrollee exceeds the stop-loss threshold. The HMO's insurance carrier pays the excess.

Rate Structure

The savings issue assumes the existence of a rate schedule for home care programs and services. The development of such a rate structure is vexing to most home care agencies. Many agencies assume that they must dis-count their existing rates to get an HMO contract. Discounting is not always necessary and is certainly the wrong conceptual starting point. Less sophisti-cated HMOs may not desire detailed financial projections and may just compare fee-for-service rate (per Medicare service or per visit or hour) of competing agency bids, look for the word *discount,* and accept the lowest bid. However, a home care agency should not assume that all HMOs react this way. Instead, the agency should design the most attractive package possible.

The key element in designing rates is a data base that allows the home care agency to know its actual cost per hour or visit by type of service or program (including direct and indirect costs) and its client profile, census, and the visit-volume assumptions on which the costs are based. Once the home care agency establishes its actual costs, as accurately as possible, it can proceed to design a rate structure for bidding with a clear knowledge of its risk (that is, its potential profit-and-loss margin).

Three key elements are used to establish the rate structure: range of ser-vices or programs, unit of service, and utilization assumptions.

Range of Services or Programs

Home care services can range from one or more of the six Medicare-reimbursable services to a host of private-duty skilled and custodial care services. However, the HMO's existing coverage policy may automatically limit this range.

Any services not in the policy require a selling job on the part of the home care agency to get the HMO to include them in the policy. Most HMO policies cover skilled nursing and one or more other services, usually therapies (physical, speech, or occupational) or home health aides. The policies do not cover programs based on diagnoses or conditions, such as the early discharge of maternity patients, home phototherapy for the treatment of jaundiced infants, or back pain care. Such programs have to be packaged and sold to the HMO as a cost-effective addition to its coverage.

The range of services or programs a home care agency offers depends, in part, on its structure and capabilities. If the agency is Medicare certified and has not segregated its private-duty and other non-Medicare services into a separate organization, it may not be price competitive because of the impact of the step-down allocation of administrative and general expenses on private-duty and other non-Medicare services.

A home care agency may consider packaging a variety of condition or diagnosis programs for the HMO either as part of a fee-for-service proposal for standard intermittent or private-duty home care services or in a separate proposal. Such programs include, but are not limited to, maternity home care, postsurgical home care, ostomy home care, home phototherapy, infant apnea monitoring, asthma home care, back pain home care, and various programs based on specific catastrophic or critical care diagnoses or conditions. Some of these programs already have been used successfully by home care agencies in servicing either HMOs or employers directly.[5] The use of diagnosis-specific or condition-specific programs not only attracts HMOs and physicians because of cost savings, but also is more understandable to them because the approach used is similar to that used in a hospital inpatient program.

Unit of Service

A variety of options can be used to establish the unit of service on which rates are based. These options can range from an individual service price (by visit or by hour) to a capitated rate (per member per month or by diagnosis or condition). As noted earlier in this chapter, the home care agency may want to offer a multifaceted package that includes a fee-for-service rate schedule for standard intermittent Medicare services and for private-duty services and a rate schedule for certain specialized programs. In establishing program pricing, the home care agency may want to offer a program price based on a certain maximum aggregate of visits, after which purchased services revert to a fee-for-service schedule. In all rate-setting situations, particularly for programs based on diagnoses or conditions, the home care agency must consider whether to include some or all medical supplies and equipment in the rate.

The overall goal in rate setting is to achieve a balance between limiting financial risk to the home care agency and providing price-competitive and cost-effective services or programs to the HMO. In general, the most predictable low-risk rate structure for the home care agency is a per hour or per visit fee for individual service, with a sliding rate scale of discounted rates based on volume.

The sliding scale encourages the HMO to use more services because the higher the volume, the lower the price. This mechanism protects the home care agency against receiving a volume of requests from the HMO that is too low to make a fixed per visit or per hour rate financially feasible. The HMO probably will not want a sliding scale because it creates an additional variable to calculate into HMO practice patterns.

If the home care agency has reliable and valid cost data and resources, it can additionally offer one or more specialized programs at a per case rate based on a number of maximum allowable hours or visits. If the home care agency is not in a position to offer such programs at the time it submits its proposal, it can include a provision in the contract under which the agency and the HMO jointly work to develop home care programs or services on a capitated basis. In such cases, the contract should be short term, perhaps one year, to allow for the development and evaluation of accurate data to be used in possible contract modification. Price structures based on a flat rate for all home care services or per patient for a specific period (that is, per member per month) seem unwise for the home care agency unless the agency has a sophisticated data base to support the setting of such rates.

The pricing of services by visit or by hour also protects the home care agency against changes in the age and clinical profile of the HMO's enrollees. Ideally, the home care agency should try to obtain age and clinical profiles of the HMO's enrollees prior to deciding if the agency wants to bid on the HMO contract. However, the HMO either may not have or may not be willing to release such data. If the home care agency designs a price on a per patient basis without such data, the result may be substantial financial losses for services to patients with multiple diagnoses, terminal illnesses, or catastrophic illnesses that require frequent or intensive skilled home care services. An extreme and potentially costly example is an HMO enrollee who contracts terminal cancer. A Medicare HMO is not required to provide hospice benefit services. Thus, to avoid costly institutional costs, the HMO may decide to provide the terminally ill enrollee with home care. If the contract between the HMO and the home care agency does not contain a price-adjustment clause for such situations or does not exclude them from the basic rate structure, the home care agency can incur a substantial financial loss as a result of the frequency and intensity of services necessary to ensure proper high-quality medical care.

Hospital-based Medicare-certified hospices should be aware that Medicare HMOs are required to advise their members if a Medicare-certified hospice is in their service area. If a Medicare HMO enrollee becomes terminally ill after enrolling in the Medicare HMO, HCFA allows the enrollee to use the Medicare hospice benefit and still retain his Medicare HMO benefit for those services not covered by the hospice benefit. In such cases, HCFA works out a reduction in the HMO's payment. Hospices and home care agencies interested in the specific billing and reimbursement procedures for such cases should contact the HMO coordinator in their HCFA regional office.

Medicare-certified home care agencies providing home care services to an HMO through Medicare should be aware that they are permitted to discount prices without affecting the *customary charge* portion of their lower-of-cost-or-charges calculation.[6] However, the income from such HMO contracts must be accounted for in the home care agency's cost report and is subject to administrative and general expense allocation by the step-down method, unless the agency has obtained an appropriate advance approval from the fiscal intermediary to use the discrete costing method (see chapter 7).

Utilization

Some home care agencies believe that contracting with an HMO is a panacea to a declining patient census or visit volume. The reasoning is that by contracting with an HMO, the home care agency gets a captive market that will increase its patient census and visit count. Also, the agency may think that such a contract gives it a competitive advantage over other home care agencies in its market area.

Such reasoning is misleading. Contracts with HMOs are not a panacea to problems caused by increased competition. In fact, a contract with an HMO actually may result in a census and visit decline. This situation is referred to as the *lock-in/lock-out phenomenon*. The lock-in/lock-out phenomenon relates to who controls the decision making on whether the patient receives care and, if so, the kind of care (home care versus other care) and the extent of care (type and frequency of visits) that the patient receives. If the home care agency is not contracting with an HMO, the patient, physician, and home care agency determine if and when a patient receives home care and how much home care is received. Once the home care agency contracts with an HMO, particularly a Medicare HMO, the HMO controls the decision-making process. The home care agency may be "locked out" of rendering care to a client or have the level of care substantially limited.

Although home care often is cost-effective for the HMO, the HMO also has other options. The primary one is referring the client to a participating physician for an office visit or to a clinic or other outpatient facility. Such noninstitutional services are less costly than hospitalization. Often physicians or hospitals may have an ownership interest or may participate in the HMO as well as having an ownership interest in a clinic, ambulatory surgery, urgent care, rehabilitation or other outpatient center. The HMO itself may also have similar interests, particularly if it is part of a larger hospital or health care system. Thus, from an overall financial perspective, using other noninstitutional care options instead of home care may be in the best interests of the HMO and its participating providers.

In the proposal, and thereafter in the contract, the home care agency should outline its participation in the decision-making process. The agency has to decide, on the basis of staff availability and cost, whether to propose any or several of the following suggested mechanisms for involvement and whether to propose them as a free service or as an additional service at a specified price:

- *Home care coordinator.* The home care agency provides a home care coordinator to work with discharge planners at the HMO's participating hospitals, clinics, or group practice locations. The home care coordinator's salary is reimbursable under Medicare.
- *Quality assurance (QA) committee.* A staff member of the home care agency sits on or works with the HMO's QA staff or committee. In turn, the agency should offer the HMO a seat on its professional advisory committee or medical advisory committee. Federal law and most state laws require that HMOs have a QA program.
- *Utilization review committee.* A staff member of the home care agency sits on or works with the HMO's utilization review (UR) committee or staff. If the agency has an equivalent mechanism, the HMO can be offered reciprocal representation.
- *Preadmission screening.* A staff member of the home care agency works with coordinating staff at the HMO's participating hospitals or clinics in the preadmission screening process.
- *Employer group screening.* The home care agency provides a staff member to screen employees of participating employers on-site and deliver appropriate care on-site. This program is the equivalent of an occupational nurse program and probably should be priced separately, perhaps as a specialized program.
- *Predischarge screening.* The home care agency provides a staff member to work with the discharge planner at the HMO's participating hospitals or clinics. Unlike the salary of a home care coordinator, the salary of such a staff member is not reimbursable by Medicare.
- *Physician education program.* The home care agency develops, with the HMO's medical director and staff, literature and educational programs for all HMO primary care and specialty physicians. This program can include marketing surveys, jointly sponsored and regularly scheduled educational programs, and educational and promotional literature identifying for the HMO's physicians the cost-savings potential of the home care program. The educational program can also include visits to the offices of participating physicians to provide information to the physician's office manager, nurses, and other relevant employees.
- *Satellite office.* The home care agency establishes a satellite office in the HMO's clinic, if it is a staff model, or in participating hospitals or clinics. The HMO provides the home care agency with an iden-

tifiable space, a phone, a desk, and related items. If necessary, the agency may pay a reasonable rent and other costs for such space and services.

- *Joint marketing.* The development of brochures, newspaper ads, television and radio spots, and community service programs describing the relationship of the home care agency and the HMO is jointly sponsored by the HMO and the home care agency, and costs are shared equally.

Perhaps the best way to affect utilization is to establish a direct financial relationship between the HMO and the home care agency. If the HMO has funds invested in the home care agency, in a related organization (for example, an agency specializing in private-duty services), or in a joint venture to establish a DME, pharmacy, or private-duty business, the HMO will probably have a greater incentive to use home care services. The same is true if the home care agency, its parent company, or its hospital (if it is a hospital-sponsored or hospital-related agency) has funds invested in the HMO.

Negotiating the Contract

By the time the home care agency reaches the contract negotiation stage, many, if not all, of the relevant issues should have been resolved. At this stage of the process, these understandings are translated into proper legal contractual form and language to protect the home care agency.

The home care agency should be aware that HMOs generally have standard participating provider contracts that are usually in two forms: one for participating physicians or groups of physicians and one for participating hospitals. The HMO may want to use the standard hospital contract. In that case, an addendum to cover specific home care issues will be necessary. Ideally, the home care agency should request a separate contract and should consult an attorney to participate in drafting and negotiating the contract.

The following are specific areas that should be included in the contract. These areas are also listed on a checklist in figure 13-1, next page.

- *Parties to the contract.* The name and location of each of the parties and the acronym by which they will be referred to in the remainder of the contract should be clearly stated.
- *Definitions.* Any relevant terms should be defined in the contract. Examples of some relevant terms that should be defined are *home care services, home health services, usual and customary charges, stop-loss, on-call coverage, homemaker, home health aide, Medicare-covered services, homebound, intermittent,* and *service area.*

Figure 13-1. Checklist of Contract Provisions in Participating Provider Contract with an HMO

☐ Description of parties to the contract

☐ Definitions

☐ Scope of services

☐ Location and service area

☐ Compensation

☐ Payment procedures

☐ Member grievances

☐ Referral, admission, and certification protocols

☐ Access to and inspection of records

☐ Confidentiality

☐ Required certifications (of HMO and home care agency

☐ Listing of providers and enrollees

☐ Marketing

☐ Insurance

☐ Indemnification

☐ Utilization review

☐ Quality assurance

☐ Relationship of parties

☐ Exclusivity

☐ Dispute resolution

☐ Term of contract

☐ Modification

☐ Termination

☐ Applicable state law

☐ Administrative cooperation

☐ Enforceability

☐ Assignability

☐ Notices

- *Scope of services.* The specific services or programs covered by the contract and the days or hours that the home care agency is obliged to provide service should be explained. Such a list may be more appropriate in an appendix to the contract. Home care agencies should also seek inclusion in the contract of noncovered services that the agency would provide and bill for separately. Also, consideration should be given to specifying coverage and procedures for emergency situations that may not be covered in the patient's plan of treatment.
- *Location and service area.* The location of the HMO and home care agency and a definition of their respective service area coverage obligations should be included.
- *Compensation.* Rate schedules should be specified, perhaps by reference to an appendix. If the rates are to be subject to renegotiation or automatic increase for any specific reasons (for example, changes in Medicare reimbursement rates or the HMO becoming a Medicare HMO), that fact should be noted in the contract. Such a clause safeguards the home care agency in case it is forced to increase its charges during the contract period as a result of an action taken by Medicare. When contracting with a non-Medicare HMO, the contract also should have a clause that requires the HMO to notify the agency if it seeks or obtains Medicare HMO status and that specifies that rates are subject to renegotiation when the HMO receives

Medicare status. This precaution safeguards the agency in case the non-Medicare client base of the HMO causes the rate schedule to be lower than the agency would charge if Medicare clients were enrolled in the HMO.

- *Payment procedures.* The home care agency's billing procedures and the time constraints on HMO payments to the agency should be specified. The contract should also include a hold-harmless clause, whereby the agency agrees not to bill HMO enrollees for any services except applicable copayments under any circumstances, including the HMO's insolvency. The type of billing forms to be used can be set forth in an appendix; the contract can simply state that the type of billing is to be mutually agreed upon. A provision should be included that obliges the HMO to pay the agency for all authorized services, pursuant to a physician's plan of treatment, even if the HMO is declared insolvent or the contract is terminated prior to completion of the treatment plans

- *Member grievances.* The home care agency should agree to participate, as appropriate, in any HMO member grievances pursuant to the HMO's grievance procedure. The HMO should agree to notify the agency of any proposed grievances and the final resolution of any grievances.

- *Referral, admission, and certification protocols.* The contract should establish protocols for and the obligations of the HMO and the home care agency in referring and admitting patients as well as in certifying for care. These protocols can be specified in detail in an appendix, or the contract can state that such protocols are to be mutually developed and agreed to.

- *Access to and inspection of records.* Both parties should have reciprocal access to administrative and health records of the HMO, home care agency, and other participating providers, as appropriate. Both parties should also be subject to federal and state confidentiality requirements.

- *Required certifications.* Both the HMO and the home care agency should specify that they are in compliance, and shall remain in compliance, with applicable federal (including Medicare) and state laws and that they will notify the other of any noncompliance action within 15 days of receipt of notice from the appropriate regulatory authority or court. The laws involved should be cited.

- *Listing of providers and enrollees.* This provision requires the HMO to provide the home care agency with a current list of all participating providers and an update of this list on at least the first day of each month. The same procedure should be provided regarding enrollees, particularly when a Medicare HMO and Medicare patients are involved. Such lists can be generated by a computer cross-referencing system.

- *Marketing.* The HMO should agree to notify all enrollees and other participating providers of the agreement between the HMO and the home care agency. Also, the HMO should allow the home care agency to distribute informational materials. The contract should provide for any joint marketing or educational activities that the HMO and home care agency agree to. The educational programs may be described in a separate provision.
- *Insurance.* Each party agrees to obtain and maintain proof, which is available to the other, of appropriate liability, malpractice, and other applicable insurance for the provider and its employees. This provision also may establish required levels of coverage.
- *Indemnification.* This provision is similar to the insurance clause and should require each provider to indemnify and hold harmless the other against any claims or liabilities that are the sole responsibility of the HMO or the home care agency, respectively. Indemnity insurance may be required. Home care agencies should check with their insurance carrier, in advance of signing a contract, to determine if their existing professional liability policy covers contractually assumed liabilities.
- *Utilization review (UR).* The home care agency should agree to cooperate in the HMO's UR procedures. This provision should include any other arrangements that the HMO and the home care agency want to agree to regarding UR. Home care agencies should be aware that Medicare HMOs are subject to review by peer review organizations.
- *Quality assurance (QA).* This provision is the same as the UR provision but is applied to QA.
- *Relationship of parties.* This provision states that the HMO and the home care agency and their respective employees are independent contractors for purposes of the contract.
- *Exclusivity.* This provision states the exclusivity arrangements, if any, between the HMO and the home care agency. Such agreements should be made with full awareness of the Medicare antifraud and abuse laws and freedom-of-choice requirements. Whether or not the contract involves any exclusive arrangements, the contract should have a clause stating that the HMO and home care agency agree to be in full compliance with the Medicare and Medicaid fraud and abuse and freedom-of-choice provisions.
- *Dispute resolution.* This provision specifies a procedure, for example, arbitration or mediation, for the resolution of contractual disputes between the HMO and the home care agency and usually specifies the specific state or other applicable arbitrative law.
- *Term of contract.* This provision establishes the applicable time frame of the contract.
- *Modification.* This provision states that modifications must be mutually agreed to by the HMO and the home care agency. The clause usually states that such changes must be made in writing.

- *Termination.* This provision allows for termination of the contract with 60 days' advance written notice of either party's intent to end the relationship.
- *Applicable state law.* This provision specifies the state law governing the contract and, if necessary, applicable federal law.
- *Administrative cooperation.* This provision specifies reciprocal general cooperation and access to specific types of data and reports on a specified or agreed-to timetable.
- *Enforceability.* This provision describes what happens to the remainder of the contract if any terms or provisions are found invalid. Usually contracts state that the invalidity of one or more terms or provisions does not affect the validity or enforceability of the other terms or provisions.
- *Assignability.* This provision should discuss the ability of either provider to assign, delegate, or transfer the contract or any portion thereof to another person or entity. Usually assignment, delegation, or transfer is prohibited unless the parties receive prior written consent, which shall not be unreasonably withheld.
- *Notices.* This provision specifies the respective names and addresses of HMO and home care agency representatives to whom any notices required by the contract must be sent. It further specifies that such notices must be sent by certified mail, return receipt requested, with postage prepaid.

As with any contract negotiations, the negotiation of a contract between an HMO and a home care agency depends on local, political, and market conditions. These conditions influence the negotiating leverage of the respective parties and the ability of each party to demand or obtain some of the contractual considerations mentioned in this chapter. If a home care agency believes it can negotiate a viable HMO contact, it should make sure the contract is short term (perhaps one or two years at most) and gives a clear statement of the liability responsibilities related to patient care. A short-term contract gives both parties an opportunity to test the arrangement. If the arrangement does not work, then the potential risk is limited. If it does work, the contract can be refined and renewed. In no case would it seem prudent for a home care agency to proceed without a contract or merely with a simple letter of understanding. The potential risk for such good-faith arrangements is high, given the uncertainties of the marketplace and the new Medicare-certified HMO structure.

Notes

1. 42 C.F.R. § 110.

2. Gail Toff, "The State-Mandated Home Health Benefit," *Caring* (1985 Oct. 4(10):56-57)

3. 42 C.F.R. § 417, Part C.

4. For examples, see data on Aetna's catastrophic accident program and ventilator-dependent home care and various pediatric home care programs (William Cabin, "The Cost Effectiveness of Pediatric Home Care," *Caring* (1985 May. 3(5)) and William Cabin, "Some Evidence of the Cost-Effectiveness of Home Care, *Caring* (1985 Oct. 4(10):62-70). For data on home care and hospice cost savings for terminally ill persons, see articles in the June 1983 (volume 2, issue 6) and Feb. 1985 (volume 4, issue 2) issues of *Caring* and also contact the National Hospice Organization.

5. Bonnie Reroder, "Diagnosis-Specific Home Care: A Model for the Future," *Caring* (1984 Dec. 3(12):39-42) and William Cabin, "Some Evidence of the Cost-Effectiveness of Home Care," *Caring.* (1985 Oct. 4(10):62-70).

6. *Medicare Provider Reimbursement Manual.* HIN-15, Section 2604.3.B.1.

Chapter 14

The Diversity of Patient Care in the Home

Dorothy Buckels
Kaye Daniels
Judith Walden

The home care market encompasses a wide array of products and services. Sixteen brief patient care histories illustrate the diversity of clients and the complexity of illnesses served in the home setting. These case histories are numbered and are categorized in figure 14-1, next page, and in the text by age group (pediatric, adolescent, and adult, which is defined as someone older than 18 years old) and then by disease and home care service.

Pediatric and Adolescent

1. Spinal and Brain Surgery

Ernie was born with spina bifida and hydrocephalus, which is a condition characterized by the abnormal accumulation of excess fluid on the brain. After repeated spinal and brain surgeries, he was still unable to hold his head upright or move his arms or legs. Ernie also suffered from continuing respiratory problems, which required a tracheostomy.

With the help of the hospital's discharge planner, arrangements were made with the MediCAL program, California's equivalent to Medicaid, to

Case histories 1, 4, 5, 6, 7, 11, and 15 were contributed by Kaye Daniels, R.N., M.B.A., vice-president, Kokua Nurses Agency, Honolulu, Hawaii. Case histories 2 and 8 were contributed by Dorothy Buckels, R.N., director, St. Clair Home Care Department, South Hills Health System/Home Health Agency (SHHS/HHA) of Pittsburgh, Pennsylvania. Case histories 3, 9, 10, 12, 13, 14, and 16 were contributed by Judith Walden, R.N., president and executive director of Hospital HomeCare, Albuquerque, New Mexico.

Figure 14-1. Case Histories Categorized by Age Group and Then by Disease

Disease Category	Home Care Product and Services
Pediatric and Adolescent	
1. Spinal and brain surgery—newborn	Respirator, nurse visits
2. Heart problems—2 month old	Tube fed, nurse visits
3. Colon surgery—4 month old	Total parenteral and intravenous (IV) antibiotics, nurse and physical therapist visits
4. Guillain-Barré syndrome (paralysis)—15 year old	Nurse and therapist visits
Adult	
5. Cancer—25 year old	Hospice care (non-Medicare hospice benefit), hospice nurse visits
6. Colon cancer—82 year old	Hospice care (Medicare hospice benefit)
7. Lou Gehrig's disease—64 year old	Ventilator, nurse and therapist visits
8. Respiratory arrest and depression—67 year old	Respiratory care therapist visits, mental health services, nurse visits
9. Respiratory and abdominal surgery—69 year old	Ventilator, gastrectomy tube, urinary catheter care, nurse and physical and occupational therapist visits, social worker visits
10. Epileptic convulsions and tracheostomy—32 year old	Respiratory equipment, nurse and therapists visits
11. Chronic obstructive pulmonary disease—81 year old	Oxygen, nurse visits
12. Cerebrovascular accident and heart failure—76 year old	Nurse and therapist visits
13. Genitourinary infection—76 year old	Nurse visits, intramuscular injections
14. Diabetes and skin graft—73 year old	Nurse visits
15. Osteomyelitis—19 year old	Intravenous (IV) antibiotic therapy
16. Liver infection—70 year old	Intravenous (IV) antibiotic therapy, nurse visits

have nurses from the Hospital Home Health Care Agency of California visit Ernie at home. Much family training and support were necessary so that this baby could finally be with his mother and two-year-old brother in their east Los Angeles home. For example, the mother had to learn how to suction the tracheostomy tube so that it remained clear.

Nurses visited weekly for nine months to assess the child's adjustment and his physical status. The nurses taught Ernie's mother, a single parent, to cope with the nearly overwhelming task of coping with a baby who has a tracheostomy and other severely limiting diseases. Today, Ernie smiles and has some movement of his arms and legs, and his mother continues to care for him.

Ernie received 15 visits by a registered nurse and three evaluations. Total costs for home care were $837.88. At $600 a day for 15 days, a hospital stay would have cost $9,000. The savings amounted to $8,162.12.

2. Heart Problems

Matthew was two months old when he was admitted to South Hills Health System/Home Health Agency, Homestead, Pennsylvania. Matthew had been born with severe heart defects. His heart was placed in the right side of his chest, and instead of the usual two atriums and ventricles of a normal heart, he had only one of each. The aorta, which is the major trunk of the arterial system of the body, was also deformed at the arch.

Everything had been done that could be done in the hospital. Matthew needed time to grow stronger and develop physically, and so he was sent home in his mother's care. His doctor ordered home care to teach and assist the mother in providing care for Matthew in the home setting. Matthew's mother was also having a difficult time emotionally coping with Matthew's condition and with all the adjustments that were required to fit his routine into her daily life.

As a result of Matthew's heart condition, he was extremely weak and unable to take nourishment from a bottle. Sucking on a nipple, even for short periods, required more energy than he possessed. Matthew was fed through a tube that was passed through the nose into the stomach four times a day. The mother learned how to do this with teaching and support from the nurse, and Matthew began to gain weight.

Matthew was admitted to the hospital in June 1982 following a reaction to an injection of diphtheria-pertussis-tetanus (DPT) vaccine. Home care services began again when he returned home. He was now being tube fed blenderized foods and 5 ounces of formula four times a day. Matthew then developed a fever as the result of an ear infection. The home care nurse worked along with his doctor and the mother, and as a result of their efforts, Matthew did not need to be hospitalized.

In January 1983, Matthew was again admitted to the hospital when he began to vomit and became dehydrated. After 12 days in the hospital, he again returned home, and home care was resumed. He continued to be fed 5 ounces of formula and blenderized foods through a tube four times a day, and his condition continued to improve.

Matthew developed congestion in his chest and was readmitted to the hospital in March 1983 with an upper respiratory infection. When he was discharged from the hospital, home care services resumed. Along with blenderized foods, he was taking 19 ounces of formula through a tube each day, 6 ounces at night, and the remainder periodically during the day. At the age of 6 months, he was strong enough to take food by mouth and suck milk from a bottle.

After being admitted to the hospital in mid-March 1983 for a cardiac catheterization, Matthew returned home after 15 days, and home care services were again requested. His condition stabilized except for recurring ear infections. His mother was taught to recognize signs of cardiac failure. When Matthew was 14 months old, his mother had a new baby. Matthew was discharged from home care about this same time.

At present, Matthew has taken his place in the family structure. He is much loved and treated as normally as possible within his limitations. Although his body has adapted to his heart's limitations, he may need surgery in the future.

3. Colon Surgery

Mike was referred by his physician to Hospital HomeCare in Albuquerque, New Mexico, when he was four months old. At that time, he was going home from the hospital for the first time since his birth. He was a twin; the other twin was healthy. The other children in the family are a healthy 7 year old and a 3 year old. Mike's mother is a nurse, and his father is in the military service.

Mike was admitted to the newborn intensive care unit at birth. He was small for his age and had a high Apgar score. He developed necrotizing enterocolitis within 24 hours, and surgery was performed to remove the large colon and one-third of the small colon. More of the small colon was removed a week later. The surgical incision became infected and required four weeks of treatment to heal. After the first surgery, a Broviac catheter was inserted, and total parenteral nutrition feedings were initiated. He had muscle hypertonicity secondary to compromised neurological function and had some seizure activity. Mike was also found to be anemic and was given blood transfusions during his stay in the hospital. He had been placed on a respirator shortly after birth and was later weaned from it with great difficulty.

Mike developed a blood infection from the Broviac catheter when he was two months old and required intravenous antibiotic therapy. A second Broviac catheter was put in place so that his parenteral nutrition feedings could continue.

Even though Mike's mother is a nurse, she required instruction regarding Mike's unique total care needs. Also, the physician thought that he needed a third-party's objective assessment of Mike's physical status, and so the physician ordered nursing visits from Hospital HomeCare. A nurse specializing in pediatric care performed these assessment functions and also drew blood specimens for prescribed laboratory tests. She further provided emotional support to an overburdened mother for a period of six weeks.

A physical therapist worked with Mike because of the hypertonicity of the muscles that resulted from the compromised neurological function. Visits were made three times a week for a two-month period. On the other days, the mother provided treatment. Therapy by a pediatric physical therapist then continued in an outpatient setting.

The home care pediatric nurse helped the family obtain respite care so that the mother could have some needed time off. The nurse also helped coordinate services from the New Mexico Medically Fragile Child Program, funded in part by a Medicaid waiver.

Services provided to Mike were paid for partly by an insurance company and partly by the family. Without these services, this child would have had to stay in the hospital or another institution, a far more costly and less desirable situation.

4. Guillain Barré Syndrome

Nickie, who is 13 years old, spent two months on a ventilator in the intensive care unit after contracting Guillain-Barré syndrome and another month in an acute care hospital. Guillain-Barré syndrome is an acute inflammation of the peripheral nerves, which causes progressive muscle weakness that starts with the distal parts of the body. This condition can progress to respiratory paralysis and death. After the acute stage and with proper long-term medical management, the prognosis for this disease is usually good.

After three months in the hospital, Nickie's medical condition stabilized, but she remained completely paralyzed and required constant care and a structured therapy program. She was to be transferred to a rehabilitation hospital, but the family and child wanted a home discharge because they believed that the child and the family would benefit emotionally if care could be continued in their suburban Los Angeles home.

The hospital's discharge planner contacted the liaison nurse at Hospital Home Health Care Agency of California. Conferences were held with the family, the physician, the insurance carrier, the physical therapists from the hospital and the home care agency, and the equipment company. By the time Nickie was ready to go home, her parents had been instructed on her personal care; the necessary hospital equipment, including a ventilator and oxygen, had been duplicated in the home; and the home care agency's therapists were familiar with the rehabilitation program started in the hospital. Five months later, Nickie was walking, had gone back to school, and was able to resume most of her previous activities. Nickie continued to be seen by a physical therapist, who worked with her on endurance, and by an occupational therapist to further her self-training toward more independent living.

Hospital Home Health Care Agency of California provided service for 265 days. Nickie received six visits by a registered nurse, 94 visits by an occupational therapist, and 161 visits by a physical therapist. The total cost, not including durable medical equipment (DME), was $16,000. For the same number of days, a rehabilitation hospital, at $600 a day, would have cost $159,000.

Adult

5. Cancer

Michael, a 25-year-old Navy man stationed in the Midwest, was diagnosed as having cancer after his wife noticed a lump on his face in the sinus area. He underwent aggressive chemotherapy and seven biopsies but eventually had to have his eye removed. After Michael's doctor explained that curative measures were at an end, he and his wife decided to go home to California so that he could be with his family in the suburbs of Los Angeles.

Because of Michael's strong desire to die at home, his doctor ordered hospice care. The hospice nurse supported the family, tried to control the patient's pain with medication, and changed head bandages. The hospice nurse also requested that a medical social worker visit the family and clarify complex insurance questions. She also discussed funeral arrangements with the wife and tried to support the family as much as possible.

Although Michael's insurance did not cover hospice care, Hospital Home Health Care Agency of California never denies a patient hospice care because of lack of funds. The total cost for eight days of hospice care was $555.30. An eight-day hospital stay without insurance coverage could have totaled approximately $4,800.

6. Colon Cancer

Bertha is an 82-year-old female who was referred to Hospital Home Health Care Agency of California with a diagnosis of cancer of the colon. She was admitted under the Medicare hospice benefit.

Bertha was diagnosed as having cancer in 1984 and treated surgically with a colostomy, which was later closed. The tumor recurred in 1985 with pulmonary metastasis. Two months later, she was referred to hospice care.

Bertha initially lived alone; but after the recurrence of the cancer, she moved in with her son and daughter-in-law. They were caring and supportive but quite stressed. At first Bertha walked with a cane and required some help with the activities of daily living. Within a week after moving in with her son, her condition had deteriorated, and she was bedridden.

When Bertha was admitted to Hospital Home Health Care, she had symptoms of diarrhea, anorexia, dysphagia (difficulty in swallowing), and weakness. A urinary catheter was inserted when she became too weak to walk to the bathroom. Nursing visits were made to instruct the family regarding the medicines prescribed, to attempt to control the symptoms, and to offer the family support. Bertha developed a sacral abrasion, which healed with treatment suggested by the nurse.

Home health aide services provided personal care for two hours each day. A social worker made one visit for supportive counseling and to help Bertha and her family prepare for her approaching death.

Bertha's dysphagia increased, and she became semicomatose within two weeks of the start of hospice care. Continuous care (round-the-clock nursing) was started at this time to control symptoms and prevent hospitalization. Three days later, Bertha died. Her death occurred three weeks after admission to the hospice care program.

7. Lou Gehrig's Disease

Harry was 64 years old and suffered from amyotrophic lateral sclerosis (Lou Gerhig's Disease), which is a slowly progressive, debilitating, and fatal disease. During his last hospitalization, he had a tracheostomy, which made him dependent on a ventilator.

His doctor's encouragement and his wife's commitment to care for him led Harry to decide to return to his home in the upper-class community of Palos Verdes, California. The seriousness of his disease required much planning by the hospital's discharge planner and liaison nurse from Hospital Home Health Care Agency of California. Harry's condition required 24-hour care, which meant that his wife had to become certified to operate and maintain the ventilator.

Harry's wife provided good care but was emotionally unstable as a result of the stress of her husband's terminal condition. For this reason, Hospital Home Health Care Agency set up a special program for changing his tracheostomy tube. To forestall any emergencies, two respiratory nurses were always present in the home when tube changes were made.

Harry received home care, which was covered by Medicare, for the final 17 months of his life. During that time, he received 18 visits by a public health nurse, 45 visits by registered nurses, 25 home health aide visits, 5 visits by a physical therapist, 6 visits by an occupational therapist, and 3 visits by a medical social worker.

The total home care costs were $6,632.00, including DME and medical supplies. A 17-month hospital stay would have totaled approximately $306,000.

8. Respiratory Arrest and Depression

Henry, a 67-year-old retired attorney, began receiving services from South Hills Health System/Home Health Agency in December 1981 after spending four months in a hospital intensive care unit. Henry had been admitted for treatment of respiratory arrest with respiratory failure as a result of pneumonia and poliomyelitis contracted in 1951. He was also severely depressed and attempted suicide in the hospital because he thought he would never be able to go home.

Significant problems were identified for home care services. Home care nursing, respiratory therapy, and mental health services were ordered, as were oxygen, a hospital bed with rails, a respirator, and a suction machine. A platform to hold the respirator was built on the back of Henry's wheelchair so that he could be more mobile about his home.

Henry was paralyzed on his right side, and he had a permanent tracheotomy. He was able to speak and feed himself with his left hand, but he needed help with dressing, toilet functions, bathing, and other activities of daily living. Although Henry weighed approximately 200 pounds, he was able to get into his wheelchair with the support of one or two persons.

Henry's wife was familiar with the respirator because he had used one at night for several years. She needed to be taught to change the tracheostomy tube and to use the newer, smaller, more portable respirator that Henry now needed constantly.

During a home care visit, the registered nurse recognized signs of internal bleeding, and Henry was admitted to the hospital in January 1982 for 51 days because of a bleeding duodenal ulcer. Henry required a subtotal gastrectomy, which meant that he had the portion of his stomach containing the ulceration removed. The incision did not heal well and reopened following surgery, causing additional problems when Henry returned home. Upon discharge, home care services that were previously provided continued, and additional nursing visits were provided to take care of the surgical wound. Henry's wife needed additional help during this period and hired a private-duty registered nurse to help at home during the day and a male helper to assist in getting Henry ready for bed at night.

In November 1983, Henry was treated in the hospital for a partial bowel obstruction. When he returned home, home care resumed. At this time, he required medication through the respirator. This medication helped to open his airway and thin out secretions, which helped Henry to breathe easier. Henry's bowel obstruction grew worse; and in January 1984, he entered the hospital to have the bowel obstruction removed. Scar tissue had apparently constricted the small bowel, and the tissue had to be released to allow normal bowel function. In July 1985, Henry was hospitalized again with chronic respiratory insufficiency as the result of an upper respiratory tract infection.

Henry remained on the ventilator continuously, with oxygen at 2 liters per minute. The tracheostomy, which required suctioning three or four times a day, was changed routinely by his wife. Henry required complete personal care because of his paralysis. His abdomen healed well, his bowels moved daily without the use of laxatives, and his voiding was normal. He was able to be up twice a day in the wheelchair, could take two to three steps with moderate assistance, and slept well at night. Henry's wife was capable of handling Henry at home due to the guidance and teaching of home care personnel regarding the many aspects of his complicated care.

Henry has received home care services intermittently since 1981. Mental health services for his depression were discontinued during his second hospital stay. Nursing, rehabilitative nursing, occupational therapy, and respiratory therapy services have been provided as needed. Respiratory therapy visits were made when recommend by the pulmonary nurse who visited Henry once a week. The nurse supported Henry and his wife as needed, identifying problems, keeping the physician informed, and providing the skilled nursing care required as his condition and nursing needs changed.

9. Respiratory and Abdominal Surgery

Louise is a 69-year-old female who has amyotrophic lateral sclerosis (Lou Gerhig's disease). She was hospitalized for three months in 1983 following respiratory failure. A tracheostomy was performed, and she was placed on a ventilator. While in the hospital, she developed a bowel obstruction and had abdominal surgery to correct this condition. She required a gastrectomy tube and urinary catheter.

Because she lived with her devoted son and daughter, she was able to be discharged to her home from the hospital, although she still needed the respirator and had the gastrectomy tube and urinary catheter in place. Although much teaching about the ventilator had been done in the hospital prior to discharge, additional teaching and reinforcement were needed at home. Visits by nurses from Hospital HomeCare in Albuquerque, New Mexico, were ordered by the physician to teach the family about the gastrectomy tube and feedings, the urinary catheter, the tracheostomy and respirator, and wound care.

Daily nursing visits were made for two weeks to teach and evaluate learning. These visits were then decreased to every other day for several weeks. Within three months, the family was fairly independent, and the 24-hour-a-day care and nursing visits were decreased to twice a week to monitor the unstable condition and problem-solve with the family. Since 1983, Louise has been hospitalized three separate times for acute complications followed with a home health referral upon each discharge. She was able to be home most of the time because she receives professional home care support and observation. A social worker assisted Louise's family with referrals to other organizations to obtain social and financial assistance, as the cost of Louise's care in the home was a heavy drain on the family resources.

Louise received weekly physical therapy visits during the first home care admission to strengthen and recondition her muscles and to prevent contractures. Family members or another caretaker were taught how to perform the exercise program that Louise needed three times a day. She also received limited occupational therapy during the first home care admission, but she was unable to tolerate the additional activity. Occupational therapy was resumed briefly on the second admission to make a hand splint for Louise. However, Louise remained totally dependent for the activities of daily living, and no further occupational therapy was attempted.

Personal care assistance was provided by home health aides through Hospital HomeCare initially and when the family was between caregivers. Even though the family was willing to provide care for Louise, they were physically unable to meet the total 24-hour demands without assistance.

Medicare paid for all of the services provided to Louise. She continues to be a home care patient, primarily for urinary catheter changes that are required monthly. The frequency of nursing visits increases after each hospitalization for another assessment of her unstable condition.

10. Epileptic Convulsions and Tracheostomy

Gary is a 32-year-old male living in Albuquerque, New Mexico. He and his wife are both mentally retarded. Although Gary has a severe speech defect, he can read short phrases slowly.

Gary's mother and sister live in Albuquerque (his mother lives only a few blocks away), but they are limited in their intervention by Gary's demand for independence. Gary was formerly employed in a sheltered workshop.

Physically, Gary is grossly obese, weighing over 350 pounds. He suffers from malnutrition because he has Prader-Willi syndrome and peptic ulcer disease. Both conditions interfere with food metabolism.

Gary was admitted to the university hospital in acute respiratory distress where he developed status epilepticus, a series of repeated epileptic convulsions without any periods of consciousness between them. He was placed on a ventilator and remained hospitalized for five months in the intensive care unit. Numerous attempts to wean him from the respirator failed. A tracheostomy had been performed, and the tracheostomy tube remained in place. He was finally transferred to a medical unit without the respirator, and rehabilitative activities were begun.

Because of the severe weakness resulting from his extended illness, which caused myopathy and deconditioning of the muscles, and the multiple medical problems, Gary was almost totally dependent on others for help with the activities of daily living. Ten days after arriving in the medical unit, he was again transferred, this time to a rehabilitation unit for two months.

Gary's physician ordered follow-up care by Hospital HomeCare after Gary was discharged from the rehabilitation unit. The care plan was developed in the hospital before discharge. Home care personnel were to teach all aspects of tracheostomy care, oxygen use, care of respiratory equipment, and nebulizer treatment. Nursing visits were also ordered for observation of the unstable respiratory condition and for dietary teaching.

All nursing visits were made by one clinical specialist in respiratory care. Continuity of care was important because Gary had a short attention span and was emotionally unstable and easily frustrated. Initially, home visits were ordered five times a week for the first week, then decreased to three times a week for two weeks, and then decreased to two times a week. Attempts to decrease visits further to one time a week failed because the patient developed pneumonia or other complications when this action was taken.

A physical therapist worked with Gary for one month. He progressed from walking five feet with supervision (while on oxygen) to walking independently for short distances and riding a stationary bicycle for 10 minutes a day. He was also able to bathe himself when physical therapy was discontinued.

Gary had developed bilateral hearing loss during his hospital stay, and so a speech therapist taught him and his wife lip reading to improve his communication skills, especially with his wife. A social worker assisted Gary by establishing long-term-care plans and arranging for a homemaker-chore service funded through the state.

As of 1986, Gary remained a home care patient. He has been seen in the emergency department of the hospital but not readmitted. He has also developed pneumonia on two occasions, but this condition has been successfully managed at home. Without home care assistance, Gary would most certainly be in a nursing home or hospital.

11. Chronic Obstructive Pulmonary Disease

Lucille is 81 years old and has a long-standing history of chronic obstructive pulmonary disease, which has required frequent hospitalizations. In 1983 she had a stroke, which left her with some weakness in her right side. So that she could return home to her daughter, son-in-law, and grandchildren in suburban Los Angeles, Lucille's doctor prescribed home care because of her respiratory problems.

Respiratory nurses from Hospital Home Health Care Agency of California taught Lucille and her family the proper use and care of her oxygen and intermittent positive pressure breathing (IPPB) equipment. The nurses also checked Lucille's vital signs and made sure her medication was taken properly because it was changed so often.

The nurses instructed Lucille's family on how to recognize signs of impending crisis relative to her disease so that they knew when to call for medical assistance and thereby prevent hospitalization. They continue to care for her and receive assistance when necessary.

During the entire month that Lucille received home care, she received 16 visits by a registered nurse, 25 visits by a home health aide, 7 visits by a physical therapist, and 1 visit by an occupational therapist. Durable medical equipment (DME) costs totaled $29.50. Total home care costs were $2,775.50, which was covered by Medicare. A hospital stay for one month would have cost approximately $18,000.

12. Cerebrovascular Accident and Heart Failure

Lou is a 76-year-old male who was hospitalized for two weeks following a cerebrovascular accident (CVA), which resulted in a muscular weakness affecting the left side of his body. He also had a history of degenerative joint disease and hypertension and was on anticoagulant therapy. After his condition had stabilized, he was transferred to a rehabilitation unit for five weeks.

Lou's physician ordered home care visits through Hospital HomeCare, in Albuquerque, New Mexico, to begin at the time of his discharge from the rehabilitation unit. He went home to a cluttered environment and a wife who was confused at times. A daughter lived nearby, and she and her children helped with Lou's care. A nurse visited on the day following discharge to assess the patient's condition. Lou was found to be short of breath, with decreased breath sounds. He had severely swollen ankles and lower legs as a result of fluid retention. The physician was notified, and Lou was rehospitalized for four more days with congestive heart failure, atrial fibrillation, and pulmonary edema.

Lou was again referred to Hospital HomeCare for home nursing followup after his discharge from the hospital. Nursing visits were ordered to teach the family about congestive heart failure, diet, and the anticoagulant therapy as well as to assess the patient's unstable cardiac condition. Close communication with the physician was maintained regarding the unstable condition. Frequent blood samples were drawn for laboratory analysis to assist the physician in monitoring the patient. Lou finally stabilized medically after five weeks of nursing visits, and nursing care was discontinued.

In addition to these nursing visits, a physical therapist worked with Lou twice a week for gait training and muscle strengthening and reeducation. After five weeks of physical therapy, Lou could walk independently on level surfaces; he required a cane only on uneven surfaces. His endurance had improved, and he became less fatigued during exercise.

An occupational therapist worked with Lou primarily to increase coordination of and sensation in the left upper body. He was found to be fairly independent in performing the activities of daily living from the time of his initial assessment. After six weeks, the occupational therapist discontinued visits when Lou's range of motion in the left upper body and arm was deemed to be within normal limits and his strength and coordination were functional. The patient was discharged feeling well and functioning on a relatively normal basis.

Medicare reimbursed the home health agency for all services provided.

13. Genitourinary Infection

Carlos, a 76-year-old male, was referred to Hospital HomeCare, Albuquerque, New Mexico, by his physician because he required intramuscular injections of the antibiotic Nebcin® every 12 hours for a genitourinary infection. He was not hospitalized but was referred by his physician for a five-day course of treatment. The family, who spoke only Spanish, was instructed regarding the effects and side effects of the medicine by a Spanish-speaking nurse. This same nurse visited at least daily. The second visit each day was made by a non-Spanish-speaking nurse, and the language barriers did make communication difficult during these visits.

By the last visit, Carlos's temperature had returned to normal. He continued to complain of frequency and urgency of urination as well as nocturia, the need to urinate during the night, but had no complaints of burning when urinating.

Two additional visits for assessment were made after the course of injections had ceased and the complaints of frequency and urgency had disappeared and the nocturia had decreased. He was discharged from Hospital HomeCare, and follow-up care was provided by his physician.

Medicare reimbursed the home care agency for the twice daily visits as well as the follow-up observation visits. Without home care services, this patient would have been hospitalized for at least one week at a much greater cost to Medicare.

14. Diabetes and Skin Graft

George is a 73-year-old male who was hospitalized for 13 days for a skin graft to an ulcer on the heel. He has a long history of diabetes, and his left leg had been amputated below the knee five months prior to this illness. He lived with a son and daughter-in-law, who both worked outside the home.

The physician requested Hospital HomeCare in Albuquerque, New Mexico, to provide home care nursing visits for daily wound care to the right heel graft, which was initially two inches in diameter, and to the donor site on the right leg. The donor site healed with no problems, but the graft was loose and eventually partially failed at the bottom. The rest of the wound healed, and the tissue appeared healthy. The diabetes appeared well controlled.

Another skin graft on the area that did not heal properly was performed. This surgery was done on an outpatient basis. Hospital HomeCare continued to provide nursing visits to the patient for follow-up wound care after the regrafting. The outpatient surgery, in addition to the home care nursing visits, allowed successful regrafting without another inpatient admission.

The agency was reimbursed for the cost of the home care services by Medicare.

15. Osteomyelitis

David, who is 19 years old and lives in Redondo Beach, California, enjoys the surf, sun, and sand. One day while walking home from the beach, he stepped on a nail. His injury resulted in the development of osteomyelitis, an infection and inflammation of the bone in his left foot. As a result of his injury, he required intravenous (IV) antibiotic therapy, which is part of the high-tech program at Hospital Home Health Care Agency of California.

David was in the hospital for four days. Because his private insurance covered home care, he could remain at home comfortably while receiving therapy three times a week for three weeks. In the past, this therapy would have required hospitalization because insurance did not cover high-tech home care. Now, with the high cost of hospitalization, insurance companies have been turning to home care as an alternative.

Nurses from Hospital Home Health Care Agency of California changed the peripheral cannula when necessary and monitored for side effects of the antibiotics. David's physician prescribed all the treatment given by the nurses.

David was able to continue surfing regularly once he was discharged from home care. By receiving therapy at home rather than in the hospital, David saved $11,839.50. Total home care costs were $760.75.

16. Liver Infection

Clara is a 70-year-old female who was hospitalized for 18 days with blood poisoning resulting from a liver abscess. She had been hospitalized nine days prior to this admission for a cholecystectomy, the surgical removal of her gallbladder.

Clara was referred to Hospital HomeCare in Albuquerque, New Mexico, by the physician who discharged her. She had a Hickman catheter in place and was receiving antibiotics intravenously. She also had a stomach tube in place for enteral feedings.

Initially, Clara was discharged from the hospital to her own home because her daughter from out of state was available to stay with her. The daughter had received instructions regarding care while Clara was still in the hospital and demonstrated an ability to administer intravenous (IV) antibiotics and care for the stomach tube without much follow-up teaching. She also learned to change dressings on Clara's abdominal wound. Daily nursing visits were made for four days to assess the patient and to evaluate the daughter's ability to perform the necessary care. Clara was then seen twice a week for two weeks for continued nursing assessment.

This daughter eventually had to return home, and Clara moved in with her son and daughter-in-law. The son and his wife were loving and willing to try to care for Clara. However, they both were unable to learn to give the IV antibiotics and do the other necessary IV site care. Because the IV antibiotic regime was short-term, with only 10 days remaining, and because Clara's situation fell well within Medicare's intermittent visit guidelines, nursing visits were made four times a day to administer the IV antibiotics, perform dressing changes and cap changes on the Hickman catheter, and assess the patient's condition. Clara was observed for one more month after the IV medicines were discontinued because the Hickman catheter still required weekly cap changes.

A social service worker from Hospital HomeCare assisted the family and the patient when the patient first moved to her son's home and later provided ongoing resource referral. Options were being explored for hired help in the home to handle the IV therapy until Medicare indicated a willingness to pay for the services through home care.

Clara was discharged from Hospital HomeCare when she regained sufficient strength and was functioning independently. She will receive follow-up care from her physician in his office.

Chapter 15

The Future of Home Care

Steven L. Griff
Dan Lerman

The rapid move in recent years toward home care and away from hospitalization is likely to accelerate as the 21st century approaches. A number of factors can be expected to affect that movement.

- Population. The elderly and handicapped population will continue to increase. The population under 65 years of age will also become increased utilizers.
- Economics. The use of prospective pricing and other payment policies to contain costs will continue to result in shortened lengths of stay in the hospital and more intensive forms of treatment provided in the home.
- Competition. As the market for home care grows, competition will increase commensurately.
- Technology. New devices and techniques will make home care a more realistic option than ever before.

Population

Approximately 12 percent of the U.S. population is over 65, and by the turn of the century, this number will increase by approximately 35 percent.[1] The

Steven L. Griff is president of Home Care Information Systems, Inc., and Home Health Associates, Totawa, New Jersey. Dan Lerman is manager of home care and hospice services in the Division of Ambulatory Care, American Hospital Association, Chicago, Illinois.

fastest growing age group in the United States, a group that is likely to increase sevenfold from 1980 to 2050, is the over 85 year olds.[2] Thirty percent of the over 85 year olds are estimated to need personal care services. Modern medicine has lengthened lifespans, and an end result will be a growing number of chronically ill and handicapped individuals.

Another group with significant potential for home care is the under-65 population, specifically pediatric and psychiatric patients, ambulatory surgery patients in need of follow-up care, maternity patients who are discharged early, well newborn babies, clients with industrial and occupational illnesses, and AIDS patients.[3] All of these persons may be better served by home care than by inpatient care.

Economics

Economics, too, will have a marked effect on the future growth of home care. Health care costs now represent 10.5 percent of the gross national product and are projected to reach $1 trillion by 1990.[4] These figures make cost containment an increasingly compelling issue. At present, hospitals account for 40 percent of health care expenditures; nursing homes, 10 percent; and home care agencies, 1½ percent. By the year 2000, the percentage of dollars expended on home care is expected to exceed 10 percent, according to the National Association for Home Care. One reason for the projected rise in home care's share of the health care dollar is the increasing pressure on hospitals to shorten inpatient stays. Prospective pricing already has had the effect of sending appropriate patients home earlier, and these patients are often in need of home care.

On a practical level, home care is cost-effective if the patient population is targeted properly. If not, home care will be an add-on, not a substitute, service. Cost savings can be achieved only if patients are carefully matched with appropriate services.

In 1986, profitable home care product lines are generally private-duty, durable medical equipment (DME), and infusion therapy. Increasing competition and decreasing payment are now contributing to declining profitability. However, sustaining that profitability will be possible only if providers efficiently control costs and if payment is adequate. Increased management skill will be required to integrate clinical and fiscal data so that managers can know exactly how much the delivery of a unit of service costs, can price services accordingly, and can make timely management decisions with this information. In addition, home care providers will need to improve documentation, record keeping, and product-line accounting. Specialized home care computer software packages, which are being more widely applied in the industry, are key tools in enhancing the management efficiency of an agency.

Like other aspects of health care, home care is, and will remain, under close government scrutiny. Government reimbursement remains problematic.

Although prospective pricing was introduced in 1983 for the inpatient sector, Medicare's home care program continues to be cost reimbursed. Concurrently, it has been the fastest growing segment of Medicare's entire program and, as a result, has been subjected to intense utilization review and the capping of reimbursement limits to control escalating costs.

The federal government is convinced that many Medicare-certified home care providers are inefficient.[5] More than 40 percent of Medicare-certified providers operated at a loss in 1983, according to a limited recent federal survey.[6] In addition, government studies claim 34 percent overutilization of the Medicare home care benefit.[7] However, these studies may have been conducted with the specific intent of producing data that would be negative for the home care industry. The industry must police itself and serve only appropriate patients. Conversely, patient care may be jeopardized if access to care for patients truly in need of services is denied, as has been reported in recent surveys of denials of claims by Medicare.[8]

In the short term, the government is likely to continue to increase utilization reviews and decrease reimbursement. Home care agencies nationwide will need to be able to prove, through careful collection and analysis of data, that they are cost-efficient and serve appropriate patients.

In addition, increased reimbursement is essential if more intensive and professional services are to be provided. The home care industry will have to work closely with the federal government to educate it as to the cost of appropriate care and to justify appropriate payment levels. If a home care prospective pricing system is established, agencies may finally have an opportunity to make a profit on Medicare home care visits if their costs for providing care are lower than the prospectively determined price. If payment is not sufficient, access to home care may be restricted. The three different home care prospective pricing methods being discussed are per visit, per illness episode, and per time period.

In any case, the expansion of home care benefits is likely in the future. More than 90 percent of Blue Cross and Blue Shield plans and nearly 50 percent of commercial health insurance plans now offer home care benefits.[9] The likelihood is that the number and kind of benefits that insurers offer will continue to increase as studies demonstrate cost savings. As benefits increase, profitable lines of home care business can then be used by organizations to support services, such as hospice, supportive care, volunteer programs, and indigent care, that are not likely to be self-supporting.

In the long term, federal funding for home care may increase if the federal budget deficit picture improves, and benefits may then be provided for maintenance and supportive care as well as for skilled care services if studies demonstrate the cost savings of implementing a comprehensive long-term-care benefit. Such additional services will require retraining the work force. Sr. Crescentia Mulvehill, senior vice-president, South Hills Health System, Homestead, Pennsylvania, predicts that allied health care workers in the future may be trained across the board to perform various aspects of occupational therapy, physical therapy, speech therapy, medical social service, and nursing.[10] This situation will have the effect of consolidating and reducing the home care skilled professional work force. Given this scenario, expanded home care benefit coverage may be offset by significant personnel expense reductions.

Competition

As the market for home care increases, so will the competition. Although hospitals and proprietary, or for-profit, programs are likely to remain the fastest growing providers of home care, 17 percent of HMOs and PPOs are now direct providers of home care, and another 60 percent indicate they are interested in directly providing, not contracting for, this service.[11] Private insurers are moving toward not only financing home care but also providing it themselves. Independent practitioners, such as physical therapists and nurses, will also be an increasing source of competition. If hospitals are to retain or increase their share of the market, they must demonstrate the quality and cost benefits of their services over the services of potential competitors.

Consumer awareness will also affect competition. Home care programs have mounted, and will continue to mount, extensive marketing, promotion, and advertising campaigns to woo consumers and differentiate high-quality home care providers from the competition. However, promotional activities will only be successful if home care programs have strong physician support. Doctors, who are a primary referral source, need to be informed of the opportunities for and advantages of home care and convinced to use this service. In addition to doctors, agencies must develop other referral sources: family and friends of current or former patients, community health agencies, religious organizations, and hospital-related or freestanding emergency departments, ambulatory surgical centers, rehabilitation programs, long-term-care programs, geriatric assessment clinics, and birthing centers. Home care needs to be perceived as an important part of the overall ambulatory care and long-term-care services provided by the hospital.

Consumers will serve as direct referral agents and will increasingly become powerful influencers, not only in where they are going to receive care, but also in the costs that will be incurred. If a voucher system is established in the future, patients will have only a stipulated amount of money or benefits to use for health care. Therefore, they may choose to be cared for in the home rather than in an inpatient facility out of economic necessity. Where care is delivered may be driven by economic considerations rather than the preferences of either the patient or the physician. Consumers of the future will have to become discriminating purchasers of health care.

As consumer awareness of home care increases, the home care organization must be sure that it is perceived as a low-cost, high-quality, truly caring alternative. Because home care is presently a highly entrepreneurial and unevenly regulated industry, strong administrative and quality control and education of hospital staff, the patient, and the family are essential if high standards of care are to be maintained and risk factors are to be averted or minimized. Hospitals must recruit top-notch management talent for their home care programs and reward them appropriately for their skills. Home care administrators must be given resources and authority to make timely decisions in this fast-paced environment. In addition, academic training programs focusing on home care management need to be expanded.

Of course, not all hospitals will choose to enter the home care market, and some will enter only a specific segment, such as DME, infusion therapy, or private-duty, rather than concentrating on the Medicare or Medicaid market. Whatever route a hospital chooses—whether it sets up its own agency, participates in a joint venture, contracts with other agencies, or simply makes referrals—it must directly provide or coordinate a comprehensive array of home care services if it is going to appropriately care for its patients.

Technology

Perhaps the most profound influence on the future of home care is the development of new technology. Health care analyst Jeff Goldsmith says that in the 21st century "changing medical technology will make it possible for the home or the residential community to reemerge as the primary site of clinical care—just as it was at the beginning of the 20th century."[12] He further notes that "technologies that took off during the 1970s—technologies such as continuous-action peritoneal dialysis and enteral and parenteral nutrition—will be joined by new generations of technologies, enabling more patients with serious illnesses to be sent home safely. Remarkable progress with implantable devices already has produced implantable insulin pumps and implantable defibrillators; combining miniaturization with advances in microprocessor technology will enable sophisticated chemotherapy to be administered safely at sites remote from the hospital."

In the future, computerized monitoring systems may allow stabilized patients and medical and clinical staff to interact on a computer screen. As a result, patients will be able to remain at home because they can be monitored by physicians and home care staff from a distance. A heart attack may trigger an alarm system at the hospital that alerts a doctor to administer, via a computerized system, a larger dose of the medication the patient is already receiving intravenously. Another alarm may prompt an ambulance to pick up the patient and rush him or her to the hospital. With such monitoring systems in place, medical and clinical staff will have a continuous flow of information that enables them to respond more quickly and effectively if a crisis situation develops.

This interactive system would also allow the patient to consult the health care professional from a distance and to order equipment and supplies by computer. In addition, videocassettes on patient education topics could be supplied for home or hospital use. Such tapes could be used to prepare the patient for the move from the hospital to home care.

As an example of sophisticated technology, advances in drug therapy will permit patients to take one daily dose of a drug, instead of multiple doses throughout the day. Also, the use of self-diagnostic tests, such as those now available for pregnancy, blood pressure, and glucose testing, will increase.

Robots will be available to do some of the tasks now performed by humans. "Many robotics companies are looking down the road to the personal robot as the total multipurpose home appliance for monitoring security, doing chores, caring for the disabled or elderly, and serving as a complete message and appliance control center."[13]

The result of all these advances in technology, Goldsmith predicts, may be that "as treatment advances divert large numbers of patients from the inpatient hospital setting, and as life-support and maintenance technologies enable patients to carry on their lives away from hospitals and nursing homes, the hospitalized population will shrink to perhaps half its current size by the early part of the next century, despite an aging population."[14]

Excellence

Predicting the future is an uncertain skill at best, especially in a field as constantly changing as home care. Nonetheless, hospitals must build the best possible home care program or coordinate the best home care network, not just for today, but for the future. No matter how competitive the environment, how the home care program is structured, what product lines the program diversifies into, or who the patients are, future success is only possible if the hospital or integrated health care system builds on what it does best.

Richard J. Mahoney, Monsanto's president and CEO, noted in a recent column about expanding a business portfolio: "Rather than merely making more, I suggest we have to concentrate on making better. Instead of mindless expansion, we must work selectively on our individual strengths. Expansion should not come because we have resources...but because expansion will put us where we want to be. We must resist fads, question dogmas, and look at each situation individually. . . . The same rules apply—excelling in fundamentals. Excellence is required, whatever the portfolio path."[15]

Hospitals need to apply Mahoney's words to their situations. The mission of all hospitals is, and must continue to be, the provision of the highest quality health care possible. Home care enables hospitals to use their "individual strengths" outside their usual environment, to go into the community and help appropriate patients maintain themselves in the comfort and security of their own homes. As stated in the AHA *Guidelines on the Role and Responsibility of Hospitals in Home Care,* home care "provides concrete evidence that the hospital is moving toward a broader concept of its role as a health and social agency in the community."[16] Home care is both a challenge and an opportunity for hospitals in their continuing search for excellence.

Notes

1. From a chart published in *USA Today.* 1986 May 27.

2. U.S. Bureau of Census. *Current Population Reports,* Series P-25, No. 952. 1984 May.

3. Non-medicare home care clients provide market opportunities. *Outreach.* 1986 Jan.-Feb. 7(1):5.

4. Halamandaris, Val. The future of home care. *Caring.* 1985 Oct. 4(10):5.

5. Medicare schedule of home health cost limits. *Federal Register.* 1986 July 5. 50(129):27734-51.

6. *Pepper Report Supports the Cost-Effectiveness of Home Care.* In: *News,* press release from U.S. House of Representatives Select Committee on Aging. 1984 Oct. 1.

7. Health Care Financing Administration, Department of Health and Human Services, Bureau of Quality Control. 1985 Spring. Unpublished data.

8. *NAHC Declares Medicare Delays Hurting Nation's Elderly.* Press release from National Association for Home Care, Washington, DC. 1986 July 12.

9. Hollander, Neal, vice-president for provider affairs, Blue Cross of Western Pennsylvania, Pittsburgh. Presentation at the National Association for Home Care annual convention in Boston. 1984 Oct. 15.

10. Mulvehill, Sister Crescentia, senior vice-president, South Hills Health System, Homestead, PA. Presentation at the International Health and Economic Institute Annual Conference, St. Thomas, Virgin Islands. 1986 Apr. 19.

11. *Home Care—HMO/PPO Perspective.* Chicago: Louden and Co., 1986.

12. Goldsmith, Jeff. 2036: a health care odyssey. *Hospitals.* 1986 May 5. 60(9):69, 74, 76.

13. Sealfon, Peggy. Resident robots. *American Way.* 1985 June 11. 60(9):74.

14. Goldsmith, p. 74.

15. Mahoney, Richard J. What to do after the consultants go home. *Business Week.* 1984 Feb. 13. No. 2828, p. 17.

16. *Guidelines on the Role and Responsibility of Hospitals in Home Care.* Chicago: American Hospital Association, 1980.

Appendix A

Hospital-Based Home Care Model

Cathy Frasca

South Hills Health System/Home Health Agency (SHHS/HHA), in Pittsburgh, Pennsylvania, is one of the largest multihospital-based home health agencies of its kind in the United States. As of 1986, the agency's total service-area population consists of 1,456,085 persons in a four-country area in western Pennsylvania. The agency has an average daily census of 2,500 to 3,000 patients, makes approximately 200,000 visits annually, and employs more than 250 professional and supportive home care staff members.

The SHHS/HHA was first established in 1963 as a home health agency of Homestead Hospital, a voluntary community hospital. In 1970, the agency reached an agreement with St. Joseph's Hospital, located in the southside area of Pittsburgh, to provide home care service on a contract basis. In 1973, these two hospitals merged to form the South Hills Health System (SHHS). A new 400-bed acute care facility, Jefferson Hospital, was then constructed. The agency's name was changed to the South Hills Health System/Home Health Agency (SHHS/HHA) to reflect the merger of these two hospitals. Prior to and during the merger process, other area hospitals contracted with SHHS/HHA through its parent, SHHS, for the purpose of offering home care services to patients discharged from their hospitals.

The agency provides a full range of services, including skilled nursing, which includes specialty nursing services such as psychiatric and mental health nursing, rehabilitative nursing, pediatric nursing, maternal infant early discharge, intravenous (IV) therapy nursing, IV chemotherapy nursing, and pulmonary nursing; home health aide services; physical therapy; occupational

Cathy Frasca is the executive director of South Hills Health System/Home Health Agency, Pittsburgh, Pennsylvania.

therapy; speech and language pathology, respiratory therapy; social work; home care volunteer services; diagnostic services; and medical-surgical supplies. In addition, the agency provides the home care component of a unique hospice program, South Hills Family Hospice. The hospice is administered by a separately incorporated organization composed of the South Hills Health System, Mercy Hospital of Pittsburgh, St. Clair Memorial Hospital, and South Hills Interfaith Ministries.

Interdisciplinary Approach

The philosophy of the agency is based on its mission statement: "The purpose of the South Hills Health System/Home Health Agency (SHHS/HHA) is to provide a full range of home health and related services with an emphasis on quality and integrated care for those individuals in need of these services in Western Pennsylvania."

Inherent in this philosophy is the interdisciplinary approach to patient care. The backbone of the service delivery model is the role of the primary nurse as stated in agency policies: "The staff nurse is responsible for the provision of primary nursing care and for assuming the role of the primary service provider when other home care disciplines are involved in the patient's care, and as such, coordinates and supervises the total care plan as defined for a primary service provider in Agency guidelines and as states in the RN Job Description and in the Pennsylvania Nurse Practice Act, and is accountable administratively to the Home Care Department Director and clinically to the patient's physician."

All other service disciplines, such as physical therapy, occupational therapy, or speech therapy, also use a *primary care approach* so that each patient relates primarily to one service provider from each discipline that provides care to a particular patient. As with nursing, substitute providers are used only when absolutely necessary to ensure continuity of care during a provider's vacation or other lengthy absence.

Even after reducing the number of providers to one for each discipline, a patient may still in fact work with many direct-service providers. In fact, the more acutely ill the patient, the more complex the patient's needs usually are, and therefore, the greater the potential for requiring multiple services.

To facilitate the communication process, the interdisciplinary team concept is essential. Each patient's interdisciplinary team is made up of those staff members who are providing the services required by the needs of that particular patient. They become a team when they plan and work together as a group for the best interests of the patient.

Because every team needs a leader, the agency designates the leader of each patient's team as the primary-service provider. In most cases, the primary-service provider is the registered nurse. The primary-service provider's responsibility is to ensure that the goals of the team are in concert with the physician's plan of treatment, the patient's priorities and wishes, and the goals of every other team member. The primary mechanism for fulfilling this responsibility is the team conference, which is explained more fully in chapter 5. Specific duties of the primary-service provider include making referrals to other disciplines in a timely manner, calling team conferences, recording the outcome of team conferences, following up on plans developed in the team conferences, and initiating the recertification process in a timely manner. When nursing is not actively participating in the care of a patient who requires multiple services, the department director assigns a primary-service provider from among the patient's allied health care providers.

Organization

The SHHS/HHA currently administers and coordinates eight satellite branch units through a decentralized organizational structure (figure A-1, next page). Six of these units are hospital based and include Canonsburg General Hospital; Mercy Hospital of Pittsburgh; St. Clair Memorial Hospital; Forbes Metropolitan Health Center and Forbes Regional Health Center of the Forbes Health System; and Jefferson Hospital. The Homestead Home Care Department is based at the Willis Center Skilled Nursing Facility, which is also a part of the SHHS. The agency also administers a community-based home care department, South Side Home Care Department, which is located in an urban area of Pittsburgh.

Under the decentralized system, the home care department of each participating hospital functions both as an integral part of the hospital's system and as a part of the total home care agency. A full complement of home care staff is assigned to each department, under the supervision of a home care department director. Home care personnel based at each home care department interact with the hospital's employees and medical staff and have access to selected resources of that participating hospital, as if they were, in fact, a department of that hospital. This unique organizational structure has been a key factor in the agency's success.

Each participating hospital's chief executive officer (CEO) appoints a member of its hospital's administrative staff to function as a liaison between the hospital and the agency. This administrative linkage helps the director of the home care department to operationally integrate the policies and procedures of the home care department with those of the participating hospital. Each participating hospital's CEO also appoints a representative to the agency's Advisory Board.

Matrix Reporting System

If this organization were to be depicted in chart form, the home care department would have a solid vertical line reflecting direct reporting to the home

Figure A-1. Organizational Structure of South Hills Health System/Home Health Agency

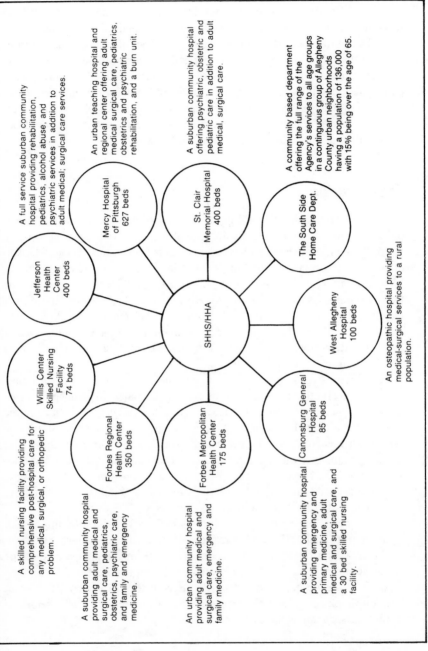

A skilled nursing facility providing comprehensive post-hospital care for any medical, surgical, or orthopedic problem.

A suburban community hospital providing adult medical and surgical care, pediatrics, obstetrics, psychiatric care, and family and emergency medicine.

An urban community hospital providing adult medical and surgical care, emergency and family medicine.

A suburban community hospital providing emergency and primary medicine, adult medical and surgical care, and a 30 bed skilled nursing facility.

An osteopathic hospital providing medical-surgical services to a rural population.

A full service suburban community hospital providing rehabilitation, pediatrics, alcohol abuse, and psychiatric services in addition to adult medical; surgical care services.

An urban teaching hospital and regional center offering adult medical surgical care, pediatrics, obstetrics and psychiatric rehabilitation, and a burn unit.

A suburban community hospital offering psychiatric, obstetric and pediatric care in addition to adult medical, surgical care.

A community based department offering the full range of the Agency's services to all age groups in a contiguous group of Allegheny County urban neighborhoods having a population of 136,000 with 15% being over the age of 65.

Willis Center Skilled Nursing Facility 74 beds

Forbes Regional Health Center 350 beds

Forbes Metropolitan Health Center 175 beds

Canonsburg General Hospital 85 beds

Jefferson Health Center 400 beds

SHHS/HHA

West Allegheny Hospital 100 beds

The South Side Home Care Dept.

St. Clair Memorial Hospital 400 beds

Mercy Hospital of Pittsburgh 627 beds

Reprinted with permission of the National Association for Home Care, from *Caring* magazine, July 1984, p. 94.

care administrative base unit and ultimately the agency's executive director. In addition, a broken vertical line would link the home care department to the participating hospital's administrative liaison. The administrative liaison reports directly to the CEO of that participating hospital, which would be reflected in this chart by another solid vertical line.

The agency's directors of allied health care are on an equal level with the department directors, as represented by a connecting solid horizontal line and are responsible to the agency's base administration as are the department directors. All department staff are responsible directly to the department director to whom they are assigned. Allied health care professionals also report to appropriate allied health directors. This reporting system is defined as a matrix reporting system.

Matrix reporting systems are well known for their ability to separate apparently conflicting accountabilities and place accountabilities where they logically belong. Each allied health care provider is responsible clinically to the director of his or her professional discipline. At the same time, each one is also responsible to the director of the assigned home care department for specific patient-related activities, including the scheduling of visits, participation in team conferences, documentation, and recertification. Staff problems are resolved through a group process involving the individual service provider, the department director, and the appropriate allied health care director.

The use of a matrix reporting system ensures that patient care decisions are made at the closest administrative level to the direct-patient care. The matrix reporting system allows individual care givers to maintain dual administrative and clinical linkages, thus allowing each professional to keep abreast of current clinical knowledge in their own discipline while ensuring that the director of the department to which the patient is assigned has full authority and responsibility for patient care. The matrix system is ideally suited to an interdisciplinary team situation because it permits flexibility in reporting relationships and thereby fosters a high degree of continuity of patient care.

The matrix system determines who prepares the individual staff member's yearly performance appraisal, commendations, or reprimands. Yearly performance appraisals are prepared by immediate supervisor, for example, nurses are evaluated by their department director; physical therapists by the director of physical therapy; social workers by the director of social work; and so on. Any department director or allied health care director involved with the staff member's performance may submit a written statement to the staffer's immediate supervisor recommending reprimand or commendation, but the actual documentation is the responsibility and decision of the immediate supervisor.

The department director is responsible for all nursing and home health aide staff. The various allied health care directors are responsible for their appropriate staff members. However, either written or verbal comments from the department directors who oversee the staff on a daily basis are secured prior to completing the documents.

Some Centralized Control

The matrix reporting system ensures that decentralized decisions regarding patient care are made effectively and efficiently. However, sometimes centralized decisions need to be made. A large, diverse agency requires centralized control over many functions, especially those that stem directly from that agency's mission, goals, and long-range strategic plan. For example, activities that require centralized control are service-areawide planning, public relations, and billing activities; coordination and dissemination of information; and exploring joint venture opportunities.

This centralized control is strengthened by the fact that each department and allied health care director is responsible to one of the two patient care directors located at the base unit. Daily verbal communication may take place when a director encounters a situation that, for example, requires clarification of policies or procedures, appears to be nonresolvable by staff, or involves issues not addressed by existing policies or procedures, or relates to budget issues. In addition to these spontaneous conferences, one-on-one meetings are routinely scheduled, usually monthly, and a joint meeting of all directors and executive staff responsible for day-to-day operations is held monthly. The two patient care directors are responsible for their assigned directors' yearly performance as well as for overseeing all activities related to that department, such as budgets, staffings, and interrelationships with the various participating hospitals. To continue the lines of responsibility, the two patient care directors are responsible to and report to the director of programs and operations, who in turn reports to the agency's executive director.

For its annual planning, SHHS/HHA uses a bottoms-up approach. On a yearly basis, each home care department and allied health care department completes an environmental assessment and outlines a plan for the next year. As the plans are reviewed at the executive level, each proposed action step is assessed in relation to the agency's mission, goals, and long-range strategic plan. At the executive level, efforts can be coordinated among departments to eliminate duplication of effort. From this activity, a detailed agency plan emerges for the following year. This arrangement enables the agency to set priorities and secure resources for the coming year so that the agency can accomplish the goals identified in its strategic plan.

From the departmental environmental assessments and plans come clear indications of service programs that are needed. These service programs may be completely new, such as the volunteer program; a redefinition or expansion of services, such as the rehabilitative nursing program; or a repackaging of services, such as the early infant and maternal discharge programs.

Often, new programs are begun as pilot programs for only a small portion of the agency's service area. Virtually all new programs are developed centrally by a member of the executive staff so that the program receives appropriate support and resources. Once the program functions well in a small geographic area, it is expanded to a larger area and eventually to the agency's entire service area.

When a program is the realization of a novel concept, a steering committee composed of members of all relevant disciplines and administrative levels within the agency may be convened. The role of the steering committee is primarily to assist the fledgling program in becoming completely integrated into the fabric of the agency and to eliminate any gaps in services that may occur without this specialized, multifaceted review.

Ensured Continuum of Care

The SHHS/HHA has proved that the hospital-based home care model can be successful and is beneficial to both the hospital and the home health agency. Hospital-based home health agencies are one of the few home care program models that can ensure for the patient an effective, comprehensive, coordinated continuum of care.

Appendix B

Home Care Network

D. Michael Elliott

St. Joseph Hospital, Flint, Michigan, set up St. Joseph Health System in 1980 with the intent of creating a continuum of health care services that would be adaptable and responsive to the rapidly changing health care industry. Through a comprehensive strategic planning process, St. Joseph decided that a hospital-based system with vertically integrated services was best prepared to meet the challenges of the fiscal environment without compromising the quality of care. St. Joseph Health System, one of the first of its kind in the United States, was developed not only to ensure the hospital's survival but also to allow it to prosper in a challenging, competitive marketplace.

St. Joseph Health System is a collection of integrated and independent services that work together so its patients and clients receive appropriate care at the least cost. The system includes 14 subsidiaries that offer a full range of care, such as acute hospital care, rehabilitative care, and home care (including skilled nursing, hospice, allied professional services, and home-based respiratory therapy). For-profit ventures, family health centers, adult day care, a nursing home, and geriatric assessment and counseling all are part of the system.

St. Joseph Home Health Network

Initially St. Joseph's home care services grew independently, each establishing its own identity within the community. However, changes in the health

D. Michael Elliott, M.B.A., was formerly executive vice-president of St. Joseph Health System, Flint, Michigan, and is now president of SelectCare, Troy, Michigan.

care market resulted in increased activities in discharge planning and home care placement, and St. Joseph Health System sought a way to solidify its position as the home care leader in the area and to better satisfy its referral sources. The development of St. Joseph Home Health Network has become a cornerstone for the success of St. Joseph Health System.

St. Joseph Home Health Network combines several of the health system's existing home care affiliates into one umbrella group. This group includes durable medical equipment, skilled care services, private-duty health services, and certified adult and pediatric hospice home care.

The goal of St. Joseph Home Health Network, a system within a system, is to offer convenient, continuous, and coordinated home care. The original structure of separate home care subsidiaries remains flexible enough to respond operationally to requests by physicians and agencies who are referring their patients and clients to St. Joseph services.

By creating the home health network, St. Joseph coordinated its home care services and created a single entry point in the system. Simplifying access to the home care services met the needs of both the general public as well as home care referrers, including discharge planners, physicians, and their office support personnel. In an effort to further coordinate home care delivery, the services share one central phone number for access to the home care delivery system. This centralization provides one-stop shopping, but the groups within the system are not legally combined.

Coordinated efforts within the home care network remain the key to much of its success and to its benefit to St. Joseph Health System. Working together allows for more cost-effective management in the areas of financial, marketing, and overall management assistance (for example, the shared use of financial systems). Working as a unit also helps promote the services of the individual home care agencies through referrals. Additional referrals to other non-home-care services in St. Joseph Health System result as well. In the area of personnel, a cooperative working relationship between agencies has resulted in more efficient use of health care professionals and support personnel and in increased employee understanding of related services.

As a whole, operating as a home care network has helped the agencies to become more efficient and financially sound and to employ personnel who are more effective. As a result, the network is attracting, and satisfying, more patients and physicians, thus improving the viability of the individual agencies as well as St. Joseph Health System. Indeed, the benchmark of St. Joseph Health System is its commitment to high quality, and each agency shares this goal. By working together, the image of the individual agencies and the entire system is further improved by association with one another.

St. Joseph Home Health Network is made up of four basic entities: a certified home care agency, a certified hospice program, a private-duty agency, and a durable medical equipment (DME) company. The following is an in-depth look at these services, and how they evolved within St. Joseph Health System.

Certified Home Care Agency

St. Joseph Health System acquired a Medicare-certified home care agency in September 1980. The agency was an existing not-for-profit corporation that was already doing a significant amount of business with St. Joseph Hospital.

Since then, the home care agency has become the dominant home care agency in a three-county area. Its services include adult nursing; pediatric nursing; physical, occupational, and speech therapy; medical social work; home health aide service; nutritional support; and Special Delivery, a program that helps care for newborns and mothers at home after a 24-hour hospital stay.

Staff members make more than 4,000 visits per month, and the number of visits continues to grow at an annual rate of 10 percent to 15 percent. As the agency has grown, so has its image as a provider of high-quality service. In fact, some of its growth has come from medical staffs of competing hospitals referring patients with unusual or difficult home care problems.

Certified Hospice Program

In 1981, the certified home care agency started a hospice program to provide home care and support for terminally ill patients and their families. The hospice program became Medicare-certified in early 1985 and became the first program in Genessee County to be licensed by the state of Michigan. In 1984, the home care agency began the first pediatric hospice program in Michigan.

Becoming both Medicare certified and state licensed has helped position the hospice program as the leader in the Flint area, and the hospice program is an ideal example of how the home care network's individual services have a positive impact on the network and on St. Joseph Health System as a whole. The hospice program not only attracts new patients to St. Joseph Health System, but it also promotes the use of other network and health systems services, including the hospital, nursing home, pharmacy, and DME agency. In addition, the hospice program also makes the system more attractive to such companies as health maintenance organizations by offering their members access to high-quality hospice care at home as an alternative to more expensive inpatient programs.

Private-Duty Agency

As the home care agency grew, it saw that it was not providing an important home care service: the private-duty services that are not Medicare certified and not generally reimbursed by commercial insurers. Because private-duty services are reimbursed and regulated differently, St. Joseph decided that the private-duty agency should not be directly associated with the certified home care agency, and so the private-duty service was established as a separate division within another existing ambulatory care, not-for-profit corporation in St. Joseph Health System. In this way, concerns about Medicare cost reports could be avoided, and wage rates and employee policies could be more consistent with other competing private-duty agencies.

The private-duty agency has experienced steady growth since it was created in the spring of 1982. Services, which include registered nursing, home repairs and maintenance, and personal care and transportation, are provided to patients at home. Temporary personnel, such as nurses and therapists, also are provided to hospitals, nursing homes, and physicians' offices. The agency also provides services to group homes for the mentally impaired and contract medical services for industrial health programs.

The private-duty agency has allowed St. Joseph to achieve much flexibility in providing home care services. The agency is also not constrained by the reimbursement guidelines and regulatory restrictions faced by other agencies in the St. Joseph Health System.

Durable Medical Equipment

As St. Joseph Health System continued to grow, it identified another missing link in its home care delivery program: equipment for patients to use at home. St. Joseph Health System was providing excellent support for patients at home but was letting other firms provide equipment. In doing so, St. Joseph Health System was creating a void in its continuum of care and therefore causing difficulties for some of its patients and their families. It also was missing out on a potential source of income.

In 1982, St. Joseph first began providing home respiratory equipment through a new division of its not-for-profit ambulatory care corporation. St. Joseph began with respiratory equipment because respiratory therapy was a strong patient service at the hospital. This activity grew rapidly, and St. Joseph soon decided to add other types of equipment, such as beds, walkers, wheelchairs, and commodes.

As St. Joseph entered the more comprehensive DME business, it became more competitive with other providers and in 1985 decided to establish a new for-profit entity because its business had grown significantly, not only in the Flint area but also in Michigan and across the country as well. This growth has allowed the company to obtain dealer status for many equipment lines, thus further enhancing cost-effectiveness and profitability.

As with its other home care agencies, quality of care is important to St. Joseph's DME activity. The respiratory division, which is staffed totally by certified respiratory therapists, provides assessment and training for patients as part of its routine services. In fact, many therapists are employees on contract from the hospital, and because of their expertise, they can perform various tests for patients right in the home. St. Joseph is one of the few DME companies to use respiratory therapists, and its level of expertise has helped to attract clients and generate interest by other hospitals throughout the state and country. The company now offers consulting and contract management services and in several cases has entered into joint venture arrangements to establish similar companies with other hospitals.

St. Joseph's DME company, which has grown significantly in the past four years, has relocated three times and is planning a further expansion soon. Likewise, personnel with new and expanded skills, such as salespersons, medical equipment repairpersons, and pharmacists, have been hired. Although all of this activity has generated significant earnings potential, it has also required large cash outlays to fund new and expanding programs. To obtain the necessary funding, all of the outstanding stock of the DME company were sold to the hospital corporation, and the hospital, in turn, pledged market-rate loans to the DME company so that it could acquire working capital.

Tips on Developing a Home Care Network

The experiences of St. Joseph Health System in developing a home care network may provide helpful advice to hospitals who want to set up a similar system. Hospitals and health care systems may provide home care services to their patients in one of three ways:

- Use existing community services and refer patients to these agencies through hospital discharge planning mechanisms
- Develop relationships with existing community agencies through cooperative arrangements
- Establish their own home care services through development or acquisition

Before a hospital or health system decides to provide its own home care services, the following questions should be addressed:

- Does the hospital or system see an unfilled need in the community?
- Does the hospital or system want to provide alternative, high-quality service?
- Does the hospital or system want to retain patients within its health systems?
- Does the hospital or system want the home care services to serve as an entry point or source for other system referrals?

Objectives

A hospital or health system should also ask the following questions to best identify its objectives for entering the home care business:

- *Does it want financial gain?* If the objective is to produce income, then the types of home care activity should be carefully reviewed in terms of profit potential. For example, the certified home care agency, under the reimbursement methods as of 1986, primarily is a cost-reimbursed provider and offers little income opportunity. On the other hand, private-duty services offer large income potential, primarily because reimbursement is paid by private individuals or by commercial insurance. However, the highest income producer in the home care field today is DME and the high-tech home care services. Margins for these services have run from 20 percent to 30 percent of total sales, although such margins may be reduced in the future to from 10 to 20 percent.
- *Does it want new patients?* A hospital should not develop a home care program if its primary objective is to attract inpatients because the vast majority of home care referrals already come from the hospital. However, a home care program offers an opportunity to maximize existing referrals to the hospital's ancillary services, such as lab and pharmacy, and potentially to other services in the system.
- *Does it want to retain patients?* If the objective is to retain patients within the system, then having the ability to refer patients to a home care company controlled by the system is important. Having a home care agency minimizes the likelihood of patients leaving the system, as professionals providing care in the home have opportunities to make referrals to other health care providers in the system.
- *Does it want control over home care activity?* If the objective is to have control over home care activity, then the hospital or system must decide whether to own and manage the home care agency itself, enter into a joint venture, or have the agency managed by an outside organization. Furthermore, the need for expediency in entering the home care business will influence the organizational structure and development and may have a long-lasting impact on the operation of the home care service.

Game Plan

When starting home care services within a system, a game plan is crucial to ensure proper growth and development. The following includes some major issues to consider when devising such a plan of action:

- *Organizational relationships* within the system must be established. For example, careful consideration should be given to whether a home care service should be part of an existing corporation, a subsidiary of an existing corporation, or a joint venture or partnership outside the existing organization. These questions become particularly important when more than one type of home care entity is being created. System management will need to address these relationships, with input from legal advisers and reimbursement experts.

- *Identifying key management personnel* early is important to the planning process so that they can participate in establishing procedures and policies and in making other decisions that will affect the company's future.
- *Having sufficient working capital* is critical to the early success of the company. Because new companies initially have greater working capital needs than their source of revenue, funding must be sufficient to cover the growth phase. Therefore, when making financial projections, conservative forecasts should be used so that boards and administrators do not prematurely criticize the new companies before they have had a fair chance to prove themselves.
- *Identifying hurdles and barriers* to starting a new agency also is important. In this way, methods for solving problems can be devised to prevent major setbacks. Some of these hurdles may be existing physician involvement, such as preference for other home care providers, or the relationships of hospital discharge planners with competitive services within the community.

Active Leadership

When developing home care services as part of a health system, the system's management must provide effective and committed guidance, direction, and leadership. Such support can come in the form of offering management, financial, and personnel expertise; providing professional support personnel; assisting and generating patient referrals; or just plain problem solving. At St. Joseph Health System, the system management division, coordinated by the system executive vice-president, serves this role.

Effective leadership may be the single most important ingredient in establishing new home care activities within a health system. System management must help address problems, encourage creativity, provide opportunities to develop entrepreneurial skills, and instill confidence to cope with the ongoing changes in the health care industry. Indeed, the most successful home care agencies are those with a good mixture of participation from system management and the individual agency.

Growing Pains

Growing pains are part of any new venture, and developing a home care service is no different. Some potential problems include:

- Politics within the organization and the health care community as a whole

- Understaffing as volume of patients grows
- Tight working capital situation as the constant demand for expansion requires greater cash flow than the receipts allow
- Changing regulations that create new challenges just as it appears old problems have been solved
- Being the new kid on the block and trying to demonstrate capabilities to get those critical new referrals

Bridge to the Future

St. Joseph Health System was created to provide programs that not only meet the needs of the community but also allow St. Joseph Hospital to respond to the changing needs of the health care market. Today, St. Joseph Home Health Network is an example of how this philosophy is working. For one thing, St. Joseph is meeting its mission by helping patients achieve optimum health in a cost-effective but caring way that reflects the dignity of the individual.

In addition, the St. Joseph Home Health Network has helped St. Joseph Health System realize operational and financial benefits through shared services, cost savings, and new income. Employees have benefited by exposure to varied health care experiences and increasingly diversified opportunities. Likewise, employee morale has improved through being associated with a new and successful venture.

Five years ago, St. Joseph Hospital set a bold, new course. Through strategic planning and corporate diversification, it has ensured its survival and renewed its mission in the community. St. Joseph Hospital recognized, and met, a crucial challenge: it had to change to survive. This philosophy is St. Joseph's bridge to the future.

Appendix C

Hospital-Affiliated Model

Judith Walden

Hospital HomeCare (HHC) originated in 1973 as a small hospital-based home care agency in Albuquerque, New Mexico. Unique among hospital-based programs, HHC was established as a joint venture between two community hospitals. The two controlling hospital corporations, St. Joseph Healthcare Corp. and Presbyterian Healthcare Services, are composed of not-for-profit hospitals located approximately 1½ miles apart in the central part of the city. The hospitals serve a population base of 460,000 persons. Although viewed by the community as highly competitive, the two hospitals share a common medical staff, jointly own an ambulance company, and plan respective expansions in a cooperative spirit. In 1985, the hospitals created Cooperative Health Care, a jointly sponsored preferred provider organization (PPO), and Health Plus, a jointly sponsored HMO.

In its early years, the home care program grew beyond everyone's expectations, experiencing a consistent annual increase of 25 percent to 40 percent in number of visits and patients served. The agency rapidly became a recognized leader in the city and state, in part because of the excellent reputations of the sponsoring hospitals.

The mission of HHC is to develop, manage, and provide high-quality patient and family-centered home health, hospice, and related support services in a cost-effective manner consistent with the expressed goals of Hospital HomeCare. The mission statement was last revised in 1985.

In keeping with this mission and to meet the home care needs of the sponsoring hospitals, the agency began adding new programs as early as 1976. The first such new service was Senior Home Care, a homemaker and

Judith Walden, R.N., is president and executive director of Hospital HomeCare, Albuquerque, New Mexico.

chore service funded through a variety of federal and state programs. This program remained an integral part of the agency until 1983 when it became a separate subsidiary corporation, HomeCare Resources, Inc.

The agency's hospice care program began in 1978 and was one of the 26 hospice demonstration projects sponsored by the Health Care Financing Administration. The hospice division of HHC became a Medicare-certified provider in April 1984. The continued financial success of the hospice care program will depend, in part, on improved Medicare reimbursement. However, HHC became Medicare certified in spite of the known constraints of Medicare and with the solid support of the medical, hospital, and lay community. The program is able to raise sufficient funds to offset losses resulting from inadequate Medicare reimbursement.

Incorporation

Prior to July 1981, HHC operated as a de facto partnership, which is essentially a nonentity. Although jointly owned, the agency functioned as a department of one of the partner-hospitals, St. Joseph Hospital. Staff members of HHC were hospital employees. The agency was governed as a hospital department, with ultimate authority residing in the board of trustees of St. Joseph Hospital.

As the agency grew and as Medicare cost-reporting regulations became less flexible, the need to formalize the structure became evident. The governing boards of both hospitals were legally responsible for this multiservice large agency, yet neither board had much direct control over operations because HHC functioned as a hospital department.

Initially, the Medicare fiscal intermediary permitted HHC to directly allocate on the cost report only those hospital costs that were specifically related to the agency. However, increased federal focus on Medicare in general and home care in particular resulted in the elimination of previously flexible cost-finding and cost-reporting methods. The agency was faced with a decision of becoming a "true" hospital-based agency affiliated with a single hospital and absorbing more hospital allocations or declaring itself a freestanding agency. As a freestanding agency, no hospital allocations would be received, and direct and increased agency administrative costs would be incurred.

Faced with cost-related decisions and the perceived need to limit governing board liability, the home care agency incorporated in July of 1981 as a not-for-profit member corporation; that is, it became a freestanding, hospital-owned agency. Under New Mexico corporation law, the members retain certain rights, such as governing board appointments and budget approval, just as do shareholders in a proprietary company. The original two partner hospital corporations are the only members of the not-for-profit corporation.

Following incorporation, HHC arranged transfer and referral agreements with four other nonrelated community hospitals in the form of a memorandum of understanding. These agreements were necessary to formalize the positive relationships between the home care agency and the hospitals, to permit access of HHC liaison staff to patient and health records, and to promote community involvement in the reorganized agency. The initial HHC governing board included representation from these hospitals; however, the member hospitals retained majority control. The chairpersons of the Professional Advisory Committee and the Medical Advisory Committee were also appointed to the agency's governing board.

With this incorporation, HHC had to establish separate accounting records, bank accounts, and payroll systems. Staff members became employees of HHC and yet were still included in St. Joseph Hospital's pension and benefit plan because of the agency's subsidiary relationship with the hospital. A formal contractual arrangement for specified management and accounting services was negotiated between St. Joseph Hospital and HHC. Following Medicare-related organization reimbursement principles, all services performed by the hospital for the home care agency were charged at their cost to the hospital. Incorporation also resulted in HHC's management having more direct control over operations. Interestingly, the Joint Commission on Accreditation of Hospitals (JCAH) considered HHC to be hospital administered, and thus the agency retained its JCAH accreditation until 1986 when the JCAH reversed its earlier decision.

The agency has a reputation of providing hi-tech, highly skilled services that have a patient education and rehabilitation focus. Nursing services for both hospice and generic home care operate on a 24-hour basis. Visits by home health aides are scheduled as late as 8 p.m. to provide personal care in the evening.

Specialty programs, such as psychiatric, pediatric and respiratory nursing, are provided by HHC staff. A Welcome HomeCare program designed for maternity patients who were discharged early was begun in 1985. Planned for 1987 is a home cardiac rehabilitation and home electrocardiogram (EKG) program.

Because of the sponsorship and support by the member hospitals, more than 75 percent of HHC referrals come from these two hospitals and from the agency's affiliated hospitals, nursing homes, and ambulatory care centers. Liaison nurses who work with the various hospital-based discharge planning units are employed by HHC to help prepare identified patients for the transition to home or hospice care. The remaining 25 percent of home care referrals come directly from physicians, who often refer patients who have not been admitted to a hospital.

Restructuring

Hospital HomeCare is a dynamic, ever-changing organization. As new opportunities are discovered, as new services and options are identified, and as management and staff expertise grow, so does HHC. As a result, another corporate restructuring was accomplished in 1985.

During 1984, HHC underwent an internal reexamination of its mission and structure to determine how to meet increasing home care needs of the member hospitals, increase autonomy, and position the agency to quickly respond to future service and product demands. A reorganization to a parent holding company model with three subsidiary companies to serve the various markets resulted.

In this reorganization, a parent holding company, Hospital Home Health, Inc., was established. The holding company had a five-person governing board appointed by the two member hospital corporations. Initially, the holding company will have no staff or separate office.

Hospital HomeCare became one of the subsidiaries although it remained essentially the same: a Medicare-certified, not-for-profit home care and hospice agency. It has also entered into contracts with preferred provider organizations and health maintenance organizations and will continue to provide intermittent home visits through other third-party payers that require home care to be provided by an agency that is licensed by the state or certified by Medicare. The pricing of its services is geared to costs.

The other two subsidiaries are HomeCare Resources, Inc., and Home-Care Enterprises, Corp. HomeCare Resources, previously a subsidiary of HHC, is further isolated from HHC's Medicare cost allocations through this restructuring. HomeCare Resources will continue as a nonregulated homemaker and chore service provider for government-subsidized clients and private-duty clients. The pricing of its services is geared to the market.

HomeCare Enterprises, a new for-profit company, has entered into two partnerships and may directly provide other services and products depending on available capital and staff expertise in various areas. Initially, a durable medical equipment service and a home infusion therapy service have been developed through partnerships with other existing companies having expertise and experience in these hi-tech areas. HomeCare Enterprises also owns a large office building that is leased at cost to Hospital HomeCare.

This latest restructuring provides an opportunity for rapid entry into new markets. In the future, new programs will be added to either of the three subsidiary corporations depending on regulatory requirements and tax implications. The new or reconstituted boards are small and autonomous. The major responsibility for strategic planning and resource allocation rests with the holding company board, which includes member hospital representation and the chairpersons of each subsidiary board. All four boards meet separately on a quarterly basis and together yearly for an annual board conference.

This multicorporation hospital-owned home care organization continues to grow. Budgeted for 1986-87 are 66,000 home care and hospice visits or units of service for HHC and 85,000 homemaker service hours for Home-Care Resources. Total revenues for all three subsidiary corporations will exceed $5.5 million during fiscal year 1986-87. Hospital HomeCare provided 53,000 home health visits to 3,050 patients and 6,000 hospice units of service to 300 patients in fiscal year 1985-86.

The agency will continue to evaluate new opportunities in the home care marketplace and may undergo another restructuring or reorganization to meet new needs in the future. This home care organization will survive the current funding constraints and constant regulatory change because of solid board and hospital commitment and management expertise. A forward thinking and creative health care organization, HHC is now well positioned to plan for and react to the evolving market.

Appendix D

Cooperative Model

Kaye Daniels

Hospital Home Health Care Agency of California was formed in 1969 as a freestanding for-profit home care agency that would serve Hawthorne Community Hospital, a 280-bed, not-for-profit, Los Angeles community hospital. The community hospital provided $65,000 to capitalize the agency. In its first year, the agency recorded 1,000 visits. The services provided included intermittent nursing, physical therapy, social services, and home health aides.

For seven years, the freestanding for-profit agency continued to grow and serve its founding hospital. During this growth period, the agency established relationships with seven other hospitals throughout the greater Los Angeles area to increase its patient base and to make the provision of its home care services more cost-efficient. Liaison nurses were hired to strengthen the relationship between Hospital Home Health Care Agency and the hospitals served. The nurses were hired by the home health agency and assigned to the hospitals. By 1974 the annual number of visits reached approximately 6,000. By 1976, visits numbered approximately 40,000; and agency revenues were in excess of approximately $700,000 (figure D-1, page 296, and D-2, page 297). This increase in number of visits can be attributed to the agency's strong hospital base.

In response to the continuous upward swing of health care costs, administrators from 10 of these hospitals, representing both religious and nonsectarian facilities, decided in 1977 that they needed to take action to reduce costs to patients while still providing continuity of care once the individual left the hospital. To meet these needs, this group and Hospital

Kaye Daniels, R.N., M.B.A., is vice-president of Kokua Nurses Agency, Honolulu, Hawaii.

Figure D-1.   Annual Visits at Hospital Home Health Care Agency of California

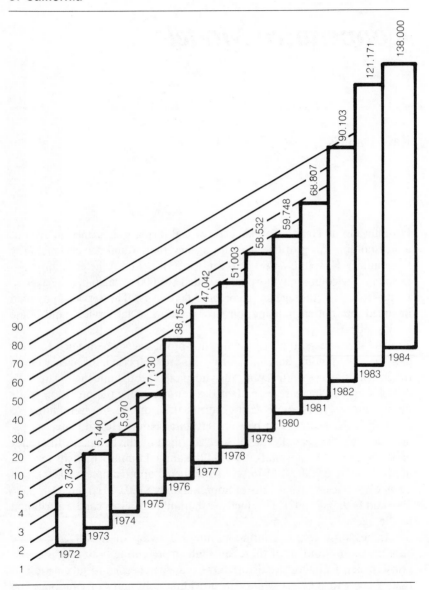

Home Health Care Agency formed the first cooperative alliance of its kind in California.

   Hospital Home Health Care Agency became a not-for-profit cooperative in 1977, and the words *of California* were added to its name. Each hospital contributed $6,500 to pay off the original $65,000 debt that the previous for-profit agency had incurred while under the ownership of the community

Figure D-2. Growth in Revenue at Hospital Home Health Care Agency of California

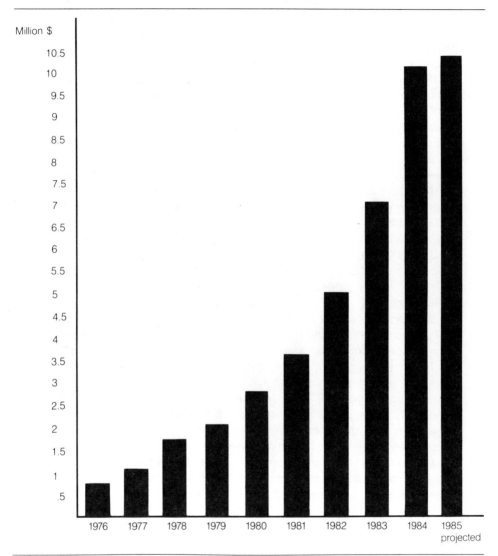

hospital. An administrator from each hospital was appointed to serve on the agency's board of directors.

Many factors were involved in the formation of the cooperative. For the first time, a united community effort on the part of 10 competing Los Angeles area hospitals would provide continuity of care for the hospitals' discharged patients. The initial capital investment was low, and the agency was no threat to the hospitals' source of income. Also, Medicare reimbursement in 1977 made it more desirable for hospitals not to operate their own agency. Besides, Hospital Home Health Care Agency was already an established viable alternative to developing their own program. Under this new arrangement, the agency saw an increase in the number of visits and revenue from 40,000 visits and $700,000 in 1976 to more than 50,000 visits and $1.7 million in 1978 (figures D-1 and D-2, pages 296 and 297). The increased revenue includes DME and homemaker services.

To meet the changing needs of the hospitals in the cooperative, Hospital Home Health Care Agency of California developed its hospice program in 1976 to aid terminally ill patients and their families. The hospice program was selected by the California State Department of Health as one of four demonstration projects to study the cost of hospice care in California. It was one of 26 programs that participated in a nationwide demonstration project, through the Department of Health and Human Services, to evaluate the quality and cost-effectiveness of hospice care. In 1977, the hospice program served 88 patients; by 1980 the number of patients served was close to 300. In 1985, a monumental year, the hospice program received full Medicare certification and served a total of 650 patients and their families.

In 1980 the agency began to affiliate with other hospitals not in the cooperative. Affiliated hospitals had no monetary investment in the cooperative and did not participate on the board of directors. However, each affiliated hospital was assigned a liaison nurse.

Agency visits reached 60,000 by 1980, and revenues were approximately $2.7 million (figures D-1 and D-2, pages 296 and 297). The agency continued to meet the needs of the hospitals in the cooperative and its affiliated hospitals by providing liaison nurses, opening two branch offices, and offering a wide variety of programs and services. These programs and services included more technical in-home procedures, such as caring for ventilator-dependent patients, changing tracheostomy tubes, and continuing intravenous therapy begun in the hospital, as well as supportive services, such as the homemaker program. The homemaker program was set up as a private-duty program under the home care agency. A consulting program was developed to assist those organizations that were interested in the development or refinement of a home care program.

By the mid-1980s the prospective pricing system (PPS), with its early discharge incentives, had a dramatic effect on how hospitals viewed home care. This system, which encouraged the cooperative hospitals to discharge patients to Hospital Home Health Care Agency, also made the opening of hospital-based programs more inviting. Because of Medicare reimbursement rules, a hospital can save money by discharging a patient to home care, and it can also shift some hospital administrative costs and general expenses to its own home care agency. Such cost shifting was a source of revenue and an incentive for the facility to open its own home care agency. Also, as of 1986, Medicare payments for home care agencies are not fixed: agencies are reimbursed for their costs, within limits, just as hospitals were reimbursed by Medicare before PPS. Also, hospital-based programs are allowed an 11 percent add-on over the cost limits to cover increased costs incurred by the agency. A freestanding agency is not allowed these add-ons.

When one of the hospitals in the cooperative proposed setting up its own agency, the agency's board of directors was forced to act. The direction the board decided to take to counter proposed moves by the member hospitals was an entirely new approach for the not-for-profit home care cooperative.

A restructuring was ordered. The new corporate structure would give the hospitals the flexibility to set up their own agencies. For the first time, hospitals in the cooperative could generate revenues through two newly formed affiliate companies: Hospital Home Health Care Ventures, Inc., and Hospital Home Health Care Shared Services, Inc.

Hospitals that are members of Hospital Home Health Care Shared Services, Inc., now deliver home care services through their own hospital-based agencies while still using the staff and services of Hospital Home Health Care Agency. The hospital-based agencies have a core staff and are licensed and Medicare certified. Hospital Home Health Agency continues to serve member hospitals that do not wish to start their own home care agencies.

Hospital Home Health Care Ventures, Inc., the for-profit affiliate, now operates the consulting services division, durable medical equipment company, and Care Connection. The Consulting Services Division was designed in response to the never-ending demands placed on the agency for expert assistance in the startup of home care agencies throughout the United States.

The durable medical equipment company has formed partnerships with several member hospitals of Hospital Home Health Care Ventures, Inc. Offices have opened within each of these facilities. These offices are staffed by employees of Hospital Home Health Care Ventures, Inc., who coordinate durable medical equipment (DME) programs of the partner hospitals. Employees of Hospital Home Health Care Agency coordinate additional services, such as intermittent and extended care.

The actual profitability of the DME program depends on its integration within the hospital. The experience of Hospital Home Health Care Ventures, Inc., has been that the partner hospitals have rapidly increased their use of DME during the first four to six months of the program's operation. This increase is attributed to the educational process that was targeted at hospital personnel and medical staff to increase awareness of the program. This type of partnership requires the full support of administration and staff within the facility.

The Care Connection, which started as the homemaker program under the not-for-profit agency, now provides all private-duty services to member and nonmember hospitals under the for-profit Hospital Home Health Care Ventures, Inc. These services include registered nurses, licensed vocational nurses, home care aides, homemakers, live-ins, and companions. In 1985, the Care Connection generated revenues in excess of $2 million a year. Of the $2 million in revenues, 50 percent is generated through nursing services, and the other 50 percent through homemaker services. As with the DME partnerships, member hospitals are also able to form revenue-producing partnerships with Care Connection. These partnerships are for private-duty services. Again, the profitability of this type of partnership depends on the integration of the program into the hospital system and the overall support of administration and staff.

The ultimate success of a cooperative arrangement depends on the ability of the agency's administration to evaluate the needs of member hospitals and their medical staffs and to meet these needs on an ongoing basis. Flexibility, a solid working relationship with hospital administration and physicians, and a responsive agency structure are the keys to this type of model. Ongoing change, development, and growth must be a part of day-to-day operation.

The cooperative model will continue to be copied and become more accepted as changes in Medicare payment rules affect home care agencies. The cooperative model of Hospital Home Health Care Agency of California is made up of competing hospitals in the Los Angeles area. In the future, the cooperative model will be made up of hospitals and alternative delivery providers, such as HMOs, that have a common focus. Competing hospitals are often reluctant to share common resources, whereas allied hospitals, such as Catholic or corporate-owned and rural hospitals that are not geographically close, are more willing to enter into these arrangements. The ultimate benefits of cooperation are satisfied patients, physicians, and hospitals and a cost-efficient, viable home care program.

Appendix E

Rural Home Care Models

Katherine Pfeifle

Home care agencies that serve rural areas of the United States face issues that may not be of primary concern to agencies in urban areas. Of primary concern is whether adequate manpower resources exist and whether available staff members have the necessary skill levels to provide adequate care to patients in the home.

The manpower problem is not an easy one to solve. Small and rural hospitals need to carefully assess what services they can initially supply and how services can be developed in the future to provide a comprehensive program for their identified service area population. In rural areas, physical therapists, occupational therapists, speech therapists, and medical social workers are frequently in short supply, and so agencies usually must contract with individuals or other area hospitals and health care facilities if they are to supply these services. Home care agencies may not want to hire professionals in these areas on a full-time basis because the number of patients requiring such services may be limited.

Other issues that are important from an administrative perspective include:

- The development of emergency plans and protocols of care for unexpected situations that occur in the home or in the process of traveling long distances to the homes of patients. Emergency planning must include procedures for visits after hours, transfer of patients from the home care setting to an inpatient facility, first aid procedures, inability to gain entrance to the home, and dangerous travel conditions.

Katherine Pfeifle, R.N., owns and operates a home care consulting firm in Grand Forks, North Dakota.

- The development of an efficient method of handling the significant amounts of downtime that occur when the staff person is traveling between patients. Accounting for the downtime resulting from staff travel may require streamlining of the agency's internal procedures, especially with regard to paperwork. Notes of home visits can be dictated, and perhaps software can be developed that would enable the mandatory forms required for Medicare-certified agencies to be handled on a computer. Also, visits to patients can be clustered so that total miles traveled is decreased.
- The provision of services to patients when few or no community resources are available.

Rural home care agencies also face problems relating to the direct provision of patient care that may require considerable improvisational ability on the part of staff members. Professional and paraprofessional staff members must be innovative problem solvers who are able to function with limited or no resources. For example, patients may not have running water, electricity, refrigeration, telephone service, or adequate heat. Many rural home care nurses and aides must haul water either from a pump or from the agency if they want to provide care and give baths. During the winter, nurses may even use melted snow.

Multiple options for pursuing the provision of home care services are available to small and rural hospitals. These options may be consolidated and categorized into the following models:

- Start-up of a program owned and operated by the hospital
- Joint affiliation between a home care provider and a hospital through a branch-office arrangement

Many issues surface as small and rural hospitals begin investigating whether they should provide home care services to their service area population. These issues, which can be organizational or environmental, political, financial, and operational, must be addressed prior to making a decision to implement any one of the possible options.

Hospital Start-up

Hospitals choose to start up their own home care programs for a variety of reasons that become apparent after an assessment of the organizational or environmental, political, financial, and operational issues that affect their particular service areas. This section looks at these issues as they relate to the start-up of a home care program by a hospital and then describes a home care program that resulted from a hospital's decision to start its own program.

Organizational or Environmental Concerns

One problem faced by a small and rural hospital is that it is frequently the sole community provider of health care services in its primary service area. This situation both creates an opportunity for the hospital and presents a possible problem. The problem is that it cannot share already established services or contract for the provision of home care services because no other organization is close enough to make such arrangements feasible. On the other hand, as the sole provider, the hospital does not have to worry about any competitors trying to capture its share of the market.

Another issue confronting a small and rural hospital is that it may have a specialized case mix that requires specific home care services. Examples of such a select target patient populations may be those persons requiring specific pediatric treatments and procedures, home dialysis patients, cardiac rehabilitation patients, or respiratory therapy clientele receiving 24-hour home ventilator care. A hospital with a specialized case mix may decide that starting up its own home care agency makes more sense financially because the expertise that already exists in the hospital can be used for caring for these patients.

Political Forces

Rural communities have a strong sense of community pride, and this pride is a significant influencing factor in a hospital's decision to develop its own home care program rather than contracting with a home care provider in its area. This sense of community pride is reflected in the attitudes of hospital administrators, board members, and physicians as well as the community at large.

Physicians frequently indicate that they support a home care program owned and operated by the hospital because they perceive that this arrangement will give them more control of the program. They perceive a loss of control if the hospital contracts with another organization to maintain a home care program. Physicians and the hospital may also fear the potential loss of patients to competing physicians and hospitals when home care is provided under contract. This fear can be a real concern, and its impact should be carefully considered before the home care program is developed.

All of these political forces need to be taken into consideration during the process of deciding whether the hospital should be involved in home care and during any negotiations with an existing home care provider. For reasons of community pride or fear of loss of hospital patients, a hospital may decide that its only viable option is to start up its own program.

Financial Considerations

Any hospital considering the development of a home care program must undergo a financial feasibility analysis of the projected financial impact and investment involved in the start-up of a federally certified home health agency as well as for other ventures planned for the agency, including private-pay services. Financial feasibility can be demonstrated by project work load and statistical units (home visits and hours of service) and projected revenue.

Private-pay services are a myriad of services provided in that home that range from private-duty nursing rendered by registered or licensed practical nurses to personal care services such as bathing, dressing, and range-of-motion exercises provided by nurse aides to handyperson service encompassing snow removal, yard work, and minor house repair. Private-pay services are complementary services to a certified home health agency, not only from the standpoint of providing comprehensive services to its clientele but also from the standpoint that revenue generated by these services contribute to the potential profit margin of a home care program.

Operational Issues

Small and rural hospitals may choose to tap into or develop the internal human and systems resources it already possesses to manage and operate a home care program. The human resources may include individuals such as registered nurses, billing and business office staff, or administrators who have previous experience working with a home care program. A home care program can also use the hospital's business office for billing and collection services, the supply and purchasing department to provide medical supplies and equipment, the laboratory for processing specimens and reporting on the results of the tests, and the nursing department for staffing the home care program. Indeed, the home care program may be totally integrated into the existing hospital operation.

Example of the Start-up of a Home Care Program

A small and rural 25-bed hospital (Hospital X) in northwestern Minnesota chose to start its own home care program after its feasibility analysis demonstrated that this option was the most viable and satisfactory of the options available to the hospital. The hospital's primary service area population (10,000) was served by four existing home care providers: two public health agencies, a freestanding proprietary home health agency, and a hospital-based home health agency operated by Hospital Z.

Hospital X is located in a small community of 1,500 persons and is the sole community provider. The next nearest hospital, Hospital Z, has 100 beds and is located 40 miles away in the same county. Hospital X provides the traditional blend of inpatient and outpatient services and operates a 48-bed long-term-care unit for nursing home clientele requiring intermediate and skilled nursing services. Its inpatient Medicare case mix utilization was significant, running at 68 percent for fiscal year 1985.

The driving political forces influencing Hospital X's decision included a medical staff of three who were quite vocal in their support of the hospital developing its own home care program. The physicians' main concerns were a perception of a lack of quality in available home care services and a lack of communication from the existing three home care providers. In addition, the hospital's governing board and administration believed that not developing its own program and entering into a joint affiliation with Hospital Z would have several disadvantages:

- Autonomy would be lost, and Hospital X could not declare to its clientele or service area that it maintained a separate identity as a home care provider for marketing and promotional purposes.
- Loss of control would result, or control would be limited in all programming aspects of the home care service including, but not limited to, the following:
  - Personnel employed
  - Personnel policies and procedures
  - Charges for services rendered in the home
  - Future goals and programs provided by the agency
  - Potential restriction on clientele admitted and served
  - Limited medical staff input
  - Marketing and promotional plan format and implementation
- Hospital X may lose patients to Hospital Z and its medical staff, resulting in Hospital Z increasing its home care, inpatient, and outpatient referral base.
- Hospital X would not realize the potential financial benefits that would result by having the hospital-based home care entity contribute financially to the hospital through revenue generated from home visits and the use of medical supplies and equipment, laboratory tests, and pharmaceuticals.

A financial analysis model was developed specifically for evaluation purposes. The components of the model included identification of estimated investments, methods of financing, statistics and work-load projections, revenue projections, expense projections, profit and loss projections, estimated capital expenses, estimated cash flow, internal rate of return, net present value, and the payback period on discounted cash flow. The financial analysis revealed that Hospital X would generate a total of 1,739 home visits by registered nurses, home health aides, physical therapists, speech therapists, and medical social workers in the third year after implementation of the program. This number of visits amounted to 65 percent of the home care marketplace. Based on the work-load projections, the hospital anticipated that it would require 2.86 full-time equivalents to adequately staff the home care program. The hospital chose not to offer occupational therapy because no therapist was available to staff this function.

Hospital X decided on an initial investment of $37,645, of which $14,000 was initial start-up expense and $23,645 was working capital for six months.

Start-up expenses included consultation fees for program development, staff orientation and training, printing expenses for the development of forms, initial supplies for the nurses' bags and small equipment, and initial promotional and marketing expenses. The hospital decided to have six months of working capital available to account for the waiting time that occurs when a new home health agency applies for federal certification with the Department of Health and Human Services. The agency cannot receive reimbursement for services provided to Medicare and Medicaid beneficiaries until it has been federally certified.

The financial analysis also revealed that Hospital X would realize an internal rate of return of 33.81 percent, a net present value of $30,901. The estimated payback period on discounted cash flow would be 3.77 years, based on the financial pro forma calculated over a six-year period.

During the feasibility study, operational issues were also considered. Hospital X determined that it could use its in-house expertise in the provision of billing and collection services, admission services, data processing and information management services, medical records support for transcription of home-visit documentation and reports, laboratory testing procedures, medical supply and equipment handling, and support staff for the provision of home care visits.

In summary, Hospital X made the appropriate decision for its needs and for the needs of its service area population. One year after implementation of its home care program, the utilization of services provided in the home surpassed the initial projections of market capture, and the agency is functioning at the level of revenue, expense, and work load projected for the third year of operation. The response by the hospital's administration and governing board, the medical staff, and the community has been positive, and significant support has been generated for the program.

Joint-Affiliation Arrangement

Joint-affiliation arrangements have many different configurations, which include the establishment of branch offices, subunits, and shared-service contracts for the purchase of mutually provided services and the creation of partnerships or corporate entities. In addition, these options may be combined in any number of ways.

Definition of Related Terms

The following definitions of terms relating to joint-affiliation arrangements in the home care industry are helpful in understanding the discussion of such arrangements:

- *Branch office:* A location or site from which a home health agency provides services to a portion of the total geographic area served by the parent agency. The branch office is part of the home health agency and is located sufficiently close so that it can share administration, supervision, and services. Thus a branch office does not have to independently meet the conditions of participation for a home health agency (Code of Federal Regulations, Title 42, Section 405.1202(c); *Federal Register,* July 16, 1973).

- *Subunit:* A semiautonomous organization that serves patients in a geographic area different from that of the parent agency. By virtue of the distance between it and the parent agency, the subunit is judged incapable of sharing administration, supervision, and services on a daily basis with the parent agency and must therefore independently meet the conditions of participation for home health agencies (Code of Federal Regulations, Title 42, Section 405.1202(w); *Federal Register,* July 16, 1973).
- *Corporation:* A legal entity created by law. A corporation is separate and distinct from the individuals or organizations that form the entity.
- *Partnership:* A voluntary association of two or more individuals or organizations who combine resources to share profit and loss in predetermined proportions.

Organizational or Environmental and Political Concerns

In some rural areas, multiple home care providers exist. Thus, the possibility for negotiating with another area hospital to share services or contract for the provision of home care services is entirely feasible.

The issues that should be addressed in analyzing all existing home care providers includes an assessment of services offered, reputation and image in the community served, financial stability and profitability, willingness to cooperate and pursue a joint-affiliation arrangement, future goals and plans for service and product-line development, physician rapport, and current share of the home care market. Another area requiring critical analysis is the extent of the home care provider's expertise and its ability to manage and operate a successful high-quality service for its clientele.

An issue that frequently confronts rural hospitals is the need to choose one home care provider over another primarily because of the relationship that the hospitals have with another local hospital that operates a home health agency. This practice is not necessarily negative or positive, but it should be viewed in context with the other factors that are investigated during the analysis of the feasibility of participating in a joint affiliation.

One political force may be the need for the rural hospital to offer home care services to its patient population. This need can satisfactorily be met by the hospital entering into a joint-affiliation arrangement, thereby enhancing its own market position and its image in its service area. Hospitals that enter into joint-affiliation arrangements typically choose a name for the home care program that is representative of both hospitals and promote the home care program jointly through such materials as brochures, patient education materials, media advertisements, and slide tape presentations.

Financial Considerations

Financial considerations may be the major influencing reason for a hospital to participate in a joint-affiliation arrangement with another area freestanding home health agency or with a hospital-based home health agency. The financial considerations may include the following:

- The feasibility analysis reveals that the small and rural hospital cannot realistically finance the development of a hospital-based home health agency, perhaps because the identified home care service area is too small to support the agency. The usual standard applied in rural areas is that the minimum service area population required to support a financially viable home health agency is 10,000 persons. Therefore, if the service area population is below 10,000, the expected annual home visits and the annual projected revenue are not adequate to support the anticipated annual expenses that are directly attributable to the home care program.
- A hospital-based home care program also incurs an initial investment at the time of start-up; and if projections of internal rate of return, net present value, and estimated payback period on discounted cash flow over a specified period of time (for example, three to five years) show no return on investment, the hospital may decide to enter a joint-affiliation arrangement. By entering into a joint-affiliation arrangement, a hospital substantially reduces the amount of its initial investment.
- The overall financial impact on the rural hospital is potentially negative and would require cross-subsidization from other hospital sources of revenue.
- The joint-affiliation option allows the rural hospital to generate revenue for home care services but does not involve major expenses or open itself to potential financial loss. These issues, of course, are dependent on the terms of the contractual agreement or joint venture.
- Various states still have certificate-of-need (CON) laws that affect the hospital's timely development of a home health agency. The CON process may require three to six months, depending on individual state requirements. Furthermore, if federal Medicare certification is pursued, the time lapse from agency development and application for certification to receipt of the provider number and notification of certification may be an additional three to six months. Thus, the hospital must fund the new operation without receiving third-party reimbursement, a situation that may result in cash flow problems for the hospital.

Operational Issues

Rural hospitals may choose to use an existing home care provider to get the necessary expertise and skills required to manage and operate a viable home care program. Many rural hospitals experience a shortage in experienced manpower or are unable to recruit and retain an adequate number of professional personnel to sufficiently staff a home health agency. Joint-affiliation arrangements minimize these problems and allow the rural hospital to implement home care services at a much more rapid pace than would be possible if it started up its own agency.

Example of a Joint Affiliation

Two small and rural hospitals located in the upper Midwest chose a partnership arrangement for the sole purpose of making a contractual agreement with the local county commissioners to assume responsibility for all public health and home health agency services provided in Canton County. Hospital A, a 40-bed hospital, is located in Abbott, a town of 2,000 persons. Hospital B, a 19-bed hospital, is located in Byron, a town of 800 persons. Both hospitals serve the same primary service area population (12,574 persons). One existing home health and public health agency known as Canton County Nursing Service also serves this area. The two hospitals are located 23 miles apart.

The hospitals retained a private home care consultant to conduct a study to determine the financial, political, organizational, and operational feasibility of acquiring the Canton County Nursing Service. The feasibility study revealed the following:

- One public health agency and home health agency existed in Canton County. This agency was administered by Canton County under the direction of the Board of Health. The Board of Health ultimately was responsible to the county Board of Commissioners.
- The local medical staff supported the hospitals taking an active role in the provision of community health services to the county.
- The county commissioners preferred that the hospitals assume responsibility for the administration of all county community health services.
- The two hospitals in Canton County were undergoing a substantial change process that was projected to affect their financial performance for many years to come. The hospitals had begun the process of vertical diversification within their own facilities and were interested in jointly pursuing projects and programs. The hospitals believed that they could benefit through joint marketing efforts and a closer tie with physicians and by mutually operating a program to decrease hospital use.

- A trend recently noted in the upper Midwest is that public health agencies operated by the county under the auspices of the county commissioners and the Board of Health are consolidating and merging with local hospitals. This trend is occurring primarily in rural areas.

The feasibility study also included a comprehensive financial analysis. The financial model used was developed specifically for evaluation purposes. Its components included identification of estimated investment, method of financing, statistics or work-load projections, revenue projections, expense projections, profit and loss, estimated capital expense, estimated cash flow, internal rate of return, net present value, and payback period on discounted cash flow.

The financial analysis revealed that by developing a partnership arrangement, the two hospitals would generate 2,872 visits by registered nurses, home health aides, physical therapists, and social workers in the third year of the operation of a federally certified home health agency. This number of visits would mean a capture of 75 percent of the home care market. An additional 2,613 visits by community aides and chore workers would be generated by the public health agency component of the proposed partnership. Other work load anticipated for the agency included early periodic screening and development testing activities; disease, prevention, and control activities; and health education activities. The anticipated revenue for this combination agency included third-party reimbursement for the visits conducted under the federally certified home health agency and a combination of federal, state, and local county subsidies administered as grant funding per fiscal year.

The partnership, to be called Canton County Home Health Care, would incur an initial investment of $90,057, of which $14,000 was identified as initial start-up and transitional expense and $76,057 was identified as the first six months of working capital. Start-up and transitional expense included consultation fees for program development and change of ownership, staff orientation and training, printing expense for form development, and promotional and marketing expenses. Six months of working capital was needed to take into consideration any delay that may occur during the transition and change of agency ownership in case the agency could not bill for services rendered during that time. The paperwork was processed with the Department of Health and Human Services.

The financial analysis also revealed that based on the financial pro forma calculated over a six-year period, the partnership would realize an internal rate of return of 15.5 percent, a net present value of $1,139, and an estimated payback period on discounted cash flow of 5.86 years.

The first step taken by the hospitals was to jointly discuss their goals and the potential for developing a joint-affiliation relationship. Early in the process, the hospital administrators met with two of the county commissioners on an informal basis to determine the county's potential interest in changing the sponsorship of the Canton County Nursing Service from the responsibility of Canton County to the responsibility of the joint venture between the two hospitals located in the county. The preliminary discussions grew into negotiations between the two hospitals and the development of a formal proposal that was submitted to the county commissioners for consideration. The proposal outlined the following key elements:

- The jointly sponsored nursing service (partnership) would act as the agents for Canton County regarding the continuation of grants and the fulfillment of obligations under the grants, except for those grants that are determined to be not cost-effective according to the mission of the partnership.
- The intent of the partnership was to continue the provision of services that are required by law and to have those services reimbursed by grants.
- The partnership would continue all services currently being provided until the services could be measured against the mission statement of the partnership.
- The county should consider its alternatives regarding the disposition of the capital equipment and accounts receivable of Canton County Nursing Service.
- The time frame for implementation must be negotiated and must take into consideration the complexity of the Medicare federal certification process and state licensing requirements.
- Canton County would no longer have direct operating authority over the nursing service, nor would it have any financial responsibilities to the nursing service except for the good-faith continuation of grants that are currently being received by the nursing service.
- Both hospitals in the joint-affiliation arrangement would have operating authority over the nursing service as well as the financial responsibility to it.

The proposal was accepted by the county commissioners. A contract outlining responsibilities was signed by the chairman of the county Board of Commissioners and by the hospital administrators. The two hospitals then sought legal counsel and formally established a partnership according to the rules of the state in which the hospitals were located.

The partnership was established and named Canton County Home Health Care. A board of directors, which consisted of the administrators of the two hospitals and representatives from both hospital boards, was appointed. The board of directors subsequently developed a mission statement and goals and objectives for the entity's first three years of operation. A home care consultant was retained to develop the implementation schedule, manage the change of ownership, and integrate the agency with both hospitals' organizational structures as well as to monitor the operations of the program throughout its initial years of operation.

The specific changes that occurred at the time of the transition included the following:

- All employees of the Canton County Nursing Service were retained during the transition.
- A new salary scale and employee benefit plan were developed and phased in at the time of the transition.
- All employees were oriented to both hospitals and to the newly formed partnership.
- All agency policies, procedures, protocols, and forms were revised.
- All existing contracts were modified and renegotiated.
- New office space was identified, remodeled, and furnished according to need.
- The partnership purchased services from both hospitals when such purchases were advantageous to the partnership financially. Such services included health record transcription services, accounting and data processing services, physical therapy services, and laboratory services.
- Internal office procedures and protocols were developed, taking into consideration existing procedures and whatever additional issues that developed as the new venture was being implemented. This process included setting staff standards for timeliness in the submission and completion of paperwork and for productivity.
- A new advisory committee that was representative of the agency's service area population was appointed.
- Two medical advisors, one from each hospital, were appointed to provide guidance and advocacy for the new entity.
- A marketing and promotional plan was developed. This plan outlined the marketing and promotion efforts for the initial year of operation as well as future plans for the partnership over a five-year time frame.

The partnership decided to locate the parent office in Hospital A, in Abbott, and to establish a branch office in Hospital B, in Byron. This decision was made because the density of population in Canton County was greater in Abbott, the existing nursing service was currently located in Abbott, and Abbott was the county seat.

The two hospitals determined their individual and mutual responsibilities for the daily operations of the agency. The parent office in Abbott is responsible for providing overall professional management, such as handling needed business and billing procedures, data processing, payment of related bills, record storage, and general administration. The branch office in Byron is responsible for the provision of direct services, discharge planning, coordination of referrals, office space, and supportive services. Services shared by the parent and branch office include quality assurance, utilization review, staff education and development activities, and promotional materials and activities.

As of December 1986, this partnership has been operational for only three months, and so success of the venture over any significant period cannot be evaluated. However, the transition or change of ownership occurred smoothly, and no major problems are anticipated. In addition, a nursing home facility located 40 miles from the parent office has requested establishment of a branch office within six months and has expressed an interest in joining the partnership in the near future.

Bibliography

Overview of the Industry

Anderson, H. J. Home care providers' business expanded rapidly during 1985. *Modern Healthcare.* 1986 June 6. 16(12):168-69.

Balinsky, W., and Shames, J. N. Proprietary and voluntary home care agency evolution: the emergence of a new entity. *Home Health Care Services Quarterly.* 1985 Summer. 6(2):5-18.

Cabin, William. The problem with independent contractors. *Caring.* 1985 June. 4(6):32-34, 63.

Frayne, Laurence. DRGs: The impact on physician home health referrals. *Caring.* 1985 Mar. 4(3):60-63.

Gaumer, G., Birnbaum, H., and others. Impact of the New York long-term home health care program. *Medical Care.* 1986 July. 24(7):641-53.

Handel, Bernard. Exploring the alternatives in health care delivery. *Risk Management.* 1985 Aug. 32(8):46-51.

Hedrick, S. C., and Inui, T. S. The effectiveness and cost of home care: an information synthesis. *Health Services Research.* 1986 Feb. 20(6):851-80.

Kaye, L. W. Measuring the extent of gerontological home care staff participation in agency policy making and planning. *Home Health Care Services Quarterly.* 1985 Fall. 6(3):19-32.

Kent, F. Miami's elderly: the future of health care? *Hospitals.* 1986 Mar. 20. 60(6):58-63.

Klane, E. M. Management development: the critical element in home care expansion. *Caring.* 1985 Nov. 4(11):28-31.

Koren, M. J. Home care: who cares? *New England Journal of Medicine.* 1986 Apr. 3. 314(14):917-20.

Kramer, A., Shaughnessy, P., and Pettigrew, M. Cost-effectiveness implications based on a comparison of nursing home and home health case mix. *Health Services Research.* 1985 Oct. 20(4):387-405.

Lange, Maxine. Blue Cross/Blue Shield cost-containment: its meaning for home care. *Caring.* 1985 Oct. 4(10):58-61.

Liu, Korbin, Manton, K., and Liu, Barbara M. Home care expenses for the disabled elderly. *Health Care Financing Review.* 1985 Winter. 7(2):51-58.

Millman, Diane. Legal liabilities for the home health paraprofessional. *Caring.* 1986 Apr. 5(4):25-27.

Moss, J. Extensions of home health services. *Contemporary Long Term Care.* 1986 June. 9(6):71, 74.

_____. In-house vs. freestanding: which is best for you? *Contemporary Long Term Care.* 1986 May. 9(5):65-67.

Pomeranz, W., and Rosenberg, S. Developing home health services in rural communities: an innovative solution to a thorny problem. *Home Health Care Services Quarterly.* 1985-86 Winter. 6(4):5-10.

Rak, K. Where is the home care industry going? *Computers in Healthcare.* 1986 Apr. 7(4):29-30, 34.

Reuben, E. B., and Hamilton, R. D. 3d. Entry and competition in the home health care industry. *Health Care Strategic Management.* 1986 Jan. 4(1):4-9.

Robinson, Nancy. Standard-setting and accreditation by the National Homecaring Council. *Caring.* 1986 Apr. 5(4):34-39.

Salvatone, T. The private nonprofit home health agency: an exploratory essay. *Home Health Care Services Quarterly.* 1985 Fall. 6(3):5-18.

Sandrick, K. Home care: cutting health care's safety net. *Hospitals.* 1986 May 20. 60(10):48-52.

Smith, H. L., and Reid, K. A. Hospital diversification into home health care: examination of strategic issues. *Health Care Strategic Management.* 1986 Jan. 4(1):17-21.

Travavella, Steve. International Insurance Seminar. Reinsurer actions may not turn market: major changes are predicted for group health coverage, risk managers blame captive woes. *Business Insurance.* 1984 July 16. 18(29):12-13.

Trubo, R. Home health care encounters growing pains. *Medical World News.* 1986 Feb. 10. 27(3):76-82, 85, 88.

Van Gelder, S., and Beinstein, J. Home health care in the era of hospital prospective payment: some early evidence and thoughts about the future. *Pride Institute Journal of Long Term Home Health Care.* 1986 Winter. 5(1):3-11.

Wagner, D. Pastoral care in home health: key issues. *Health Progress.* 1986 Mar. 67(2):21, 71.

Wood, J. The effects of cost-containment on home health agencies. *Home Health Care Services Quarterly.* 1985-86 Winter. 6(4):59-78.

Physician Issues

deUlibarri, M. J. Involving physicians in home care. *Home Healthcare Nurse.* 1986 Jan.-Feb. 4(1):11-14.

Richard, D. M. How the home health care movement will affect your practice. *Physician Management.* 1985 Dec. 25(12):123-24, 127-31, 134.

Hot Topics

Baker, D. Managing a hospital-based home health information system. *Computers in Healthcare.* 1986 Mar. 7(3):21-26.

Barrera, M. E., Rosenbaum, P. L., and Cunningham, C. E. Early home intervention with low-birth-weight infants and their parents. *Child Development.* 1986 Feb. 57(1):20-33.

Bender, J. H., and Faubion, W. C. Parenteral nutrition for the pediatric patient. *Home Healthcare Nurse.* 1985 Nov.-Dec. 3(6):32-39.

Burda, D., and Powills, S. AIDS: a time bomb at hospitals' door. *Hospitals.* 1986 Jan. 5:60(1):54-61.

Bonstein, R. G., and Mueller, J. Improving agency productivity. *Caring.* 1985 Nov. 4(11):4-9.

Cohen, D. Getting under your skin [P.F. Lorde, Jr., of Ulster Scumtifie, diabetes testing service]. *Venture.* 1985 Dec. 7(12):14.

Freishtat, H., Gortmaker, S., and others. The corporate reorganization survey: management indicates satisfaction. *Caring.* 1985 Nov. 4(11):40-42, 44-45.

Jackson, P., and Goldman, C. AIDS: caring for your home care patient. Can nurses overcome the fear surrounding this disease to give competent care at home? *Canadian Nurse.* 1986 Mar. 82(3):18-22.

Light, M. J., and Sheridan, M. S. The home apnea monitoring program for newborns: the first 300 patients. *Hawaii Medical Journal.* 1985 Nov. 44(11):419-20, 423-24.

Martinson, I. M., Moldow, D. G., and others. Home care for children dying of cancer. *Research in Nursing Health.* 1986 Mar. 9(1):11-16.

Schraff, S. H. Value of computerization: home health executive viewpoints. [interview by Mary Elizabeth McIlvane] *Computers in Healthcare.* 1986 Feb. 7(2):38-43.

Stefanchik, M. Networking technology interest for home health. *Computers in Healthcare.* 1986 July. 7(7):46.

Traska, M. R. No home means no home care for AIDS patients. *Hospitals.* 1986 Jan. 5:60(1):69-70.

Infusion Therapies, High Tech, Pharmacy

Austin, E. Records review (in case of) litigation. *Home Health Journal.* 1985 Dec. 6(12):13, 19.

Borfitz, D. Mercy killing issues ripples: affects homecare. *Home Health Journal.* 1985 Dec. 6(12):3-4.

Bowyer, C. K. The complex care team: meeting the needs of high-technology nursing at home. *Home Healthcare Nurse.* 1986 Jan.-Feb. 4(1):24-29.

Clarke, R. G., and Quayle, A. R. Home artificial nutrition. *ACTA Gastroenterologica Belgica.* 1985 May-June. 48(3):214-23.

Connaway, N. I. The legalities of home care: Documenting patient care in the home: legal issues for the home health nurse. *Home Healthcare Nurse.* 1985 Sep.-Oct. 3(5):6-8.

_____. Documenting patient care in the home: legal issues for the home health nurse. (Part 2). *Home Healthcare Nurse.* 1985 Nov.-Dec. 3(6):44-46.

_____. The legalities of home care: should a home health nurse carry her own professional liability insurance? *Home Healthcare Nurse.* 1986 Mar.-Apr. 4(2):7-8.

_____. The legalities of home care: what would you do in the following situations? *Home Healthcare Nurse.* 1986 Jan.-Feb. 4(1):35-36.

Detsky, A. S., McLaughlin, J. R., Abrams, H. B., and others. A cost-utility analysis of the home parenteral nutrition program at Toronto General Hospital: 1970-1982. *Journal of Parenteral and Enteral Nutrition.* 1986 Jan.-Feb. 10(1):49-57.

Dickerson, J. Parenteral nutritional support. *Hospital Material Management Quarterly.* 1986 Feb. 7(3):37-49.

Greenberg, R. B. Legal implications of home health care by nonprofit hospitals. *American Journal of Hospital Pharmacy.* 1986 Feb. 43(2):386-91.

Hoppe, M. C. Nutritional support in the home. *Hospital Material Management Quarterly.* 1986 Feb. 7(3):72-79.

Lennard-Jones, J. E., and Wood, S. The organization of intravenous feeding at home. *Health Trends.* 1985 Nov. 17(4):73-75.

Payment, Pricing, Costing, Accounting

Special report: coding with Medicare cost limits: agencies must tighten belts to stay below new cost caps. *Hospital Home Health.* 1986 July. 3(7):85-88.

Special report: coding with Medicare cost limits: agencies use discrete costing to cope with new Medicare cost caps. *Hospital Home Health.* 1986 July. 3(7):89-91.

Bishop, C. E., and Stassen, M. Prospective reimbursement for home health care: context for an evolving policy. *Pride Institute Journal of Long Term Home Health Care.* 1986 Winter. 5(1):17-26.

Borfitz, D. Elderly barter for service credits, or homecare IRA. *Home Health Journal.* 1985 Dec. 6(12):8, 12.

Curtiss, F. R. Financing home health-care products and services. *American Journal of Hospital Pharmacy.* 1986 Jan. 43(1):121-31.

_____. Recent developments in federal reimbursement for home health care. *American Journal of Hospital Pharmacy.* 1986 Jan. 43(1):132-39.

Firshein, J. Payment squeezes home health care. *Hospitals.* 1986 Apr. 20. 60(8):26, 28.

_____. Prepaids' use of home health services booming. *Hospitals.* 1986 Apr. 20. 60(8):66-67.

Grazier, K. L. The impact of reimbursement policy on home health care. *Pride Institute Journal of Long Term Home Health Care.* 1986 Winter. 5(1):12-16.

Traska, M. R. Case management is just the ticket for home care. *Hospitals.* 1986 Mar. 20. 60(6):80-81.

Durable Medical Equipment

Suppliers: Should hospitals get involved in ADL? *Hospitals.* 1986 May 20. 60(10):83.

Cohen, D. Serving handicapped athletes [Motion Designs, Inc.] *Venture.* 1985 May. 7(5):17.

Kacmarek, R. M., and Spearman, C. B. Equipment used for ventilatory support in the home. *Respiratory Care.* 1986 Apr. 31(4):311-28.

Pierson, D. J., and George, R. B. Mechanical ventilation in the home: possibilities and prerequisites. *Respiratory Care.* 1986 Apr. 31(4):266-70.

Prentice, W. S. Placement alternatives for long-term ventilator care. *Respiratory Care.* 1986 Apr. 31(4):288-93.

Marketing

Pappas, J. P. Marketing home care: organizational posture and positioning. *Caring.* 1985 Nov. 4(11):48-50.

_____. The marketing audit and communications. *Caring.* 1985 Dec. 4(12): 54-59.

Petre, P. Marketers mine for gold in the old. *Fortune.* 1986 Mar. 31. 113(7):70-78.

Medicare/Skilled Care

Benjamin, A. E. State variations in home health expenditures and utilization under Medicare and Medicaid. *Home Health Care Services Quarterly.* 1986 Spring. 7(1):5-28.

Callahan, W. Medicare use of home health services. *Health Care Financing Review.* 1985 Winter. 7(2):89-91.

Liu, K., Manton, K. G., and Liu, B. M. Home care expenses for the disabled elderly. *Health Care Financing Review.* 1985 Winter. 7(2):51-58.

Risk Management

Borders, C. R. Practice trends: avoiding poor outcomes in home care. *Patient Care.* 1986 Feb. 15. 20(3):139-41, 145-46, 148-149.

_____. Reducing liability risk in home care. *Patient Care.* 1986 Mar. 15. 20(5):57-59, 62, 66-67.

Butt, B. Use of protocols in home care: an innovative approach to meet today's needs. *Home Healthcare Nurse.* 1986 Mar.-Apr. 4(2):37-40.

Fletcher, M. Trend toward home care poses new liability worries. *Business Insurance.* 1985 Sept. 16. 19(37):10.

Gould, Joyce E. Standardized home health nursing care plans: a quality assurance tool. *Quality Review Bulletin.* 1985 Nov. 11(5):334-38.

Grey, A. Personal emergency response systems. *Contemporary Longterm Care.* 1986 Jan. 9(1):40, 42.

Griffith, D. Blending key ingredients to assure quality in home health care. *Nursing and Health Care.* 1986 June. 7(6):301-302.

Hospital-based home care requires strong risk management. *Hospital Risk Management.* 1986 Mar. 8(3):29-33.

Tehan, J., and Colegrove, S. L. Risk management and home health care: the time is now. *Quality Review Bulletin.* 1986 May. 12(5):179-86.